Coming of Age

Revised Edition

**A 60-Year History of the
American College of Healthcare Executives
and the Profession It Serves
1933–1993**

by Duncan Neuhauser

with the assistance of Steven Neuhauser

Health Administration Press
Ann Arbor
1995

98 97 96 95 94   5 4 3 2 1

Library of Congress Catalog Card Number: 93-081268

ISBN: 1-56793-009-3

The paper used in this publication meets the minimum requirements of American National Standard for Information Sciences—Permanence of Paper for Printers Library Materials, ANSI Z39.48-1984. ∞™

Health Administration Press
A division of the Foundation of the
   American College of Healthcare Executives
1021 East Huron Street
Ann Arbor, Michigan 48104-9990
(313) 764-1380

The Mission of the American College of Healthcare Executives is to be the professional membership society for healthcare executives; to meet its affiliates' professional, educational, and leadership needs; to increase the effectiveness of healthcare management; and to advance healthcare management excellence.

July, 1989

Contents

Foreword to the 1995 edition of *Coming of Age*

We are proud to present this new edition of *Coming of Age*, a history of the American College of Healthcare Executives. Few other professions have experienced the kind of rapid growth and evolution that has occurred in the field of healthcare management. Thanks to the diligent and dedicated work of Duncan Neuhauser, the College's contributions to healthcare management over the past 60 years have been richly preserved. As in the initial version of this book, published in 1983, Dr. Neuhauser once again skillfully analyzes the role and impact of the College in response to major developments in healthcare delivery and management education. He makes it abundantly clear that the College has had a significant impact both within the profession and on the nation's healthcare delivery system.

In this current edition of *Coming of Age*, Duncan Neuhauser and Steven Neuhauser present a chronology of the profession along with "memoirs" of our professional society. They have gathered historical information from archives, studies, surveys, and personal interviews. The end result is an impressive testament to the College's rich tradition of excellence and innovation in healthcare management and its strong leadership role in the healthcare field.

This is a book for everyone with an interest in the management of healthcare services. *Coming of Age* will give you a feeling of pride in your professional society and in your chosen profession. The present volume is an important contribution to the fulfillment of the College's mission to preserve and acknowledge its past, to revitalize its present, and to creatively shape its future. We are confident that the American College of Healthcare Executives will continue to provide, as it has over the past 60 years, outstanding leadership in the field of healthcare management.

Ronald G. Spaeth, FACHE
Chairman

Col. William C. Head, USAF, MSC, FACHE
Chairman-Elect

Robert R. Fanning, Jr., FACHE
Immediate Past-Chairman
American College of Healthcare Executives

Thomas C. Dolan, Ph.D., FACHE
President/CEO
American College of Healthcare Executives

1

Introduction and Overview

Most internally generated (corporate) histories are too superficial, too low in thematic content, and too low in their levels of abstraction to be either useful to managers or trusted by historians. Most company histories deal with the contents of a corporation's past, rather than with its essence. They should rather concentrate on the dynamic accumulation of past events and decisions that have abiding significance for the present and the future.

Corporate history can be a way of thinking about the company, a way of comprehending why the present is what it is, and what might be possible for the future.

Once managers recognize the value of the corporate past, they can enhance their ability to diagnose problems, reassess policy, measure performance, and even direct change.[1]

The American College of Hospital Administrators (ACHA) was founded in 1933. It led to the creation of a profession out of an amorphous occupational group that often fell into supervising hospitals by chance.

Hospitals became more complex with the growth of technology and division of labor. Formal education for hospital management grew so that the College's role changed from primary educator to continuing education. As hospitals became parts of ever larger delivery systems, hospital administration became too narrow a definition, so in 1985 the College changed its name to the American College of Healthcare Executives (ACHE). In this book, the current name will be used except for citations, references, and direct quotations.

The words "profession" and "professional" have been used so widely that they have lost much of their original meaning. However, there is a meaning which the founders of the College had in mind over 60 years ago.[2] They sought to define the profession of health care administration through College Membership and Fellowship.[3] This emphasis

1

on professionalism requires a body of relevant knowledge (Chapter 7), the development of formal education and continuing education (Chapter 5), judgment of excellence by peers (Chapter 6), the development of a code of ethics (Chapter 3), a professional association (Chapters 2, 8, 9, 10), and scholarship through publication (Chapter 7).

The history of the College cannot be understood through a narrow review of its internal organization. That would ignore the close link between the ACHE and the changing field of hospital administration and health care management (Chapters 3 and 4). Nor can the College be considered as a single, distinct entity. It has been—and continues to be—composed of extraordinary and unique leaders of the field. Their individuality is not easily expressed in the minutes of College committee meetings. Above all, it can never be forgotten that the College is only as effective and innovative as its leadership and affiliate body. The College is people.

The evolution from hospital superintendency to hospital administration to health care management can be separated into five distinctive eras since 1873. These five eras are outlined in Table 1.1. These dates represent model cresting of eras and not sharp splits from one time to the next.

Between 1873 and 1915, the number of hospitals grew from approximately 200 to more than 5,000.[4] Many new hospitals were founded by practicing physicians as a place to care for their patients, or by Catholic sisterhoods or other religious and ethnic groups. The content of hospital administration theory focused largely on hospital architectural design.

Between 1915 and 1945, the average hospital remained small and uncomplicated. Even in 1945, 45 percent of general hospitals had fewer than 50 beds and almost 70 percent had fewer than 100 beds.[5] Superintendents came to their positions by chance, not through career planning. Professional "stepping stones" included nursing, medicine, or religious administration. Superintendents were expected to know all the details of hospital work, including sterile technique, food preparation, sanitation, and keeping medical records.

From 1945 to 1965, hospitals became more complex.[6] Administrators no longer worked with details. Instead, they recruited technically skilled workers to accomplish the work of the hospital. This era saw the growth of graduate programs in hospital administration and the creation of a separate profession chosen—and not fallen into—as a career by its members. The College's nondegree "Institutes" were replaced by degree programs, regional meetings, and an annual Congress on Administration.

The introduction of Medicare and Medicaid in 1966 parallelled

TABLE 1.1
Five Stages in the Evolution of Hospital and Healthcare System Management

Date	The Hospital and Healthcare	The Theory of Hospital and Healthcare Management	The Healthcare Executive's Career
I The Creation 1873–1915	The community hospital becomes universal Era of public health	Hospital architecture, military style discipline	Trustees, nurse, sister, or practicing physician owner directs the hospital
II The Hospital 1915–1944 IIa Standardization 1915–1933	The small independent uncomplicated hospital with little division of labor	Knowing all the details, classical management theory, standards	The administrator often comes by chance from medicine, nursing, or religious administration
IIb Superintendent 1933–1944			The beginning of a profession with the founding of the College
III Technology and Increased Access 1945–1978 IIIa The hospital administrator 1945–1965	Growth of hospital-based technical and professional personnel and private insurance	Working through people, human relations	The growth of graduate schools in hospital administration and a separate profession
IIIb The Medical Center Manager 1966–1978	Medicare, Medicaid, government regulation, and organizational differentiation	The Complex external environment	A growing number of healthcare managers working outside hospitals
IV Cost Containment and Organization 1979–1990 The CEO and the Multi-Institution System	A competitive environment in the healthcare industry	The corporate model	Lengthening careers in middle management and the growth of specialization within healthcare management
V Quality driven systems management 1991–	Managed competition	Systems thinking, continuous quality improvement, process improvement	Master's preparation the norm, lifelong learning expected

rising costs and government regulation. It also brought other organizations like neighborhood health centers, planning agencies, consultants, and large third party payers, health maintenance organizations (HMOs), preferred provider organizations (PPOs)—all requiring health managers. More of the hospital manager's time was occupied with external affairs, particularly regulatory agencies. With increasing hospital size and the attractiveness of hospital management as a career, a longer portion of the manager's career was spent in middle management. Specialized healthcare management also grew in importance.

Although they existed for years before, by 1979 multi-institutional systems were the center of attention. The Chief Executive Officer (CEO) became increasingly concerned with marketing, competition, corporate reorganization, and financing.

The change of the College's name from hospital administration to healthcare executive (effective July 29, 1985) reflected the change of focus to healthcare systems, where College members held positions in many different organizations and the hospital became a part of a continuum of care. By 1990, systems thinking and continuous quality improvement/total quality management brought a new vision. Time will tell whether this is a momentary enthusiasm or a major turning point.

The First, the Average, and the Last

Historical trends have a beginning, crest, and often, an end. The founding members of the College were not average administrators . . . they were leaders. The ideas generated by the College were a vanguard for the field. A study of hospital costs and budgeting in 1929 did not imply that all hospitals carried out cost analysis with the same sophistication at the same point in time.[7] The large hospital of 1945, staffed with medical specialists and skilled managers, existed simultaneously with hospitals staffed by physicians with inferior education (received in grade C medical schools, which the Flexner reforms of 1910 eventually closed by 1940). Although x-rays were used in 1896, there were still hospitals without x-ray machines in the 1940s.

In an era of multi-institutional systems, fewer managers report directly to boards of trustees. Instead, they work in organizations which include tens—and even hundreds—of hospitals under one corporate umbrella. Today there are more assistant administrators, vice presidents, and middle managers.[8]

In this evolution, the skills acquired in previous eras have not been abandoned. Hospital administration still requires knowledge of architecture, operations, and human resources, as well as concern for the external environment and quality improvement. The College has fostered and paved the way by being a forum for these evolutionary stages.

In many ways, the founding members of the College were more like their colleagues in 1945 than like their peers in 1933. By 1983, it was quite possible for one regional vice president of a single multi-hospital system to be responsible for a larger dollar volume of work than that of the College's entire group of founding members in 1933. Thus has been the change in hospital administration over the years.

In 1980, it could be written that "The history of hospitals exists primarily as introductory chapters in textbooks, while the history of hospital administration is virtually non-existent."[9] This void began to be filled when the 50-year history of the College was written.[10] Since then a lot has changed. In conjunction with the American Hospital Association (AHA), the College created the Center for Hospital and Healthcare Administration History in 1984.[11] This Center has collected over 400 published hospital histories[12] and supports the Lewis Weeks Oral History series of interviews with leading healthcare executives.[13] See Table 1.2 for highlights of the College's role in pro-

TABLE 1.2
The College Promotes the History of Healthcare Management: A Chronology

1955	J. Dewey Lutes Chairs College History Committee responsible for the publication of Ira Kipnis's[25] 25th Anniversary History of the College.
1978	Stull, Richard, "Historical Perspective," ACHA *1977–1978 Annual Report*.
1983	Colleges publishes four-volume set of "Commemorative Editions," *Challenging the Profession, Foundations for Excellence, Coming of Age, Judgment in Administration* (Ray E. Brown).
1984	Paul Starr, *The Social Transformation of American Medicine*, wins James A. Hamilton Award.
1984	Start of the Center for Hospital and Health Administration History, AHA/ACHE Ad Hoc Historical Committee (Andrew Patullo chair).[26]
1984	Lewis Weeks Oral History Series managed by the Center (Series started 1978 by AHA and Hospital Research and Educational Trust (HRET).[27]
1987	George Bugbee autobiography published by HRET.
1989	Friends of the Center for Hospital and Health Administration initiated.
1990	The Center produces first list of histories of individual U.S. hospitals.
1990	Rosemary Stevens, *In Sickness and in Wealth: American Hospitals in the Twentieth Century*, wins the James A. Hamilton Award.
1991	*Ray E. Brown: Lectures, Messages and Memoires*, published by Health Administration Press.
1992	ACHE historical archives organized.[28]
1994	Sixtieth Year College history published.

moting health administration history. Twenty years ago there was only one social history of hospitals: Brian Abel-Smith's history of London hospitals.[14] Now there are a number of outstanding works by Geoffrey Rivett (London),[15] Paul Starr,[16] Charles Rosenberg,[17] (American hospitals in the nineteenth century) and Rosemary Stevens,[18] (American hospitals in the twentieth century).

In 1980, the book about Henry M. Hurd, first administrator[19] of Johns Hopkins Hospital (1920), was the only one that came close to being a biography of a hospital administrator. George Bugbee's autobiography (1987)[20] and Ray Brown's memoirs (1991) finally followed.[21] Some major organizations still do not have histories. The last American Hospital Association history was written in 1937;[22] that of the Association of University Programs in Health Administration (AUPHA) in 1959.[23] The Joint Commission on the Accreditation of Health Care Organizations is without any written history, as is the case for university degree programs in health administration.

This book is part of the College's effort to promote the study of the history of healthcare management.[24]

NOTES

[1] Smith and Steadman, 1981, pp. 164–165.
[2] Greenwood, p. 206, Carr-Saunders and Wilson, 1933. Abbott, 1988, argues that professions can best be understood by their boundary battles such as lawyers and accountants, psychology and psychiatry, optometry and ophthalmology. Healthcare management has been remarkably free (but not totally) from such battles over turf and employment.
[3] In 1948 the College defined a profession by citing a definition proposed in 1915 by Abraham Flexner in an address at the National Conference of Charities and Correction. A profession (a) "involves essentially intellectual operations accompanied by large individual responsibilities;" (b) "is learned in nature and their members are resorting constantly to the laboratory and seminar for a fresh supply of facts;" (c) "they are not merely academic and theoretical. Indeed, they are definitely practical in their aims;" (d) "they possess a technique capable of communication through a highly specialized educational discipline;" (e) "they are self organized with activities, duties and responsibilities, which completely engage their participants and develop group consciousness;" and (f) "they are likely to be more responsive to public interest than are unorganized and isolated individuals, and they tend to become increasingly concerned with the achievement of social ends," ACHA, *Hospital Administration: A Life's Profession*, 1948, pp. 40–41.
[4] Toner, 1873.
[5] The Commission on Hospital Care, 1957, p. 312.
[6] Wesbury, "Toward a Broader View of Health Care," in Sloane and Sloane, 1992.
[7] Sawyer, 1929.

[8] Although the typical titles have changed over the years, this history will usually use the words "administrator" and "manager" interchangeably. It will primarily use the word "administrator" because this was the word first used in the College's name. In February 1935, the Executive Committee of the College "determined to make 'administrator' the common designation for the executive head of a hospital," Kipnis, 1955. "Various titles have been given to the chief executives of the hospital, such as superintendent, manager, business manager, director, executive director and medical director, but the more commonly accepted designation is administrator," ACHA, *Hospital Administration: A Life's Profession*, p. 29. The titles of hospitals have also changed, to health centers and medical centers and to multi-institution systems.

[9] Wren, 1980, p. 31.

[10] Neuhauser, *Coming of Age*, 1983. This second edition includes nearly all the content of and updates the first edition.

[11] Center for Hospital and Health Care Administration History, Annual Reports.

[12] *Ibid.* "United States Hospital Histories," AHA Resource Center, 1992, p. 37.

[13] *Ibid.* Lewis Weeks oral history series. There are over 80 such interviews.

[14] Abel-Smith, 1964.

[15] Rivett, 1986.

[16] Starr, 1982.

[17] Rosenberg, 1987.

[18] Stevens, Rosemary, 1989. Other histories include Rosner, 1982; Vogel, 1980; Risse, 1986; and Dowling, 1982.

[19] Cullen, 1920 (*Henry M. Hurd of Johns Hopkins Hospital*). Other partial exceptions are *Michael M. Davis: A Tribute*, 1972; Goldwater, Chapter 1, 1947; and Codman, 1934, Chapter 1. So far as I know, only one hospital administrator in this century kept a daily diary of his work running a hospital, but this diary is lost. Goldwater, 1949, p. xxxiii, and personal communication, Mt. Sinai Medical Center archivist.

[20] Bugbee, 1987.

[21] Blanks et al., *Ray E. Brown: Lectures, Messages and Memoirs*, 1991. The College republished his *Judgment in Administration* in a College Fiftieth anniversary edition in 1983. It was originally published in 1966.

[22] Caldwell, 1937.

[23] James Stephan in *Ray E. Brown*, 1959.

[24] In addition to those thanked in the first edition, thanks also go to Pat Wakeley, Michael McCue, Eloise Foster, Art Strobeck, Frankie Perry, Peter Weil, Lynn Kahn, Thomas Dolan, Daphne Grew, and once again Stuart Wesbury.

[25] Lutes, "HM Salutes," 1956. Kipnis, "Preface," 1955, lists the members, which included A.C. Bachmeyer, Maurice Dubin, Ernest Erickson, Gerhard Hartman, Malcolm MacEachern, Robert Neff, Joseph Norby, and Dean Conley.

[26] Center for Hospital and Health Care Administration History, Final Report to the W.K. Kellogg Foundation, 1991, AHA, Chicago, p. 1.

[27] *Ibid.*

[28] ACHE, "Archives Inventory, 1992," 10 pp.

2

The Birth of the College

There were five objectives when the College was founded in 1933:
1. *To elevate the standards of hospital administration.*
2. *To establish standards of competency for hospital administrators.*
3. *To develop and promote standards of education and training for hospital administrators.*
4. *To educate hospital trustees and the public to understand that the practice of hospital administration calls for special training and experience.*
5. *To provide a method of conferring Fellowships in Hospital Administration on those who have rendered or are rendering noteworthy service in the field of hospital administration.*[1]

PART I

Historical Overview

The College is a product of the changing healthcare field—an evolving organization shaped by historical events. Table 2.1 summarizes nearly 100 years of both U.S. and healthcare history, and 60 years in the development of the College.

The Eras of Creation and Standardization: 1873–1933

In 1873, there were approximately 178 hospitals in the entire U.S.[2] By 1915, there were more than 5,000. Aseptic and antiseptic surgery and x-ray machines made it necessary to bring the ill to the controlled environment of a hospital. Especially in the north and east, philanthropy, fueled by industrial development at the turn of the century, led to the endowment and funding of voluntary hospitals. In the south and west, where philanthropy was less available, doctors created their

9

TABLE 2.1
Chronology of Events: General History, Health Services, and the College 1900–1993[3-7]

Date	General	Health Services	ACHE[9]
1900	1901: J. P. Morgan forms the United States Steel Corp.	1896: X-Rays used in USA	
	1901: Theodore Roosevelt becomes President	1899: Founding of what became the American Hospital Association	
		1903: New York City outbreak of typhoid fever. "Typhoid Mary," a carrier, is named	
1905		1906: Pure Food and Drug Act defines pharmaceutical industry.	
1910	1909: W. H. Taft President	1910: Flexner Report[8]	
		First university-based School of Nursing (Minnesota) opens	
	1912: Woodrow Wilson elected	1913: American College of Surgeons founded	
	1913: Federal income tax		
	Jul., 1914: World War I starts		
1915		1915: More than 5000 hospitals (up from about 178 in 1873)	
	Nov. 11, 1918: Armistice Day ends World War I	1918–1919: Worldwide influenza pandemic (estimated 500,000 deaths in USA)	
		1918: American College of Surgeons starts hospital accreditation	
1920:	Aug. 26: Woman's suffrage adopted W. Harding elected President		
1921	Aug. 2: C. Coolidge becomes President	1922: Insulin discovered by Banting and MacLeod, Canada	
1925	1928: Herbert Hoover elected President	1928: Penicillin discovered by Alexander Flemming in England	

10

	Date	Event	Date	College Event
1930	Oct. 28, 1929:	The Great Stock Market Crash		
	1929:	Blue Cross concept starts at Baylor University		
	1932:	Franklin Roosevelt elected President	1932:	Dewey Lutes and three other administrators meet to plan association
	1931:	First Randomized Clinical Trial in Medicine[10]	Feb. 13, 1933:	Palmer House Meeting starts College
	1934:	University of Chicago starts first graduate degree program in hospital administration	Feb. 13, 1933–37:	Dewey Lutes General Director (CEO)
			Sept. 12, 1933	First Annual Meeting
			Mar. 26, 1934:	College Incorporated
1935	Aug. 14, 1935:	Social Security Act signed by Roosevelt	1935:	227 total college affiliates
	1935:	Antibacterial activity of sulfa drugs discovered	Nov. 25, 1936:	Local committees for geographical regions appointed
	1935:	Wagner Labor Relations Act	1937:	First permanent hdqtrs.
	1938:	Harold Cox grows typhus microbes in chick embryos, leading to development of an effective vaccine available for World War II.	1937–41:	Gerhard Hartman, Ph.D., Executive Secretary (CEO) College;
1940	Sept. 1, 1939:	Hitler invades Poland	1939:	Total affiliates 853
			1940:	First examinations conducted for entrance to College
	Dec. 7, 1941:	Pearl Harbor		
	1941:	Penicillin first used on a human patient. Only widely available after the war.		
	1942:	Kaiser Permanente formed from earlier capitation plan started in 1938.		

TABLE 2.1
Continued

Date	General	Health Services	ACHE[9]
1941		1941: Effect of rubella on fetus during early pregnancy shown	1941: Code of Ethics adopted 1942–65: Dean Conley, Executive Director (CEO)
1945	Apr. 12, 1945: Atomic bomb dropped FDR dies; Harry S. Truman becomes President May 7, 1945: V.E. Day Aug. 6, 1945: Hiroshima bombed Sept. 2, 1945: V.J. Day ends World War II United Nations formed	1944: Streptomycin discovered 1945: Fluoridation of water introduced in USA 1946: First version of Benjamin Spock's *Baby and Child Care* 1946: Hill Burton Program	1944: Total College affiliates 1,317 1945–8: Joint Commission on Education of ACHA and AHA
1950	1947: Taft Hartley Act 1948: Transistor discovered 1950–53: Korean War	1951: Joint Commission on the Accreditation of Hospitals formed 1952: Isoniazid introduced effective chemotherapy for tuberculosis	1949: Arthur Bachmeyer Memorial Annual address start
1955	1953: Dwight D. Eisenhower elected President Oct. 4, 1957: Sputnik I launched	1953: Discovery of DNA structure by Watson and Crick 1955: Peak in number of mental inpatients 1955: Salk polio vaccine	1952: *Hospitals Visualized* published 1954: New office 620 N. Michigan Ave. 1955: Total College affiliates 3,467 1956: Journal *Hospital Administration* starts Feb. 13, 1958: Observance of the 25th Anniversary, Ray Brown, Chairman: Founding of the Annual Congress

Year	General History	Medical / Health History	Association History
1960	Jan. 20, 1961: John F. Kennedy inaugurated President	1960: Ultrasound used to diagnose brain damage	1958: James A. Hamilton Hospital Administrators Book Award started
1961	Nov. 22, 1963: President assassinated: Lyndon Johnson became President	1962: The limitations of broad spectrum antibiotics appear after 20 years of use	1961: Malcolm MacEachern Memorial Lecture started
	1964–66: Lyndon Johnson and "New Society" legislation	1963: Government expenditure on medical research exceeds one billion dollars	1964: Start of Gold Medal Award for Excellence in Hospital Administration
1965	Apr. 4, 1968: Martin Luther King assassinated	1964: New York passes first Certificate of Need law	1965–71: Richard J. Stull, Executive Vice President (CEO)
		1965: Medicare and Medicaid legislation passed	1965: Reorganization Council of Regents and Board of Governors; Total College affiliates 5,276
		Apr. 21, 1966: Michael DeBakey implants first artificial heart	1967: Dean Conley Award starts
		Dec. 3, 1967: Christian Bernard performs heart transplant	1967–80: *Administrative Briefs* published
	1969: Richard Nixon inaugurated President	1967: First coronary artery bypass surgery at Cleveland Clinic	Aug., 1967: The British National Health Service Tour (published 1969)
	Jul. 20, 1969: First moon landing		1969: Robert S. Hudgens Memorial Award for Young Hospital Administrator of the Year starts
1970	Jan. 27, 1973: Vietnam peace treaty signed	1973: HMO Act (PL93-222)	1970: 8,147 affiliates
	Aug. 9, 1974: Nixon resigns; Gerald Ford becomes President	1974: Nonprofit Hospital Amendments to the National Labor Relations Act (allows unions to organize in hospitals)	1971–79: Richard J. Stull, President (CEO)
		Smallpox eradicated world-wide	1972: Computerized Membership Data Profile
1975	Nov. 2, 1976: Jimmy Carter elected President	1972: Computerized axial tomography	1974: End of special recognition of the administrative residency
		c.1975: Number of patients in nursing homes exceeds patients in hospitals for the first time	1976: ACHA Journal becomes *Hospital and Health Services Administration*
		1979: Hospital Corp. of America exceeds 1 billion dollars in revenue and total assets	1979: Stuart A. Wesbury, Jr., Ph.D., President (CEO)

13

14

TABLE 2.1
Continued

Date		General	Health Services		ACHE[9]	
1980	Nov. 2, 1980:	Ronald Reagan elected President			Jul., 1980:	Accord with AHA on public policy[11]
			1981:	AIDS identified	Aug., 1981:	"Programmatic Thrusts"
					Feb., 1982:	25th Annual Congress on Administration
1983			1983:	Jarvik artificial heart	Jan. 1, 1983:	College dues paying affiliates 16,433
			1983:	Medical care 10% of gross national product		
			1983:	Creation of first artificial chromosome	1983:	50th Anniversary Professional Assessment Program Starts Committee on Public Policy
1984		K. Chernenko declared head of USSR	Oct. 1:	First successful surgery on a fetus DRG payment method starts	1984:	Delphi Study with Arthur Anderson ACHE/AHA Washington Contract; Strategic Plan
	Nov.:	Ronald Reagan elected 2nd term	Dec.:	3,000 cases of AIDS reported		
		Indira Gandhi assassinated				
1985				HMO enrollment 21 million people in 480 plans	Jul. 29:	Name changes to ACHE
1986	Jan. 28:	Space Shuttle Challenger explodes		FDA approves first genetically engineered Vaccine (Hepatitis B)	1986:	Ambulatory Care Simulation Book evaluation
		Iran Contra scandal		33 million Americans without health insurance		Survey of Members about access to care
1987			Apr. 4:	19,181 cases of AIDS; 37% died	May 21:	Statement on Access to Health Care
					Jan. 1:	18,967 affiliates
					Feb. 9–13:	30th Congress on Administration
					Feb. 9:	Statement on Medical Records confidentiality
1988		George Bush elected President			Jul. 18:	College Strategic Plan

Year		World Events	Healthcare Events	College Events
1989	Nov. 9–10: Dec.: Dec. 25:	Berlin Wall comes down Invasion of Panama Romania's Ceausescu shot	JCAHO starts Agenda for Change	Revision of Professional Assessment
1990	Feb.: Mar. 11: Mar. 13: Apr. 24: Oct. 3:	Nelson Mandela released Lithuania declares independence Communist Party monopoly ends in USSR Sadam Hussein invades Kuwait Michael Milken "Junk Bond King" fined $600 million Reunion of Germany formalized		Amended code of Ethics
1991		Desert Storm		Jan. 1: 21,048 affiliates Jan.: Faculty Practice Fellowship Program Guidelines Feb.: First Ethical Policy Statement Jun. 2: Robin Burki, M.D., dies; last founder Aug. 31: Stuart Wesbury steps down; Thomas C. Dolan, Ph.D., becomes President (CEO) Dec. 31: College Assets $9.9 million Expenses $12.2 million[14]
1992	Nov. 3:	William Clinton elected President Healthcare reform a major issue	RBRVS payment changes Outpatient surgery exceeds inpatient surgery for first time	Aug. 1992: Code of Ethics Revision Jul. 31: 63 officially designated Healthcare Executive groups (70 total); 105 student chapters; 20 Women's Healthcare Executive Networks (14 officially designated)
1993		Clinton health plan proposed		60th Anniversary

own proprietary hospitals to care for patients. As they grew, and as their original founders retired, many of these proprietary hospitals were transformed into voluntary institutions. However, even today, acceptance of the proprietary hospital remains greater in the sunbelt states than in other parts of the country.[15]

In the years 1890 to 1920, there was widespread agreement on the value of public health measures like sanitation, vaccination, pasteurization, and clean water supply.[16] These programs would ultimately result in a declining death rate from infectious disease, and in the prolongation of life.

In the old voluntary hospitals, supported by contributions from trustees and others,[17] philanthropy provided the power to admit patients.[18] Only at the turn of the century did trustees abandon their involvement in selecting "the deserving poor" for admission.[19] After that time, the decision to admit became the sole province of the physician. The hospital thus became an institution of medical science rather than social welfare.[20] When trustees paid all the bills, their power was predominate.[21] The decline of trustee influence meant the rise of medical influence.

Founded in 1899, the LaCrosse Lutheran Hospital in Wisconsin had no administrator until 1921, only a nurse-matron and a chief physician. Their first superintendent in 1924 was a general store manager before he started work as a hospital administrator.[22] It was not until after World War II that professionalization of hospital administration, along with the growing complexity of the hospital and the external environment, signaled a rise in the administrator's influence.[23]

The 1920s saw important advances in medical care: insulin for diabetes in 1922, and penicillin in 1928. In 1935, sulfa drugs were shown to have antibacterial effects. Although the impact of these changes extended over decades, they greatly enhanced the role of medical care and the hospital. Although penicillin was discovered in 1928, it was first used in humans in 1941, and was not widely available for the civilian population until after World War II.

The stockmarket crash of 1929 and the subsequent Great Depression that led to President Roosevelt's New Deal also brought changes. The Blue Cross concept began at Baylor University in 1929. The Depression encouraged the growth of this idea even more as hospitals sought to reduce their bad debts.[24] The Social Security Act of 1935 became the greatest landmark in twentieth century American social legislation. And the 1935 Wagner Act gave a boost to the union movement, laying the ground work for negotiated healthcare benefits through collective bargaining.[25]

With the exception of health insurance, the major building blocks of the healthcare system were in place by 1915. The hospital became universal. The 1906 Pure Food and Drug Act further defined the pharmaceutical industry by declaring that a large number of powerful drugs could only be sold with a doctor's prescription.

German scientific medicine, brought to the U.S. by way of Johns Hopkins Medical School, became the standard of excellence in medical education proposed by Abraham Flexner in his famous 1910 report. In 1873, the first nursing schools in the U.S. opened, based on Florence Nightingale's principles. This was an essential step in the development of nursing as a profession.[26]

The 1918 worldwide influenza pandemic cost the lives of millions of people. Health insurance, as we know it, was only economically possible without the great epidemics which could otherwise bankrupt even the largest insurer.[27]

The Idea of a College

In 1518, King Henry VIII chartered the Royal College of Physicians in London.[28] The idea of such a college suggested an educated gentleman as compared with the merchants and tradesmen of the London companies and guilds. A higher education was synonymous with the knowledge of Latin, and in the case of physicians, knowledge of the classical medical writers. Like those of the other learned professions of barrister (the law) and the clergy, the gentleman physician did not work with his hands. He was distinct from uneducated or apprentice-trained barber-surgeons, midwives and apothecaries.

In 1745, the London surgeons separated from the barbers; by 1800, they had achieved sufficient status to transform their company into the Royal College of Surgeons.[29] Although the Royal College of Physicians did not encourage this change, the surgeons no doubt built on this earlier concept. It was only after the discovery by Laennec of the stethoscope in 1819 that these physicians actually began to "lay hands" on patients.[30]

From the start, these colleges were exclusive; they selected only elite practitioners for fellowship. Table 2.2 shows the founding dates of professional colleges and other organizations from 1518 through 1933.

The American College of Surgeons (ACS), founded in May, 1913, was modeled directly on its British counterpart. In August of that year, Doctors George Crile, Harvey Cushing, William Mayo, and John Murphy received honorary fellowship in the Royal College of Surgeons. These leaders of American surgery were all to become presidents of the American College of Surgeons,[39] and in November, 1913, Sir Rickman Godlee, the President of the Royal College, gave the dedicatory address at the first convocation of the ACS.[40]

TABLE 2.2
Founding Dates of Professional Colleges and Other Organizations[31-33]

1518	Royal College of Physicians (of London) founded by King Henry the Eighth
1540–1745	The Company of Barber-Surgeons
1745–1800	The Company of Surgeons
1800	The Royal College of Surgeons
1847	American Medical Association
1872	American Public Health Association
1899	The Association of Hospital Superintendents formed (to become the American Hospital Association)[34]
1913	Founding of the American College of Surgeons (The First of the American Medical Specialty Colleges)
1915	Founding of the American College of Physicians
1915	Founding of the Catholic Hospital Association[35]
1917	Founding of the American Board of Ophthalmology (The First of the Medical Specialty Boards)
1919	Founding of the American Protestant Hospital Association[36]
1920	Society of Medical Administrators[37]
1929	Founding of the Royal College of Physicians and Surgeons of Canada by Act of Parliament[38]
1931	Founding of the Canadian Hospital Council
1933	Founding of the American College of Healthcare Executives

The ACS had three initial concerns. Through fellowship designation, they sought to demonstrate to the public the distinction between well-qualified surgical specialists and other physicians who performed some surgery as part of a general practice. They also worked to eliminate fee splitting between surgeon and referring physician and to improve hospital services through a program of hospital standardization.

The first chairman of the hospital standardization committee was Dr. Ernest Amory Codman, a Boston surgeon, who owned and managed his own proprietary hospital from 1909 to 1917.[41] He called it "The End Result Hospital" because he kept meticulous records of patient care, including notations of errors in skill and judgment. He also retained follow-up on every patient's condition after discharge, allowing for comparison of the end results of care with possible shortcomings in practice.[42]

For several years, he published these end results, patient by patient, in the annual report of the hospital, including notations of error. He challenged every other hospital in the country to do the same.[43]

The ACS was concerned with improving hospital management. According to the report of Arthur C. Bachmeyer, M.D., to the American Hospital Association:

> During the meeting of the American College of Surgeons of October, 1917 . . . at which time the campaign for improving the efficiency of hospitals was launched, the question of establishing a course of instruction for hospital executives was discussed. Many prominent men, both hospital administrators and surgeons participated in the discussion. Dr. A. J. Ochsner of Chicago finally introduced a resolution which provided that a committee be appointed to report . . . in the fullest practical detail on the organization of a school for the training of hospital superintendents . . . The resolution was unanimously adopted but the appointment of the committee was deferred" [indefinitely].[44]

Surgery could not be performed outside of an appropriate hospital setting, and the record of a surgeon's experience and skill could not be demonstrated without complete medical records.[45] The first cohort of ACS fellows was chosen on the basis of reputation. But future candidates for fellowship would be required to submit records of 100 surgical cases. Davis writes of the problems that arose:

> Few candidates, however, could comply with this requirement inasmuch as hospitals in the United States and Canada seldom kept records which provided accurate data. It was also discovered that the average hospital lacked laboratory, x-ray and other essential diagnostic and therapeutic facilities necessary to the surgeon in making a proper pre-operative study of his patient. Furthermore, medical staffs of hospitals were not organized; the professional work generally lacked supervision; most hospitals were deficient from the standpoint of scientific efficiency. The need for improvement was evident.[46]

The first hospital survey in 1918 covered 692 hospitals of over 100 beds. Only 12.9 percent were approved. By 1933, 1,603 hospitals of over 100 beds were surveyed, and 93.9 percent were approved.[47] The hospital standardization program was a great success and eventually was transformed into the Joint Commission on the Accreditation of Hospitals (JCAH).

The growth of this program was so rapid that the ACS decided to find a single individual to direct it. On October 25, 1921, the Regents of the ACS authorized an agreement with Malcolm T. MacEachern, M.D., to devote a third of his time to the direction of this program. He would receive a total of $400 for four months a year to do this work. On June 2, 1923, he became an Associate Director of the ACS in charge of the program. He held this post for the next 28 years.[48,49]

MacEachern graduated from McGill Medical School in 1910, trained in obstetrics. He became Superintendent of the Montreal Maternity Hospital in 1911. In 1913, he became General Superintendent of the Vancouver General Hospital. J. Dewey Lutes remembers "Mac" as being known throughout the country:

> Everyone loved him, and he did everything he could to help the College—an unusual man. I remember one meeting where MacEachern was in the back of the room asleep. (He sometimes slept during meetings.) I was speaking and I said, "I am sure you would like to hear from Dr. MacEachern." He woke up and came up front and gave a superb talk.[50]

Throughout his many years in Chicago, MacEachern regularly commuted to his home in Montreal where his wife and child resided.[51]

He became an internationally recognized expert on hospital administration as a result of his work for the ACS, and was one of the driving forces in the ACHE. Thus, from its inception, the ACHE had the American College of Surgeons to look to as a prototype organization. Dr. MacEachern was a bridge between both colleges.[52] In its own time, the ACHE became a prototype for other organizations of health management specialists.

The first published prospectus of the ACHE said:

> There is no field which requires the recognized specialist more than hospital administration. It is to this end that the *American College of Hospital Administrators* is proposed.
>   So that hospital administration may be improved and eventually fully established and recognized as a profession, the *American College of Hospital Administrators* is proposed. The organization would bear a relationship to the American Hospital Association as the American College of Physicians bears to the American Medical Association.[53]

PART II

The Eras of the Superintendent and Administrator: 1933–1965

How the College was Created

In September, 1932, Paul H. Fesler, Superintendent of the Wesley Memorial Hospital in Chicago,[54] and President of the American Hospital Association, told the AHA at its Detroit convention:

It is deplorable to notice that some of the best hospitals in this country are administered by men with no experience or training in hospital administration. It seems that it would be for the benefit of our patients if a college of hospital administration could be created to train hospital executives. These trained executives would be known as fellows of hospital administration. A board of regents should be created, and admission to the college be on a similar basis as fellowship in the American College of Surgeons. A candidate to be accepted should have at least five years experience in a private and acceptable hospital and should be admitted by examination on the basis of a thesis. It is ridiculous to think that men without any training whatsoever are permitted to head institutions responsible for the saving of lives and representing millions of dollars. This would not be possible in any business organization.

We regret little or no definite progress is being made in the training for the work of hospital administration. As a result, many are entering the hospital field as superintendents with little or no preparation or fitness for such important work. Some are succeeding, some are failing, and all are blundering for many of their early years in this work.[55]

Fesler, an ACHE Charter Fellow, was regent during 1937–1938.[56]

In 1932, Matthew O. Foley, Editor of *Hospital Management*, an advocate of improving the education and qualifications of administrators, approached Dewey Lutes about creating an association of hospital administrators. Ira Kipnis wrote:

Foley and Lutes envisioned an organization which would define the qualifications of hospital administrators, recognize those who qualified by admitting them to membership, educate hospital governing boards to the need for qualified administrators, and elevate the practice of hospital administration to the status of a profession.[57]

Lutes approached Dr. MacEachern, who gave the project his immediate support.

On October 7, 1932, Lutes invited four Chicago administrators to lunch at the Hotel Sherman to discuss criteria for establishing an American Institute of Hospital Administrators. These were: Maurice Dubin, Superintendent, Mount Sinai Hospital; Ernest I. Erickson, Superintendent, Augustana Hospital; and L. C. Vonder Heidt, West Suburban Hospital. Unable to attend was Charles A. Wordell of St. Luke's Hospital.[58] They were all to become Charter Fellows of the College.

They agreed to create an organization of hospital administrators, where great care would be taken in the selection of members. The organization was to be nonpolitical and nonsectarian, open to men and women, and lay and religious administrators—if they could meet the qualifications.[59] Lutes proposed three classes of members: Members, Senior Members (Members of three years, plus evidence of ability), and Fellows (open to Senior Members after three years). There were also to be Honorary Members. Policy for the organization was to be determined by a Council of Regents, which was to be elected by the Fellows and Senior Members.

A month later, Lutes invited this group to dinner at Ravenswood Hospital. This core group selected 48 administrators to be invited to start the organization.[60] The group consisted of 42 men from 20 states and 6 men from Canada. Twelve were physicians.

The American College of Surgeons also started by selecting a founding group in this way. The ACS produced a prolonged hostile reaction from many physicians who practiced some surgery and who objected to an elitist organization which would put some surgeons ahead of others.[61]

The ACHE was no such economic threat. It met with very little hostility except from some physician administrators of larger eastern hospitals who felt that the College was trying to preempt hospital administration for non-physician managers.[62]

On February 2, 1933, MacEachern, Lutes, Erickson, Wordell and Fesler met at the Chicago office of the American College of Surgeons. Responses of the administrators were reviewed. It was decided to call a meeting to officially create the organization. Wordell was appointed Chairman of the organizing committee.[63]

On February 13, 1933, 18 administrators, including MacEachern, Matthew Foley (*Hospital Management*) and John McNamara (*Modern Hospitals*), attended the meeting which created the college at the Palmer House in Chicago. This meeting was held during the meeting of the Council on Medical Education and Hospitals of the American Medical Association (AMA).[64]

MacEachern "gave many reasons why we should have an organization to elevate the standards of hospital administration," and a motion to form such an organization was unanimously adopted. The name of American College of Hospital Administrators was chosen by a large majority and the slate of officers was unanimously elected.

President	Charles A. Wordell
First Vice President	Robert E. Neff
Second Vice President	Joseph G. Norby
Director General	J. Dewey Lutes
Executive Committee	Reverend Herman Fritschel, Maurice Dubin, and John Smith[65]

Among the objectives of the College were: Elevation of the standards of hospital administration; establishment of a standard of competency for hospital administrators; development and promotion of standards of education and training for hospital administrators; education of the public and of hospital trustees to the fact that the practice of hospital administration called for special training and experience; and provision for a method of conferring fellowships in hospital administration on those who had done or were doing noteworthy service in the field of hospital administration.[66]

These objectives have been pursued throughout the 60-year history of the College. Chapter 5 describes the evolution of hospital administration education and the accompanying role of the College. Chapter 6 explains how standards were developed by the College to define excellence in hospital administration. Chapter 7 explores how the College conveyed the complex nature of hospital administration by defining its intellectual content through College publications. Chapters 8, 9, and 10 probe the evolving organization of the College.

In the first annual report of the Director General in 1934, Dewey Lutes reported that during the September, 1933, meeting of the College in Milwaukee, 70 names were approved for Charter Fellowship and 11 for Charter Honorary Fellowship. By the date of the first anniversary meeting, this number had risen to 103 Charter Fellows and 17 Charter Honorary Fellows.[67] Lutes reports:

In a few instances fear was expressed that the College should have been organized by the American Hospital Association and that we would duplicate the work of that organization. In these cases, it was clearly pointed out that the American Hospital Association could not, by virtue of its own constituency, show any distinction of standards of competency for hospital administrators and that the trustees of the AHA were agreed on this point.[68]

On February 12, 1934, Wordell and Lutes met with the AHA trustees to present the plans and objectives of the College. Adds Lutes:

This was a most friendly meeting terminating in the clear understanding of the relationships between the two organizations and with their best wishes for the success of the College. To quote the exact words of the Chairman of the Board of Trustees on that occasion, "Is there anything the American Hospital Association can do at this time to help?"[69]

The relationship between the College and the AHA was to be a close one, as was reflected by the number of Charter Fellows who became or had been presidents of the AHA.[70] See Table 2.3.

TABLE 2.3
Administrators who were Charter Fellows, Chairmen (formerly called Presidents) of ACHE, and/or Chairmen of AHA and AUPHA and their Dates of Office[72]

Name	Charter Fellow (CF) or Honorary Charter Fellow (HCF) or Fellow (F)	ACHE Chairman (Date)	AHA Chairman (Date)	AUPHA Chairman (Date)
Charles Wordell	CF	1933–34		
Robert Neff	CF	34–35	1938	
Fred Carter, M.D.*	CF	35–36	40	
Basil MacLean, M.D.*	CF	36–37	42	
Howard Bishop	CF	37–38		
Robin Buerki, M.D.*	CF	38–39	36	
James A. Hamilton	F	39–40	43	1951–53
Arthur C. Bachmeyer, M.D.*	CF	40–41	26	48–49
Lucias R. Wilson, M.D.*	CF	41–42		
Joseph G. Norby	CF	42–43	49	
Claude W. Munger, M.D.*	CF	44–46	37	
Frank R. Bradley, M.D.*	F	46–47	55	54–55
Jessie Turnbull	CF	48–49		
Frank J. Walter	CF	50–51	44	
Ernest Erikson	CF	51–52		
Merrill Steele, M.D.	CF	54–55		
Dewey Lutes	CF	55–56		
Arthur Swanson	CF	56–57		
Frank S. Groner	F	57–58	61	
Ray Brown	F	59–60	56	66–67
Melvin Sutley	CF	60–61		
Tol Terrell	F	61–62	58	
Thomas Howell, M.D.	HCF		14	
Asa Bacon	CF		23	
Malcolm MacEachern, M.D.	HCF		24	49–50
G. Harvey Agnew, M.D.	HCF		39	53–54
B. W. Black, M.D.*	CF		41	
Donald C. Smeltzer, M.D.*	CF		45	
Peter D. Ward, M.D.*	CF		46	
D. Kirk Oglesby	F	86–87	92	
James O. Hepner, Ph.D.	F	90–91		75–76

*Members of the Society of Medical Administrators.

24

Of the 103 Charter Fellows and 17 Honorary Charter Fellows of the College, 17 became chairmen of the ACHE; 15 became chairmen of the AHA. Eight were all three: Charter Fellows, chairmen of AHA, and chairmen of ACHE. Frank J. Walter was the last ACHE chairman to be all three. Six additional people, although not Charter Fellows, have been heads of both ACHE and AHA: James A. Hamilton, Frank Bradley, Frank Groner, Ray Brown, Tol Terrell, and D. Kirk Oglesby, Jr. However, AHA chairmen have usually been Fellows of the College up to the present time.[71]

Of the early administrators, several held major academic positions in health administration programs during their careers: James A. Hamilton (Minnesota), Arthur Bachmeyer, M.D. (Chicago), Ray E. Brown (Chicago, Duke, Northwestern), Frank Bradley, M.D. (Washington University, St. Louis), G. Harvey Agnew, M.D. (Toronto), and Malcolm MacEachern, M.D. (Northwestern). Since 1967, there has been an increased division of labor between practicing administrators and professors of hospital administration (see Chapter 7).

More recently, Everett Johnson, Ph.D., and James Hepner, Ph.D., have directed health administrtion degree programs. Hepner was president of AUPHA in 1975–1976 and Chairman of the College in 1990–1991.

Here is how John R. Mannix remembered a few of the Charter Fellows: George O'Hanlon, M.D., of the New Jersey Medical Center in Jersey City, was loyal to Mayor Hague, who ran that city the way Richard J. Daley ran Chicago. Bryce Twitty, a devout Methodist, was at Baylor University Hospital when Justin Ford Kimball started prepayment there for teachers, thus precipitating Blue Cross.

Melvin Sutley was a lawyer who taught commercial law in Japan before becoming an administrator. Most of his administrative career was at Delaware County Hospital in Drexel Hill, Pennsylvania.

Eighteen of the founders were Canadian, including A. J. Swanson, Muriel Anscombe, Peter Ward, George F. Stephen and Donald Smeltzer, M.D.

Joe Norby was Administrator of the Fairview Hospital in Minneapolis. His son, Morris Norby, was associated with Blue Cross of Pittsburgh and was given the Justin Kimball award.

Basil MacLean, M.D., was another Canadian and served with the Touro Infirmary in New Orleans. Later, he became President of the National Blue Cross Association prior to Jeb Stuart, who preceded Walter McNerney.

Arthur C. Bachmeyer was a real dean and the great administrator of this century. As the father of Bob Bachmeyer, he helped form the only father and son pair who would both be presidents of the College.

E. M. Bluestone (he never used anything but "E.M."), was Administrator of Montefiore Hospital in New York and trained by Dr. S. S. Goldwater. He was one of the first people interested in geriatrics.

Albert G. Hahn, Administrator of Deaconess Hospital, Evansville, Indiana, was the only blind man in the founding group. His wife, Grace, was always with him. Mannix never saw them apart and met Hahn several times before he realized he was blind. The College made Grace an Honorary Charter Fellow in 1953.

John R. Mannix remembered Asa Bacon as always remaining young "I always came away with a great deal of sound advice from him."

According to Mannix, Bob Buerki was one of the all-time greats, as was Claude Munger, M.D.

Bob Jolly, a Texan from Houston, was a close friend of MacEachern.

Jesse Turnbull was a nurse and a real leader of the Hospital Association of Pennsylvania. "All of the 103 Charter Fellows were outstanding leaders," Mannix noted.[73]

The last living Charter Fellow, Robin Buerki, M.D., died in 1992 bringing the founding era to a close.

The Eras of the Manager and CEO: 1966–1993

The Eisenhower years, 1954–1961, saw the Supreme Court's decision to end school desegregation, the launch of Sputnik starting the space race, and the introduction of the Salk polio vaccine. By 1955, the College had 3,467 affiliates. The College journal, *Hospital Administration*, began in 1956. The twenty-fifth anniversary of the College saw the start of its annual Congress on Administration.

As part of the "Great Society" legislation of Lyndon Johnson, the Medicare and Medicaid amendments to the Social Security Act took effect in 1966. A growing complexity in the healthcare environment followed: health maintenance organizations, neighborhood health centers, health planning agencies, nursing homes, and increasing government involvement in regulating health services. As a result, a higher proportion of College members than ever before were managing health organizations other than hospitals.

Rising hospital costs created the need for Medicare and Medicaid, which in turn allowed rising costs to continue. Total expenditure on medical research in 1949 was only $45,000,000. Government expenditure on medical research was $1.008 billion, out of a total of $1.545 billion in 1963. By 1977, the government paid for $3.612 billion, out of a total of $5.526 billion for medical research.[74] Not only did this large investment in research lead to improved medical care such as heart surgery and diagnostic devices, it also helped increase medical care costs.

Not all new treatments increased costs. Drugs to control tuberculosis emptied the once numerous tuberculosis hospitals. Nineteen fifty-five was the peak year for the number of mental hospital inpatients. Effective drugs and community mental health centers led to the era of deinstitutionalization. Polio vaccines replaced the costly iron lung. As the proportion of the population over the age of 65 grew, the number of residents in nursing homes increased. By about 1975, there were, for the first time, more people in nursing homes than in hospitals.

No precise date hails the era of the multi-institutional hospital system, but 1979 was the first year that the Hospital Corporation of American (HCA) exceeded a billion dollars both in revenue and assets.[75] In 1983, the College's fiftieth year, membership was a record 16,433 affiliates, reflecting both the size of the health field, which then consumed 10 percent of the gross national product, and the continuing value of the College to the profession of hospital and health services administration.

The 1990s brought new ideas of quality improvement as reflected in the Joint Commission on Accreditation of Healthcare Organization's "new initiative" and the College's 1990 Standards of Excellence for Staff (Table 2.4) and the start of its own internal continuous quality improvement effort in 1992.

Throughout these years the College's growth has been constant, as Table 2.5 shows.

PART III

The Organization of a Profession

From the very beginning, Dewey Lutes and the AHA Trustees saw a clear distinction between the AHA and the ACHE. The AHA would seek to represent all hospital superintendents, while the ACHE would work to single out more qualified superintendents for designation as Fellows, thereby raising the standards of the profession.

In order to understand the role the College has selected for itself and its relation to other professional organizations, it is useful to consider types of organizations, as well as their relationships and functions.

TABLE 2.4 [handwritten: Internal Quality Improvement]
ACHE Standards of Excellence for Staff (adopted August 1990)[76]

Service: We are committed to exceeding the expectations of our affiliates and our co-workers in a helpful and courteous manner.

Quality: We do things right the first time.

Integrity: We can be trusted to perform our jobs with honesty, sincerity, and respect for others.

Timeliness: We promptly respond to affiliates because they are our highest priority; we meet or exceed all deadlines and help our co-workers to do the same.

Reliability: We can be trusted to do what we say we are going to do and to follow through on tasks to successful completion.

Teamwork: We work harmoniously with others to get the job done.

Competitiveness: We do not stand alone in the marketplace—healthcare executives have other organizations to which they can turn for professional services. Therefore, we must always be responsive to our affiliates' needs.

Professionalism: We consistently demonstrate behavior that is worth emulating and reflects well on the organization.

Fiscal responsibility: We use our resources wisely and efficiently to achieve our goals.

Staff development: We constantly work to enhance our knowledge and skills.

Organizational Types

One feature of a profession is the presence of one or more national organizations. Within the healthcare field, there are basically four general types of organizations for each profession:

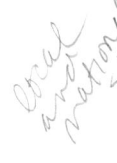

1. An inclusive organization open to all, often called an association.
2. An exclusive organization whose fellowship is open to the qualified elite, usually called a college.
3. An association for educators in the profession.
4. Specialized organizations for professionals with focused interests.

The first two are likely to have local and national organizational components.

In this century, there has been a continuous division of labor in health, and subspecialization both in medicine and administration, resulting in a growing number of "subspecialty" organizations.

In medicine, the inclusive organization welcoming all physicians is the American Medical Association. The exclusive organizations are primarily the specialty colleges. The organization of medical educators is the Association of American Medical Colleges. Specialized organizations abound.

TABLE 2.5
**Active (Dues-Paying) Affiliates of the ACHE as of January of
each year[77]**

Year	Fellows	Members	Nominees	Students	Total
1933	104				104
1935	147	80			227
1937	188	198	33		419
1939	286	424	143		853
1941	317	530	218		1065
1943	288	624	258		1170
1945	272	731	366		1369
1947	268	867	619		1754
1949	280	1035	949		2264
1951	304	1220	1083		2607
1953	429	1413	1205		3047
1955	540	1687	1240		3467
1957	681	1852	1291		3824
1959	872	2049	1449		4370
1961	1070	2286	1808		5164
1963	1209	2141	1649		4999
1965	1125	2567	1584		5276
1967	1388	2980	1749	480	6597
1969	1519	3304	2371	993	8187
1971	1604	3752	2476	1059	8891
1973	1580	3861	2765	1395	9603
1975	1471	4258	2556	1414	9699
1977	1519	4687	2730	2254	11185
1979	1606	5181	3302	2556	12645
1981	1653	5565	4612	3602	15432
1983	1761	6084	5412	3176	16433
1985	1801	6511	5542	5656	19510
1987	1761	7044	5870	4292	18967
1989	1936	7419	6775	4755	20885
1991	1649	6351	8050	4998	21048
1993	2431	7101	10370	5389	25291

In hospital management, the inclusive organization is the American Hospital Association. The exclusive organization is the ACHE, although it reaches out beyond hospitals. The relevant association of educators is the Association of University Programs in Health Administration. A number of the specialty national health organizations are listed in Table 2.6. Some of these are inclusive; others are exclusive; and some may be a mixture of the two.

TABLE 2.6
Other Health Management Professional Organizations in Existence in 1992[81]

Date of Founding	I—Inclusive E—Exclusive	Name (comments)
1926	I	Medical Group Management Association[82]
1930	I	National Executive Housekeeper's Association[83] (members both in and out of health field)
1942	I	Association of State and Territorial Health officials
1946	I/E	Healthcare Financial Management Association (formerly Hospital Financial Management Association)[84]
1948	I	Association of University Programs in Health Administration (incorporated 1950)[85]
1948	I/E	American Association of Healthcare Consultants[86]
1954	E	College of Osteopathic Healthcare Executives[87]
1956	E	American College of Medical Practice Executives (affiliated with Medical Group Management Association[88]
1957	I/E	The American Academy of Medical Administrators[89] (all areas of health management, plus fellowship)
1957	I	National Association of Hospital Purchasing Materials Management
1958	I	National Association of Hospital Central Service Personnel (in 1969 changed to International Association of Hospital Central Service Materiel Management)[90]
1959	E	Association of Mental Health Administrators[91]
1960	I/E	Association for Volunteer Administration[92]
1962	I/E	American College of Health Care Administrators (formerly American College of Nursing Home Administrators)[93]
1962	I	American Society for Hospital Materials Management (of the AHA)[94]
1965	I	American Society for Healthcare Human Resources Administration (formerly American Society for Hospital Personnel Administration) of the AHA[95]
1967	I	American Society for Hospital Food Services Administrators of the AHA[96]
1967	I	Association of Nurse Executives (of the AHA)[97]
1968	I	National Association of Health Services Executives[98]
1970	E	Canadian College of Health Service Executives[99]
1971	I	American Health Planning Association[100]
1971	I	Clinical Laboratory Management Association
1972	I	American Healthcare Radiology Administrators Inc.[101]
1975	I	The American Academy of Medical Directors[102]
1978	E	The American College of Physician Executives (Merged into the American Academy of Medical Directors Jan. 1, 1989)[103]
1978	I	Society for Healthcare Planning and Marketing (AHA)

Relationships between Professions

Early writers on the professions worked with the model of the private practicing physician or lawyer functioning as an independent entrepreneur. Independent practice called for licensure as a means to define both the profession and exclude unqualified practitioners. With the growth of organizations, hospitals and medical group practices, professionals are also organizational members and employees, their work being defined by a position in an organization chart.

To the degree that organizational position defines the profession, licensure recedes in importance. Overwhelmingly, the healthcare executive is defined by such an organizational position rather than by licensure. For a number of years, hospital administrators were licensed in Minnesota, but this is no longer the case.[78]

Specialties in healthcare management are defined by organizational position. The growing division of labor in the field had led to the growth of the health management specialty organizations listed in Table 2.6.[79] The inclusive associations were created before the exclusive colleges. Healthcare professions can have numerous relationships, which in turn affect their national organizations. These are summarized in Table 2.7. They can be parallel, independent, and noncompetitive like medicine and dentistry. Or, they can be parallel, independent and competitive like podiatry and medicine.

Relationships can also be vertical, in that one profession can define the activities of another. This can occur through required membership in the general profession before becoming a specialist.

Vertically related healthcare management specialty areas are largely connected through organizational dominance (#4) rather than through professional dominance (#3), primarily because of the absence of licensure in healthcare management. The single licensed healthcare management profession is nursing home administration, because of a federal legislation mandate.[80] Since nursing homes and medical group practices evolved separately but parallel with hospitals, they have developed separate organizations for managers.

Up to 1945, the average community hospital had only one administrator, thus allowing no division of managerial labor. The growth of the hospital in size, cost, and complexity occurred largely after 1966, requiring more specialist managers.

By 1979, with the development of multi-institutional systems, there were proportionately fewer CEOs and more specialized middle managers and staff specialists.

Up to 1945, the hospital was almost the only large organization in the healthcare field. After 1966, the growth and diversity of other organizational forms, including Blue Cross, planning agencies, HMOs,

TABLE 2.7
The System of Profession Typology of Parallel and Vertical Relationships between Health Professions

I. Parallel Relationship between Professions
  1) Not overlapping parallelism
    Example: Dentistry and Medicine are separately licensed and organized with a general agreement as to task boundaries.
  2) Overlapping parallelism
    Example: Osteopathic and (General or Allopathic) Medicine or Psychiatry and Psychology.
II. Vertical Relationships between Professions
  1) A Specialty achieved only through membership in the larger specialty
    Example: One must be a physician in order to be a surgeon.
  2) Specialty within a larger profession with independent entry.
    Example: Nursing Home Administration is a specialty of health administration with independent entry. See Table 2.6 for other examples.
  3) Professional Dominance[104]
    The dominant profession of pathology defines the certifying examinations for cytotechnologists.[105]
  4) Organizational Dominance
    General hospital administrators supervise executive housekeepers.
III. Combinations of the above relationships
  Hospital Administration is parallel with medicine, but some managers supervise physicians and physicians supervise some managers.

and neighborhood health centers, was rapid. As a result, managers could increasingly move to varied types of organizations during the course of their careers.

These changes have, from the beginning, posed two organizational issues for the ACHE: how to relate to specialized managers and how far down the organizational hierarchy to move in accepting members.

In 1934, the College voted not to accept executives of healthcare associations as members and instead to be an organization of hospital administrators. But by the 1940s, it was apparent that occasionally, Fellows who had been hospital administrators would become Blue Cross plan managers or professors of hospital administration. In 1959, 16 of 17 graduate programs used "hospital administration" in their titles. By 1969, 9 of 28 AUPHA member programs were using the phrase "health administration" to reflect their graduates' employment in other health service organizations as well as in hospitals.[106] In 1976, the College's journal changed its name from *Hospital Administration* to *Hospital & Health Services Administration*.[107]

In 1981, a motion to change the title of the College from "Hospital" to "Health" was defeated,[108] although 20 percent of the College membership was working in organizations other than hospitals throughout the 1970s.[109] In 1985, the vote went the other way and the organization became the American College of Healthcare Executives. The Regents and Governors were nearly all managers of hospitals (94 percent in 1981–82).[110]

In medicine, the professional boundary is defined by state licensure. The National Board of Medical Examiners coordinates these efforts. Because medicine was a self-employed occupation independent of an organization in its formative years, licensure was required.

By contrast, hospital administration is defined by an organizational position. This, in turn, requires that a hospital be defined. Initially, this was done by the AMA and later through the AHA list of hospitals, and by state hospital licensure. Like the AMA, the AHA is inclusive, welcoming all hospitals as institutional members and interested individuals as personal members.

Inclusive professional organizations tend to develop a stable central leadership, reflecting the senior, elite members of the occupation. For both the AMA and the AHA, this is accomplished through the leadership of state constituencies that comprise the national house of delegates.

In medicine, specialization and elite organizations are combined in the specialty colleges like the American College of Surgeons. In hospital administration, the elite organization—the ACHE—came before managerial specialization.

Professional educators have sufficiently distinct interests that they created their own organizations: the Association of American Medical Colleges for physicians, and the Association of University Programs in Health Administration for hospital and health administration educators. However, the practitioner organizations have a continuing interest in education and do not leave these concerns solely to the educators. There is a partial overlap between these educational and practitioner organizations.

The first generation of hospital administration program directors were usually accomplished hospital administrators and College Fellows. Later on, many faculty were full-time academics who were not qualified to manage hospitals, but instead were sociologists, economists, and such. Into the 1960s, these academics were ineligible for College Fellowship, which stood for high competence in hospital management. After 1967, College admission requirements were broadened to allow full-time academics to become College affiliates. However, they are still expected to demonstrate a broad understanding of health management as reflected in the College examinations.

The growth of healthcare management specialty societies has not stopped the growth of the ACHE. By joining the ACHE, the healthcare management student declares an aspiration toward leadership and general management. To achieve this goal, the student might begin a career in specialized management and progress toward general management. The College has therefore grown steadily in an increasingly specialized healthcare management world. In the last few years, the College has developed even closer contact with various specialized associations.[111]

In the field of medicine, becoming a generalist precedes specialization. In health administration, specialization often occurs before promotion to a generalist position.

With the growth of the college has come increased organizational complexity based on region, education and research, special interests, and international links. These are summarized in Table 2.8. The size of the college has led to the creation of seven regional districts covering the USA and Canada. In addition, there are local healthcare executive groups. As of 1992, there were 70 local groups of which 63 were "officially designated."[112] Other special interest groups include 20 women's healthcare executive networks of which 14 are officially

TABLE 2.8
Typology of Relationships within ACHE

National Organization	ACHE
I. Regional Affiliates	1) Districts (7)[113]
	2) State chapters (few)
	3) Local Groups (Healthcare Executive Groups)[114]
	a) officially recognized
	b) listed
II. Education and Research	1) Student affiliates, Student Chapters[115]
	2) Faculty affiliates[116]
	3) Research Division[117]
	4) ACHE Foundation[118]
III. Special Interest Groups	1) Physician Executives, Nurse Executives, Long Term Care Executives, Managed Care Executives, Women's Healthcare Executive Networks[119]
	2) Specialization
	3) Other
	a) Uniformed Services (District 8)[120]
	b) Regents-at-large
IV. International	1) Canada (included in 7 districts)
	2) Other[121]

designated. There are student chapters associated with about 100 degree programs in health administration. There are both Student Associates and Faculty Associates. Research is carried out within the College. Specialization in management is reflected not in organizations, but in component parts of the College's competency evaluations.

The U.S. Military medical service officers have long been active in the College and College advancement is recognized for promotion in military rank. The uniformed services members constitute District 8. In addition, the position of regent-at-large, created in 1989, represents people or areas underrepresented among the districts regents. International links with Canada have been close from the start because a number of leading healthcare executives in the United States were originally from Canada. Unlike research and medical societies there is little linkage with organizations of healthcare executives in other countries, although the College several times organized study tours of the medical care systems of other countries and published reports about them. Perhaps one reason for this is that the knowledge of hospital management depends on the reimbursement and regulatory system of the country. A British textbook on hospital management has little relevence in the United States and vice versa.

The Functions of Professional Societies

Nearly all professional societies have a core of functions and activities they implement for their membership. These are listed in Table 2.9.

The Definition of Boundaries

The first function required for the existence of the society is definition of the profession's boundaries. Licensure or certification makes these boundaries easier to define. However, hospital and healthcare administration is largely defined by organizational position rather than licensure.

The College has a program for credentialing and certification, as described in Chapter 6. It also participates in the accreditation of university-based degree programs in hospital and health administration through voting representation on the Accrediting Commission on Education for Health Services Administration, founded in 1968.[122] The other voting members are the American College of Medical Practice Executives, the American Hospital Association, the American Public Health Association (APHA), the Association of University Programs in Health Administration, and the joint Canadian Hospital Association–Canadian College of Health Service Executives membership.[123]

Directories of society membership also help define the profession. The College has published such directories since 1938.

TABLE 2.9
Functions of Professional Societies[126]

  I. Definition of the Boundary of a Profession and Membership
    —Professional licensure
    —Organizational position
    —Certification
    —Accreditation of professional schools
    —Publication of membership directories
  II. Liaison
    —With other organizations of the same profession
    —With government (Public Policy)
      —development of position papers
      —lobbying
      —political action committees (PAC's)
    —With other relevant organizations
 III. Definition of Excellence based on peer judgment rather than the marketplace
    —Fellowship examination
    —Awards
 IV. Publications
    —Journals, Books
    —Newsletters, Audio and Video Tapes
    —Technical Reports, Policy Statements
    —Publicity, News Releases
  V. Continuing Education
    —Short courses
    —Conferences
    —Correspondence courses and material
    —Accreditation of continuing education
    —Self-assessment of members
 VI. Research and Consulting
    —Research conferences for society members
    —Research carried out directly by the staff of the Society
    —Historic Archives
VII. Socio-Economic Issues
    —Colleagueship
    —Codes of Ethics, ethical standards
      —adjudication
    —Job Placement Service
    —Advice and Consultation to individual members
    —Insurance for members
    —Surveys of working conditions
VIII. Maintenance of the Society's internal organization
    —Staff
    —Finances

Liaison and Public Policy

Professional societies must relate to other organizations within the same profession. In recent years, the College has pursued these liaison activities on a more regular basis.[124] Government relations, however, are typically more important for the inclusive organization, which has a broader political base due to a larger membership. In medicine, the AMA spends more energy on lobbying than the medical Colleges. The AHA and the AMA both have political action committees (PACs), while the ACHE does not.[127]

Any society that assumes an active liaison role with government must have a mechanism for developing consensus on policy issues. For the first 40 years of its existence, the College chose not to take positions on government legislation and regulation, leaving this activity to the AHA. This changed in 1973 with the acceptance of the Report of the Board of Governor's Special Task Force, "The Role of the ACHA in the Legislative Process," by Everett Johnson (chair), Boone Powell, Frank C. Sutton, M.D. and R. Zach Thomas, Jr. (See Table 2.10.) This report recommended that the College not become involved in lobbying nor open a Washington, D.C., or Ottawa office. It should introduce position papers and assure that they be brought to the attention of appropriate legislative bodies.[128]

In 1974, the College developed position papers on national health insurance resulting from a Board of Governors' Special Study Commission chaired by Peter Terenzio.[129] At the same time, Professor Odin Anderson was commissioned to write a position paper on the implications for hospital management of national health insurance.[130]

A major departure from the College's past philosophy of political inactivity also occurred in 1980 in an accord reached with the AHA. The two organizations agreed to "have mutually supportive roles in the development and advocacy of policy affecting health care institutions and the professional management of these institutions."[131] This document reflects a continuing close relationship between these two organizations. It appears as an appendix to this chapter.

The College's first venture in this area was to deliver testimony before the U.S. Treasury Department on deferred compensation for managers in nonprofit organizations.[132]

In 1982, the College also produced a press release and backgrounder on the ethical conflicts arising through healthcare rationing.[133] "The question of whether life should be preserved at all costs will be the most difficult ethical decision facing hospitals in the 1980s," the material stated.

In 1983 a standing committee on public policy was started and a policy analyst hired. In 1984 a ACHA/AHA agreement was signed, whereby AHA would provide Washington representation for the Col-

TABLE 2.10
ACHE Public Policy Chronology[134]

June 7–8, 1973	Acceptance of the Report "The Role of the ACHA in the Legislative Process."[135]
1974	Special Study Commission on national health insurance.[129,130]
April 24, 1980	Statement on deferred compensation.[132]
July, 1980	ACHE/AHA Accord approved (see Appendix)
1981	Programmatic Thrusts approved, Public policy objectives added to ACHE Bylaws.
1982	Statement on Ethical Conflicts[133]
1983	Committee on Public Policy approved and appointed, Policy analyst hired.
1984	ACHE/AHA Washington Contract signed; Strategic Plan Drafted.
July, 1985	Policy Statements: Healthcare Coalitions, Voluntary Credentialing, Institutional Ethical Mechanisms, Educational Training in Ethics for Healthcare Executives.[136]
1986	Policy Statements: Access to Healthcare; Death with Dignity, Organ Donation
Feb., 1987	Policy Statement: Medical Records Confidentiality
July, 1989	Policy Statement: Community Service Ethic
July, 1990	Policy Statement: Enhancing Minority Opportunities in Healthcare Management
1991	Washington contract ends; public policy activities subsumed by current staff
July, 1991	Strategic Plan calls for enhanced public policy
May, 1992	Policy Statements: Strengthening Healthcare Employment Opportunities for Persons with Disabilities; Age Discrimination and the Healthcare Executive.[137]
1992	Public policy columns introduced in *Healthcare Executive* magazine
	Government Relations Director hired

lege.[138] The AHA would focus on institutional concerns while the College would focus on professional and societal concerns. Starting in July 1985, the College has produced a series of policy statements relevent to health care executives. The policy committee monitors issues and develops, with the help of the staff, position statements which go to the Board of Governors for approval before release.[139] In 1992, the position of Director for Government Relations was created and filled, and in 1993 a public policy plan was developed.

The Definition of Excellence

Professionalism assumes a learned body of skills and knowledge aspired to and known by members of the profession. This expertise is defined by the profession's leadership and is not necessarily identical to actual performance. Physicians, for example, have long believed that the best physician—as defined by his or her peers—is not necessarily the one that earns the highest income. Exclusive professional societies therefore often use peer judgment of expertise as the definition of fellowship.

Hospital governing boards (non-experts) define the organizational role of hospital managers by hiring them and fixing their salaries. However, the governing board's opinion and peer opinion have not always been consistent. This was an early issue raised within the College. Should the College come to the aid of a Fellow who has been dismissed from his position by a hospital board for reasons that appear to be arbitrary to his peers? The College decided not (see Chapter 6).

Publications
Professional societies must communicate with their members and the College is no exception. They do this through journals, newsletters and magazines, technical reports, policy statements, news releases, audio and video tapes, and announcements of educational programs and publications. In the last decade the College began a book publishing program by acquiring Health Administration Press (see Chapters 7 and 8), and by initiating a magazine, *Healthcare Executive*.

Continuing Education
Continuing education embraces seminars, conferences, books, self-study courses, and materials such as audio cassettes available by mail. A professional society can become involved in accreditation or approval of continuing education programs. The College is committed to life-long learning and continuing self-assessment of its affiliate body (see Chapter 5).

Research and Consulting
Meetings to exchange current research findings are often a feature of professional societies, but more likely those of academics than of practitioners. Research on health administration is more often presented at meetings of the APHA and/or the AUPHA rather than at those of the AHA or the ACHE. However, the College's journal has been an important source for reporting research in recent years. The College's Division of Research and Development issues each year a number of reports; sometimes these are funded by external sources.

Socio-Economic Issues
The opportunity to renew old acquaintances, make new ones, and talk with like-minded peers is an important part of a professional society.

Professional societies are also concerned with the ethical conduct of their profession. The AHA and the AMA both have codes of ethics. The American College of Surgeons was concerned with stopping fee splitting from its inception. The ACHE code will be discussed in Chapter 3.

Societies also provide job placement services. Sometimes this is accomplished formally through a job clearing house where written offers and requests are received and distributed. More often, it is accomplished on an informal basis at society meetings. The College now regularly lists available positions in *Career Mart*, which is available by subscription.

Some societies also offer individual consultation for members. College affiliates have available the services of Career Decision, Inc., a subsidiary firm, that offers complete outplacement services and other counseling services related to career development.

The College has also published reports and studies about working conditions in the field.[140]

Finally, professional societies must maintain a stable ongoing staff and funding to carry out their objectives and continue their existence (see Chapter 9).

APPENDIX
Proposed Accord on the Roles and Responsibilities of the American Hospital Association and the American College of Hospital Administrators in the Development and Implementation of Public Policy
approved by the Board of Trustees of the American Hospital Association and the Board of Governors of the American College of Hospital Administrators
July 1980

The American Hospital Association (AHA) and the American College of Hospital Administrators (ACHA) have mutually supportive roles in the development and advocacy of policy affecting healthcare institutions and the professional management of those institutions.

Coordination of ACHA and AHA in policy development is achieved at a number of levels, through both formal and informal means. The president of ACHA is invited to attend the AHA Board of Trustees meetings, and governors of the College are invited to attend Regional Advisory Board meetings. The president of the AHA is invited to attend ACHA Board meetings. In addition, affiliates of the College are involved at every level of AHA: Board, council, Regional Advisory

Board, and staff. Regular contact between top management of the two associations further enhances coordination in policy development.

Their roles, as agreed to by the Board of Governors of ACHA and the Board of Trustees of AHA, are described in this document for the purpose of delineating the respective responsibilities in policy development and policy advocacy of the two organizations.

POLICY DEVELOPMENT ACTIVITIES

A. American College of Hospital Administrators' Role.
1. The ACHA will play a key role in the development of policies personally affecting the affiliates of the College as distinguished from institutional issues. Some examples are:
   a. Education
   b. Compensation
   c. Credentialing
   d. Manpower/Management Research
   e. Managerial Effectiveness
2. It is considered appropriate for the ACHA to take the initiative in the development of policies in the above areas. Close coordination with AHA and other allied associations is assumed to be necessary.
3. During the ACHA policy development process, ACHA affiliates will also represent, concurrently, AHA institutional interests on the Council of Regents, Board of Governors and committees. This dual representation will keep communications open between the two organizations.
4. The ACHA will assist AHA in promotion and operation of the AHA's Political Action Committee wherever legally and operationally feasible and appropriate.
B. American Hospital Association's Role.
1. The AHA's policy development role will concentrate primarily on those issues affecting the institution as distinguished from those affecting individual College affiliates connected with the institution. Examples are:
   a. Financial Requirements of the Institution
   b. Institutional Regulation
   c. Environmental Forces Affecting the Institution
   d. Institutional Management Effectiveness
2. During the AHA policy development process, ACHA's Board, affiliates, and staff will maintain contacts through services on the AHA Board, Regional Advisory Boards,

council, and committees. Through this mechanism, communications will remain open and active at all levels.

POLICY IMPLEMENTATION ACTIVITIES

A. American College of Hospital Administrators' Responsibilities.
1. The ACHA recognizes both the separate and joint responsibility roles in governmental policy implementation as well as the importance of cooperation and coordination of its activities with the AHA on national health issues.
2. The ACHA will attempt to increase the effectiveness of implementation in a number of ways, including but not limited to the following activities:
   a. Encouragement of affiliate involvement in the allied associations (AHA/state/metro) "Partnership for Action."
   b. Playing a supportive role to AHA in issues for which that organization has primary responsibility for implementation.
   c. Playing a primary implementation role in issues for which ACHA has a recognized primary responsibility, with close AHA coordination.
B. American Hospital Association's Responsibilities.
1. Because national and mutually vital issues must be prioritized and balanced and because subtle shifts in policy are often necessary to accommodate changes in the political environment, the AHA must, in most cases, play the primary role in implementing national policy.
2. These activities pertain to the implementation of policy in the legislative, executive and judicial branches of government.
3. In policy implementation, the AHA recognizes the need for broad support and cooperation from ACHA and participation of affiliates in the "Partnership for Action."

CONTINUING EVALUATION

The roles and responsibilities described in this accord will be subject to annual review by the chairman officers and presidents of both organizations in joint meeting.

NOTES

[1] Carter, 1936, p. 67, based on the College's Articles of Incorporation, March 26, 1934. Also ACHA, *1960 Directory*, p. 11.

[2] Toner, 1873.

[3] Morris, 1953, pp. 541–546.

[4] Wilson and Neuhauser, 1982.

[5] *Information Please Almanac*, 1981, U.S. Department of Health, Education and Welfare; *Health in America, 1776–1976*, 1976, pp. 195–211.

[6] Steinberg, 1949.

[7] *The Timetable of Technology*, 1982.

[8] Flexner, 1910. Also see Burrow, 1977.

[9] ACHA documents, Kipnis, 1955.

[10] Amberson, McMahon, and Pinner, 1931.

[11] White, 1985.

[12] *The World Almanac*, 1991, New York, pp. 41–68.

[13] *The New York Public Library Book of Chronologies.*

[14] ACHE, *1991–1992 Annual Report and Reference Guide.*

[15] Steinwald and Neuhauser, 1970.

[16] Dowling, 1977.

[17] Starr, 1982, p. 150.

[18] *Ibid.*, 1982, p. 153, Abel-Smith, 1964.

[19] Starr, p. 161.

[20] *Ibid.*, p. 147.

[21] Even at the turn of the century, voluntary hospitals received financial support from local and state government. Stevens, Rosemary, 1982.

[22] Sims, 1981.

[23] Perrow, "Goals and Power Structure: A Historical Case Study," pp. 112–146 in Freidson (editor), *The Hospital in Modern Society*, 1963.

[24] Anderson, 1975.

[25] Wilson and Neuhauser, 1982.

[26] Kalisch and Kalisch, 1978.

[27] The 1918 influenza epidemic lasted only six weeks, and hospital bed days in 1918 were 16 percent greater than in 1917. John R. Mannix was challenged with this problem of epidemics when he advocated prepayment in the 1930s. He said that prepayment could have coped with the 1918 influenza epidemic with a 16 percent buffer in premiums (interview March 1983).

[28] Reader, 1966.

[29] Cope, 1959.

[30] Reiser, 1978, pp. 26–30. The physician's gold-headed cane was also a symbol that the physician of 1800 did not work with his hands. Veblen, 1953.

[31] *American and Canadian Hospitals*, 1937.

[32] Cope, 1959.

[33] Davis, Loyal, 1960.

[34] Caldwell, 1937. The AHA was founded in 1899, but the AHA symbol shows 1898. This is not correct, but the AHA has found it too expensive to change its symbol. Quoting from a letter from John Sullivan of the American Hospital Association to John R. Mannix dated October 1, 1979:

"You are right of course. The founding date [of the AHA] is 1899 no doubt. The error was made half a century ago or however long ago the seal was designed. The story I have heard is that the individual designing the seal assumed that the first annual meeting occurred at the end of the first year. In any event, because the seal has been registered as a service mark for over 30 years, no one wants to correct the error. I think, too, it would be more confusing to the field than living with the error."

[35] Shanahan, 1965.

[36] American and Canadian Hospitals, 1937.

[37] Society of Medical Administrators, 1955, 1967. This society of physician administrators met once or twice a year from its precurser in 1909 through 1966 and beyond. Up to 1966, it only had about 120 members. However, out of this group, 38 members became presidents of the American Hospital Association between 1907 and 1969, and 13 became Chairmen of the ACHE, Madison Brown, M.D., personal communication, April 8, 1983. According to several people interviewed for this history, some of the members of this Society opposed the founding of the College, saying "the politics" were "dirty." The members of this Society were all physicians and administrators of general hospitals, typically on the east coast. Malcolm MacEachern was not a member. "There was intrigue and warfare between MacEachern and Bachmeyer," Lewis Weeks' interview of Gerhard Hartman, p. 10. Bachmeyer was a leading light of the Society of Medical Administrators.

[38] Soderstrom, 1978.

[39] American College of Surgeons, 1963.

[40] Davis, Loyal, 1960. Stevens, Rosemary, 1971, Chapter 4. Stephenson, 1990.

[41] Codman, *The Shoulder*, 1934. Neuhauser, 1990.

[42] Codman, 1917.

[43] Typical of Dr. Codman's style is his attack on Dr. F. A. Washburn when he was president of the AHA. Comments by E. A. Codman. *Transactions of the American Hospital Association*, Vol. 15, 1913, p. 180. However, this attack appeared to have its effect. See Washburn and Bresnahan, 1915.

[44] Bachmeyer, Arthur C. "A Course in Hospital Administration," 1919, pp. 279–280.

[45] John G. Bowman (Director, ACS), 1916. "In another hospital of approximately 200 beds [large for the time] the leading surgeon recently explained to me that they had always got along very well without case histories [medical records] of any description. 'Why,' he asked, 'should we disturb our success now by introducing this new stuff,'" p. 290.

[46] Davis, Loyal, 1960, p. 5.

[47] American College of Surgeons, 1938.

[48] Davis, Loyal, 1960. Stephenson, 1990, American College of Surgeons Archives on MacEachern and Codman, Jan. 1993.

[49] See *Hospitals JAHA*, Vol. 30, Feb. 16, 1956, p. 88; *Hospital Management*, Vol. 80, Aug. 1955, p. 80, Vol. 82, Aug. 1956, p. 82. Prestori, Charles B., 1956 Wolverton, Charles A., *Congressional Record* 1954 declaring August 16 as Malcolm MacEachern day. "Health Care Hall of Fame" *Modern Healthcare*, Sept. 9, 1988, p. 48. "Management in Health, The MacEachern Legacy: The Next 100 Years," April 30–May 1, 1981. Program in memory of Malcolm T. MacEachern, M.D. (1881–1956), founder of the Program in Hospital and Health Services Management, Northwestern University 1981. Four-

page printed brochure, "Malcolm Thomas MacEachern," listing his life accomplishments, no date; American College of Surgeons archives.

[50] Dewey Lutes interview, April 20, 1982.

[51] Dean Conley interview, April 1983.

[52] John R. Mannix interview, 1982; Dewey Lutes interview, 1982.

[53] "American College of Hospital Administrators," 1933. Signed by Dewey Lutes, Robert E. Neff, Joseph A. Norby, and Charles A. Wordell, "provisional committee," p. 3. Also see Dewey Lutes, "Why the College of Hospital Administrators?" 1933.

[54] Paul Fesler was formerly superintendent of the University of Minnesota Hospitals. He started Dean Conley and Ray Amberg in their careers in hospital administration, and Amberg replaced him at Minnesota. Dean Conley interview, April 1983.

[55] ACHA Minute Book, Vol. 1, Oct. 7, 1932.

[56] Kipnis, 1955, p. 1.

[57] *Ibid.*, pp. 9–10.

[58] ACHA Minute Book, Vol. 1, Oct. 7, 1932.

[59] *Ibid.*

[60] Kipnis, 1955, p. 12.

[61] Davis, Loyal, 1960.

[62] John R. Mannix, interview, 1982.

[63] Kipnis, 1955, p. 12.

[64] Lutes, "To the Members of the Board of Regents," First Annual Report of the Director-General of the ACHA, 1934, in ACHA Minute Book, Vol. 1.

[65] ACHA Minute Book, Vol. 1, Feb. 13, 1933.

[66] Kipnis, 1955, p. 13.

[67] *ACHA 1981 Directory.* Lutes (1934) includes 100 Charter Fellows and 16 Charter Honorary Fellows in his report. However, he was probably not counting exactly. According to John R. Mannix, 114 administrators were elected to become active Charter Fellows. Of these, 102 accepted (32 of these were physicians) and 12 declined (of these, nine were physicians). Of the nine physicians who declined, six were later made Honorary Members: Drs. Christopher Parnall, William H. Walsh, John M. Peters, S. S. Goldwater, Frederic Washburn, and Winford Smith. Of the three lay administrators who declined, two later joined. And, Mrs. Albert C. Hahn was made an Honorary Charter Fellow retroactively.

[68] Lutes, 1934.

[69] *Ibid.*

[70] In 1943 and 1944, there was serious consideration of merging the College into the AHA. A joint commission developed recommendations for merger, but they were rejected by the College Regents in February 1944, who voted for a continued independent existence. An agreement was made that the College would be concerned with continuing education for administrators and the AHA for departmental groups in the hospital (see Tables 1–4), Kipnis, 1955, pp. 83–87.

[71] "Among the past Chairmen of the American Hospital Association, it would appear that obtaining ACHA Fellowship is almost a prerequisite to assum-

ing this leadership role," Wesbury, ACHA, April 1981, p. 6. In recent years, to become president of the AHA (like the AMA for physicians), has required years of active work at the state level, which makes becoming head of both organizations very difficult. Further, the growth in the number of hospital administrators has increased the pool of people to draw leadership from (Wesbury interview, 1983).

72 Sources: AHA *Guide Issue*, 1982, p. B4; Kipnis, 1955; ACHA, *1981, 1992 Directory*; AUPHA 1948–1973, *Twenty-Fifth Anniversary Dinner*, 1973; Society of Medical Administrators, 1967, p. 73. Other members of the Society of Medical Administrators who became Chairmen of the College were Robert H. Bishop, M.D., 1943–1944; Wilmar M. Allen, M.D., 1949–1950; Fraser D. Mooney, M.D., 1952–1953; Albert C. Kerlikowski, M.D., 1954–1955; and Frank C. Sutton, M.D., 1962–1963. Madison Brown, M.D., personal communication, April 8, 1983.

73 John R. Mannix interview, October 1982.

74 Mushkin, 1979, p. 37, citing U.S. Department of Health, Education and Welfare, *Basic Data Relating to the National Institutes of Health*, 1962, 1966, 1978, Washington, D.C., U.S. Government Printing Office.

75 Hospital Corporation of America, Annual Report 1980, Nashville, Tennessee.

76 ACHE, *1991–1992 Annual Report and Reference Guide*, p. 63. In 1989, the College established an award honoring the memory of Alton E. Pickert, chairman 1983–1984, that each year recognizes employees who have demonstrated significant service.

77 ACHE "Fact Sheet," February 1993. The 1993 affiliate census of Feb. 2, 1993, comprised the following: 1,741 Fellows; 690 Recertified Fellows; 956 Life Fellows; and 61 Honorary Fellows (total Fellows 3,448); 5,283 Members; 1,818 Recertified Members; 531 Life Members (total Members 7,632). In addition there were 218 Faculty Associates and 190 Candidates for Nomineeship. Altogether, there were 19,902 Full-Dues-Paying Affiliates and 7,345 Non-Full-Dues-Paying Affiliates.

78 Stuart Wesbury interview, January 1983.

79 Abbott, 1988, proposes that current professional boundary disputes are often with organizations encroaching on their domain. Healthcare managers are often involved in boundary issues between other professions (for example, the role of nurse midwifes and obstetrics) rather than in fighting off other professions encroaching on management. The boundaries of health management have not been major battlefields.

80 Under the Social Security amendments of 1967 (PL 90-174).

81 *AHA Guide to the Health Care Field*, 1982, 1992; *Encyclopedia of Associations*, 1988; AUPHA *Health Services Administration Education*, 1983–85, pp. 329–335, and 1989–1991 edition, pp. 329–336; Bellin and Weeks, 1981. Associations included in the College's computer-coded member information are added to the list in the first edition.

82 Medical Group Management Association, 1982. Stevens, Edward, 1976. *Encyclopedia of Associations*, 1988, p. 1193.

83 National Executive Housekeeper's Association, 1980.

[84] Healthcare Financial Management Association, n.d., *Encyclopedia of Associations*, 1988, p. 1192.

[85] Hartman, Gerhard, *et al.*, "The Impact of Graduate Programs in Hospital Administration," *Hospital Administration*, Vol. 7, Spring 1962.

[86] Briggs, "History of the American Association of Hospital Consultants," The Association, 1984.

[87] American College of Osteopathic Hospital Administration, 1980, 1981.

[88] American College of Medical Group Administrators, 1981, 1982. Graham and Wright, 1981, *Encyclopedia of Associations*, 1988, p. 1192.

[89] American Academy of Medical Administrators, 1982, *Encyclopedia of Associations*, 1988, p. 1191.

[90] International Association of Hospital Central Service Management, n.d.

[91] AUPHA, 1989, pp. 333–334.

[92] Association for Volunteer Administration, n.d.

[93] Becker, Carl A., 1982. AUPHA, 1989, pp. 331–332.

[94] American Society for Hospital Purchasing and Materials Management, n.d.

[95] American Society for Hospital Personnel Administration, n.d.

[96] American Society for Hospital Food Service Administrators, 1992.

[97] Janine A. Swent, R.N., personal communication, 1982.

[98] See Bellin and Weeks, 1981. AUPHA, 1989, p. 336.

[99] Canadian College of Health Service Executives, 1975. AUPHA, 1989, p. 334.

[100] AUPHA, 1989, pp. 331–332.

[101] *Radiology Management* (American Hospital of Radiology Administrators), 10th anniversary issue, Vol. 4, No. 3, June 1982. There is also a Radiologists Business Managers Association founded in 1968, *Encyclopedia of Associations*, 1988, p. 1193.

[102] The American Academy of Medical Directors. The American College of Physician Executives AAMD/ACPE, Falls Church, Virginia, n.d. (circa 1982). Personal communication with Shattuck Hartwell, M.D., 1982. *Encyclopedia of Associations*, 1988, p. 1191.

[103] Stuart Wesbury interview, January 1983. *Encyclopedia of Associations*, 1988, p. 1192.

[104] Friedson, *Profession of Medicine*, 1970; *Professional Dominance*, 1970.

[105] Wilson and Neuhauser, 1982, pp. 95–96.

[106] Wesbury, 1972, AUPHA *Program Notes*, No. 49, Oct. 1972, pp. 48–50 and No. 55, Sept. 1973, pp. 19, 26–27.

[107] Vol. 21, No. 1, Winter 1976. *Hospital & Health Services Administration*. In 1973, the Association of University Programs in Hospital Administration changed to the Association of University Programs in Health Administration, its current name. *Program Notes*, loc. cit.

[108] ACHA, "Background Information Concerning the Proposal to Change the Name and Objects of the ACHA." Stuart Wesbury, April 1981. La Violette, 1981, p. 77.

[109] ACHA, *op. cit.*, April 1981.

[110] ACHA, *1981–1982 Annual Report and Reference Guide*. Of 66 Officers, Governors, and Regents for this convocation year, only four were not then hospital directors: Edward McCauley, North Carolina Hospital Associa-

tion; James Hepner, Professor and Program Director, Washington University; Major William Head, USAF, Chief, Medical Computer Systems; and Jerome Peck, Associate Dean, University of Hawaii Medical School.

[111] See ACHA, *1980–1981 Annual Report*, p. 7, and *1981–1982 Annual Report*, p. 35.

[112] ACHE, *1991–1992 Annual Report and Reference Guide*.

[113] ACHE, *1991–1992 Annual Report and Reference Guide*, pp. 50–57. AUPHA, 1989, p. 332.

[114] ACHE, *National Directory of Healthcare Executive Groups*, 1992.

[115] ACHE, *Directory of Student Chapters*, 1992.

[116] ACHE, *1991–1992 Annual Report and Reference Guide*, p. 43.

[117] *Ibid.* p. 62.

[118] *Ibid.* pp. 35–37.

[119] ACHE, *National Directory of Women's Networks in Health Administratiion*, 1992.

[120] ACHE, *1991–1992 Annual Report and Reference Guide*, p. 57.

[121] For example, the Healthcare Executives of Okinawa, Japan, pp. 57–58 in the ACHE *National Directory of Healthcare Executive Groups*, 1992. U.S. Military Members constitute the officers.

[122] Accrediting Commission on Education for Health Services Administration, 1982.

[123] Graham and Wright, 1981, p. 66.

[124] The College published a critique of JCAH principles on hospital management in 1974. William S. Brines was chairman of the task force.

[125] Felch and Greene, 1981.

[126] ACHA, "The Proceedings of the Board of Regents Conference on Future Program and Policy," 1955.

[127] Feldstein, Paul J., 1977. Wesbury interview, 1983.

[128] ACHA, "The Role of the American College of Hospital Administrators in the Legislative Process," circa 1974. White, 1985.

[129] ACHA, "National Health Insurance . . . ," 1974.

[130] ACHA, "National Health Insurance," 1974.

[131] ACHA, "Accord on the Roles and Responsibilities . . . ," July, 1980.

[132] ACHA, "Statement of the ACHA on Deferred Compensation," April 24, 1980. Wesbury interview, 1983.

[133] ACHA, "Healthcare Executives Must Prepare for Serious Ethical Conflicts," 1982.

[134] White, 1985.

[135] *Ibid.* ACHA Council of Regents Meeting Minutes June 7–8, 1973, pp. 18–21, 36.

[136] ACHE Public Policy Statements, circa 1989.

[137] ACHE, 3 single printed pages, July 27, 1990; May 4, 1992.

[138] White, 1985, p. 9.

[139] ACHE Public Policy Statements, circa 1989.

3

From Cottage Hospital to Health Care System

Any study of the work, responsibilities and qualifications of the present day Hospital Administrator would be quite incomplete without some introductory reference to the character of the institution with which he is associated in his daily tasks. Some knowledge of its relationships, problems, objectives and characteristics of growth is essential to an understanding of the position of its executive officer.

ACHA, 1935[1]

What the hospital is defines what its hospital administrator does.[2] What the hospital administrator does defines the College. We therefore look at the state of hospitals at the College's inception, along with some major ways hospitals have evolved in the last 60 years.

In this chapter, we explore the changing hospital. In the next chapter, we examine the changing administrator. As the administrator has changed, so have the appropriate education (Chapter 5), qualifications for excellence in administration (Chapter 6), and the intellectual content of administration (Chapter 7).

Genesis: 1873–1915

"And so it came to pass eventually that all mankind needed the hospital."

John A. Hornsby, M.D., 1913[3]

In 1873, there were slightly more than 178 hospitals in this country[4] (see Table 3.1). These years featured rapid growth. The total number of hospitals mushroomed in response to the availability of aseptic and antisep-

TABLE 3.1
Number of Hospitals by Year and Ownership[6]

Era	Year	Total Number of Hospitals	Total Beds (000's)**	Percent Investor Owned (Proprietary)
Creation	1873	178+		22% (estimated)
1880–1915	1878	442		
	1903	2500		
	1909	4359	421	
	1910			56% (estimated)
	1914	5047	532	
Standardization	1918	5323	612	
1915–1933	1923	6830	756	
	1928	6852	893	36%
Superintendent	1938	6166	1161	27%
1933–1945	1941	6358	1324	25%
Administrator	1946	6125	1436	18%
1945–1965	1950	6788	1456	18%
	1956	6966	1607	14%
	1960	6876	1658	12%
Manager	1966	7160	1679	12%
1966–1978	1968	7137	1663	11%
	1978	7015	1381	10.4%
CEO 1979–	1981	6933	1362	10.5%
	1991	6634	1202	—

tic surgery, x-ray, and laboratory tests. The hospital, therefore, became essential to the private practice of medicine. In fact, in the absence of philanthropic capital some of these new hospitals were started by physicians on a proprietary basis. Later, many of these hospitals eventually closed; others were transformed into nonprofit institutions.[5]

Most of these hospitals were very small. The larger ones were typically built in the pavilion style of architecture, usually on one level, with long corridors between wards in order to control infection.[7] Even from the vantage point of 1935, the turn of the century hospital was so simple as to be called a "boarding house for the sick."[8]

Along with an increase in the number of hospitals, the number of nursing schools also grew from 34 in 1880 to 1,755 in 1920. By 1927, there were 2,286 schools.[9] In 1925, the model nursing school had its students on duty from 55 to 64 hours a week.[10] This explosive era of hospital growth resulted in a wide variation in quality of services.

Standardization: 1915–1933

The standardization movement was not limited to the hospital field. The National Bureau of Standards, located in the U.S. Department of Commerce, was established in 1901 for the development, construction, and maintenance of references and working standards in science, engineering, industry and commerce. It started with 14 employees, increasing to 850 by 1928.[11] A major boost to this Bureau occurred after World War I when Herbert Hoover served as Secretary of Commerce under President Warren G. Harding.[12]

John R. Mannix remembered that 1,000 different surgical needles were available in the 1920s; 300 of these were in stock at his hospital, where only 50 different operations were performed. According to Mannix, it was finally agreed that only 17 different needles would fulfill every need—a startling example of the rewards of standardization in hospitals.[13]

In 1910, the Hospital Bureau of Standards and Supplies was started as an independent organization. By 1938, it was performing joint purchasing for 211 member hospitals in 24 states. It standardized and tested products used by hospitals and still exists today.[14] Judging by the number of articles in its *Transactions* on standardization, the AHA was actively involved in this effort from 1914 into the 1930s.[15]

In 1918, the American College of Surgeons' minimum standards for hospital accreditation were minimal indeed (see Table 3.2). That so many institutions failed to meet these standards documents the negative state of most American hospitals of this time. The ACS's minimum standards—the same in 1938 as in 1918—are reproduced in Table 3.2.

Between 1918 and 1936, the ACS conducted over 40,000 hospital surveys.[16] In 1918, only 12.9 percent of the largest hospitals surveyed could meet these minimal standards. By 1936, nearly all of the largest ones and many smaller ones could meet these basic standards of good organization (see Table 3.3.)

The Catholic Hospital Association, founded in 1915, enthusiastically took on the task of increasing the proportion of Catholic hospitals qualifying for accreditation.[17] Concurrent with hospital standardization was an effort driven by the Flexner report of 1910 and supported by the Rockefeller Foundation. This effort brought medical schools up to the standard of full-time faculty and research, set in the U.S. by the Johns Hopkins Medical School. By 1929, this foundation had granted $78 million to standardize medical education.[18]

In 1923, the Goldmark report on nursing education proposed improvement by emphasizing "the fundamental need to recognize the hospital school as a separate educational department, dedicated to giving students, not a course of training, but a thorough liberal education in nursing."[20]

There were several reasons that hospital standardization was so enthusiastically adopted. For the patient, approval of standardization was an assurance of efficient and competent care; for the physician,

TABLE 3.2
ACS Standards 1918[19]

Minimum Standard for Hospitals

1. That physicians and surgeons privileged to practice in the hospital be organized as a definite medical staff. Such organization has nothing to do with the question as to whether the hospital is "open" or "closed," nor need it affect the various existing types of medical staff organization. The word staff is here defined as the group of doctors who practice in the hospital inclusive of all groups, such as the "regular medical staff," the "visiting medical staff," and the "associate medical staff."

2. That membership upon the medical staff be restricted to physicians and surgeons who are (a) graduates of medicine of acceptable medical schools, with the degree of Doctor of Medicine, in good standing, and legally licensed to practice in their respective states or provinces; (b) competent in their respective fields; and (c) worthy in character and in matters of professional ethics; that in this latter connection the practice of the division of fees, under any guise whatsoever, be prohibited.

3. That the medical staff initiate and, with the approval of the governing board of the hospital, adopt rules, regulations, and policies governing the professional work of the hospital; that these rules, regulations, and policies specifically provide: (a) that medical staff meetings be held at least once each month; (b) that the medical staff review and analyze at regular intervals their clinical experience in the various departments of the hospital, such as medicine, surgery, obstetrics, and the other specialties; the medical records of patients, free and pay, to be the basis for such review and analysis.

4. That accurate and complete medical records be written for all patients and filed in an accessible manner in the hospital, a complete medical record being one which includes identification data; complaint; personal and family history; history of present illness; physical examination; special examinations, such as consultations, clinical laboratory, x-ray and other examination; provisional or working diagnosis; medical or surgical treatment; gross and microscopical pathological findings; progress notes; final diagnosis; condition on discharge; follow-up and, in case of death, autopsy findings.

5. That diagnostic and therapeutic facilities under competent medical supervision be available for the study, diagnosis, and treatment of patients, these to include at least (a) a clinical laboratory providing chemical, bacteriological, serological, and pathological services; (b) an x-ray department providing radiographic and fluoroscopic services.

the security of a proper working environment; for the hospital, a well-functioning operation; for the intern and student nurse, a level of organization, equipment, and personnel to assure good education and facilitate licensure and registration; and for the community, pride in

TABLE 3.3
Hospitals Surveyed, by Size and Percent Approved by The American College of Surgeons 1918–1936[21]

	Large 100+ Beds		Medium 50–99 Beds		Small 24–59 Beds	
	Number Surveyed	% Approved	Number Surveyed	% Approved	Number Surveyed	% Approved
1918	692	12.9	—	—	—	—
1922	812	83.4	812	41.3	—	—
1924	961	86.2	973	52.2	307	15.9
1928	1204	93.1	941	62.2	491	18.1
1933	1603	93.9	1044	63.1	907	24.2
1936	1745	94.2	1049	67.5	775	29.0

a hospital that was meeting universally recognized standards.[22]

Both standardization of hospitals and professional education contributed to the mobility of professional workers. A physician or nurse trained in one area of the country could quickly adapt to work in another region. This similarity of tasks, relations, and organization across thousands of independent hospitals was a remarkable social achievement.

1933–1945

With the Depression came the disappearance of nearly 700 hospitals (from 6,852 in 1928 to 6,166 in 1938). Still other hospitals faded from the scene, but were replaced by new ones. When the ACHA was formed, hospital standardization was an accepted fact and needed no additional support from the College. However, the growing complexity of hospitals required better management.

The architectural landmark of this era was the appearance of the vertical hospital, an alternative to the earlier pavilion style.[23] Vertical hospitals were technically possible after the use of the Otis elevator in 1857,[24] and the creation of the skyscraper office buildings of the Chicago school of architecture in the 1880s.[25] Growing hospital size and urbanization were also necessary preconditions.

However, it was the understanding and control of hospital infections which made the vertical hospital acceptable.[26] This change in thinking about hospital architecture (vertical skyscraper versus horizontal pavilion) was noted by S. S. Goldwater in 1929.[27] Goldwater was made an Honorary Fellow of the College in 1938.

> For the thoughtful hospital planner the most significant contrast is not one between hospitals with vertical and horizontal lines of com-

munication, respectively, but between hospitals in which interdependent departments are conveniently and those in which they are inconveniently grouped.[28]

The multistoried hospital was proposed as early as 1905 by Dr. A. J. Ochsner, yet, it was only after the control of hospital infection and the disappearance of the miasmic theory of infection that the vertical hospital became a reality, according to E. H. L. Corwin, an Honorary Charter Fellow of the College.[29]

Goldwater's concept of conveniently grouping interdependent hospital departments came from the classical school of management theory. It was this change in consciousness that created the climate for the founding of the ACHE.

In 1935, Franklin Roosevelt's Public Works Administration financed a business census of hospitals to collect information about "the financial structure of hospitals and opportunities for employment within them." This was part of a larger census of all American business.

According to the annual "Hospital Number" of the *Journal of the American Medical Association*,[30] there were 6,246 registered hospitals containing 1,076,350 beds. Five thousand nine-hundred forty-four hospitals responded to this government study directed by Elliott Pennell, Joseph Mountin, and Kay Pearson with the advice of Michael M. Davis and C. Rufus Rorem.[33]

This was the era when tuberculosis was treated by years of stay in specialized hospitals, a time before chemotherapy in the 1950s emptied these institutions. Statistical information about hospitals in this era is shown in Tables 3.4 to 3.13.

TABLE 3.4
Hospitals, Type and Ownership 1935[31]

5,944 hospitals		
	4,841 general and special	261 federal
	597 mental	569 other government
	506 tuberculosis	2,469 voluntary
		1,542 proprietary

TABLE 3.5
Non-federal Hospital Beds per 1,000 Population by Hospital Type, 1935[32]

Area	All Hospitals	General + Spec.	Mental	Tuberculosis
USA	7.62	3.13	3.97	0.52
Massachusetts	12.28	4.96	6.33	0.99
Mississippi	3.59	1.34	1.99	0.26

In 1935, hospital beds per 1,000 population were maldistributed by state (see Table 3.5). Annual per capita payments (expenditures) on hospital care averaged $3.37 for the country as a whole. Per capita payments varied tenfold from the highest ranked state to the lowest. Well over half of the payments came directly from the patient paying out-of-pocket. Taxes supported government hospitals. Of the rest, endowment income was important in areas like Massachusetts (see Table 3.7).

In 1935, both nonprofit general and special hospitals were losing money. For every dollar spent by voluntary general hospitals in 1935, only 96 cents was returned from all income sources. The smallest hospitals had the greatest deficits per bed (see Table 3.8).

Although this was a small expense per bed by today's standards, it was large when compared to the yearly expense per bed at that time in southern mental hospitals ($211 per year or 58 cents per bed per day). The income for nonprofit general and special hospitals came from patients (70.9%), taxes (10.3%), endowment (6.3%), and others (12.5%). On an average day, only 64 percent of all general and special hospital beds were occupied. For the proprietary hospitals, it was 45 percent. This low occupancy rate was in part related to the small size of these hospitals. Expenses of these hospitals went for payroll (48.9%), supplies and maintenance (47.2%), and other (3.9%).

TABLE 3.6
Hospital Size and Type, 1935[34]

Number of Beds	General & Special	Number of Beds	Mental	Tuberculosis
Less than 25	1,287			
25–49	1,177	Less than 50	144	135
50–149	1,580	50–499	189	231
150+	797	500+	264	140
Total	4,841		597	506

TABLE 3.7
Annual Per Capita Payment for General & Special Hospitals by Area, 1935[35]

Area	Per Capita Payment	% From Patients	% From Taxes	% From Other
USA	$3.37	61.8	24.3	13.9
Massachusetts	7.05	55.9	21.2	22.9
Mississippi	0.67	73.5	25.1	1.4

For these general and special hospitals, average plant assets per bed were $4,682 per bed. They were comprised of land (9.5%), buildings (73.4%), equipment (14.8%), and other (2.3%). For general and special hospitals, the endowment per bed was $1,090. However, 78 percent of all hospital endowments were in the northeastern quarter of the U.S. (north and east from—and including—Pennsylvania and Maryland).

Hospital Employment 1935

Five thousand eight-hundred thirty-six reporting hospitals with 1,035,503 beds employed 461,884 employees. For nonprofit general and special hospitals, there were .89 employees per bed. Of these, 80.8 percent were paid full-time, 3.5 percent were paid part-time, and 15.7 percent provided maintenance (room and board) only. Workers receiving maintenance only were predominantly student nurses and resident physicians. Both of these groups provided a substantial amount of labor, particularly in the larger hospitals.

For all general and special hospitals, this work force consisted of physicians (4.8%), nurses (40.8%), technical and other professionals (5.4%), administrative and clerical (7.2%), and orderlies and other nonprofessional workers (41.8%). The average monthly pay for these workers was $55.53.

When Dewey Lutes helped start the College in 1933, he was administrator of the 150-bed Ravenswood Hospital in Chicago. He knew every employee by name, and walked through the hospital every day. "Anyone could come into my office without an appointment," he said. "There was more feeling for patients and fewer electronic things." He remembered tears in the eyes of nurses caring for dying cancer patients. Added Lutes, "That doesn't happen so much now."

Virtually every room was a patient room on the nursing floor. There were only three nonpatient rooms: one for housekeeping, a floor kitchen, and a supply room. There were no nursing stations, and hospital housekeeping was no different from that practiced in a home. The administrator's major problems were keeping the hospital in good repair and collecting bills.

TABLE 3.8
Annual Income and Expense Per Bed Per Year for Nonprofit General and Special Hospitals, 1935[36]

Average Income per bed per year	$1,180
Average Expense per bed per year	1,221
Average *loss* per bed per year	$ 41

The latest technology was a new EKG on rollers. "It was really something," Lutes said. The Ravenswood lab had one part-time pathologist. Technicians were trained on the job, and the whole lab was located in one little room. "We didn't know what a social worker was," said Lutes. In 1933, there was no problem finding nurses either. The graduates of the hospital nursing schools stayed on to work in the hospital. "Nursing students really worked then," said Lutes.

The hospital's funds were in a local bank. "I took all the money out of this bank in cash and put it in a safety deposit box," Lutes reported. "Two weeks later the bank failed. The Board of Trustees gave me a pat on the back for that." While some hospitals closed during the Depression, Lutes noted of his hospital, "We all took pay cuts."[37]

Even as late as 1946, in hospitals of 200 to 299 beds (larger than average), a survey of 155 hospitals revealed that 62 had "no assistant administrator, medical director or the like"; 65 had one assistant; 23 had two assistants; and five had three or more assistant administrators.[38]

In summary, in 1935 the average general hospital administrator presided over a small hospital with a small number of unskilled employees. Very likely, the hospital was running at a deficit even though expenses were very low and patients had to pay out of their own pocket. The threat of hospital closure was real. Many of these small hospitals were not unlike nursing homes of today. Although endowments and philanthropy were important, these funds were even less evenly distributed across the country than were all hospital services per capita.[39]

The Era of the Administrator: 1945–1965

At the beginning of this era, the typical hospital was, by today's standards, a low cost operation. Plant assets per bed were $4,814. Although the great majority of hospitals had x-ray equipment, only 45.5 percent in Utah did. Although the great majority of hospitals had clinical laboratories, only 62.5 percent in South Dakota did.[40] In 1945, staffing per patient day was not intensive (see Tables 3.9 and 3.10).

But hospitals were becoming larger.[43] They were adding more staff per patient day; hiring a wider range of professionally trained specialists; increasing their scope of services; and becoming more expensive. All of the changes called for more skilled management.

After World War II, healthcare expenditures grew (see Table 3.11). Personal health expenditures actually fell by half a billion dollars from 1929 to 1935, but rose from 3.5 percent to 4 percent of the gross national product, reflecting the massive impact of the Depression. Private health insurance played a negligible role prior to World War II. During the war, wage freezes encouraged the growth of fringe ben-

TABLE 3.9
Personnel Per Patient Day By Type of Hospital in 1945, 1960, 1991[41]

	Personnel per Patient Day 1945	1960	1991
General Hospitals, Community Hospitals	1.43	2.26	4.31
Mental	.17		
Tuberculosis	.59		
Chronic & Convalescent	.47		
Federal Civilian (VA)	.57		

TABLE 3.10
Total Employees, Costs Per Patient Day, and Staffing in General Hospitals by Size in 1945[42]

Size/Beds	Total Employees	Cost per Patient Day	Personnel per Patient Day
−49	28,904	$7.99	1.06
50–99	54,682	8.01	1.22
100–249	158,027	8.60	1.45
250+	188,987	8.96	1.57

efits such as health insurance. By 1950, private health insurance paid 9 percent of personal health expenditures. Government expenditures rose steadily, with the largest jump occurring during the 1960s with the start of Medicare and Medicaid. The cumulative result was that direct payment for healthcare fell from 88.4 percent in 1929 to 26.8 percent in 1980, by which time the hospital was confronted not only with reimbursement from patients directly, but also from private insurers and governments, resulting in a vastly more complex external environment. The percent of gross national product spent on health went from 3.5 percent in 1929 to 9.8 percent in 1982 and to 11.1 percent in 1988.

The uneasy relationships between compassionate humane care, medical technology, and hospital economic survival have existed throughout the life of the College. Sister John Gabriel, writing in 1935, said:

> In these hectic times of rapid progress and new discoveries, with more and more provision available for accurate diagnosis, a physician is very much tempted to become so absorbed in the study of the disease itself as to ignore the object of the disease. The x-ray pictures may be discussed, the laboratory findings talked over, the physiotherapy

TABLE 3.11
Personal Health Expenditures 1929–1988[44]

	Amount (billions)	Out of Pocket Payment %	Private Insurance %	Gov. %	National Health Expenditures as % of GNP
1929	$3.2	88.4	—	9.0	3.5
1935	2.7	82.4	—	14.7	4.0
1940	3.5	81.3	—	16.1	4.0
1950	10.9	65.5	9.1	22.4	4.5
1960	23.9	55.9	21.0	21.4	4.4
1970	64.9	39.5	23.4	34.6	7.3
1980	218.3	27.1	29.7	39.7	9.1
1988	478.3	24.7	31.9	39.9	11.1
1990	585.3	23.3	31.8	41.3	12.2
1992	838.5(est.)				14.+
1993	939.9(est.)				—
1994	1000.0(est.)				—

treatment analyzed, the diet therapy methods inspected—all these without the least reference to the patient only inasmuch as he furnishes the material to show the efficiency of these departments.[45]

And S. S. Goldwater, M.D., wrote in 1938:

> A balanced hospital budget may be something to be proud of or it may be a callous testimonial of unfelt shame. If a balanced budget has been attained through the heartless sacrifice of adequate medical care, if it has been effected by disregarding the patients' best interests, it is worse than an unbalanced budget unavoidably resulting from an honest effort to supply genuine needs.[46]

In 1940, a million people were employed in health services. By 1979, this had grown to 4.95 million workers, of whom 3.84 million worked in hospitals. Not only did the total number of hospital-based employees increase; they increased per 100 patients in the hospital from 226 full-time equivalents (FTEs) in 1960 to 302 FTEs in 1970, and 388 FTEs per 100 patients in 1979[47] (see Table 3.12).

The College has seen the average general hospital of 1933 with about 50 beds with fewer than 50 employees evolve by 1983 to an average of 200 beds and 750 employees and then to the multi-institution systems of 1993. The hospital of 1933 could be managed by a nurse with some on-the-job experience.

Investment in hospitals in 1928 at current prices was $3.5 billion; in 1935, $3.74 billion; in 1947, $5.88 billion; in 1956, $13 billion; in

TABLE 3.12
Health Services Employment (millions)[48]

Year	Total Employment	Employment in Hospitals	Employment in Nursing Homes
1940	1.0	—	—
1950	1.5	1.0	—
1960	2.5	1.5	—
1970	4.25	2.69	.51
1980	7.34	4.04	1.20
1989	9.11	4.57	1.52

1960, $17.7 billion.[49] In 1935, there were 800,000 births in hospitals; by 1959 there were four million births in hospitals.[50] In 1928–31, the average American went to see the doctor 2.6 times in a year. In 1954–1959, that statistic grew to five times a year.[51]

This growth in hospital and medical services created a demand for health insurance coverage. In 1940, 12 million people had some type of health insurance. Of these, six million were covered by Blue Cross/Blue Shield plans. By 1950, 76.6 million people were covered; by 1960, 122.5 million; and by 1970, 158.8 million. By 1978, 166.8 million people under the age of 65 had hospital insurance protection.[52]

The availability of health insurance fueled the rise in national health expenditures (see Table 3.13). It also helped concentrate medical care in the hospital.

In 1935, 37 percent of live births occurred in hospitals. By 1953, 93 percent of live births were in hospitals. Maternal mortality fell from 58.2 per 100,000 live births in 1935, to 6.1 per 100,000 in 1953. Infant mortality fell from 55.7 per 1,000 live births in 1935 to 27.8 in 1953. In 1935, 18 states had less than 30 percent of live births in hospitals. By 1953, 36 states had over 90 percent of live births in hospitals. In 1945, the average work week for untrained hospital employees was over 48 hours. By 1954, it was down to 43 hours. In 1954, the average short-term general hospital had 102 beds and 18 bassinets, and 149 full-time equivalent personnel.[54]

Table 3.15 compares some of the services provided by nonprofit general hospitals from 50 to 99 beds in 1954 and 1981. In 1954, 89 percent of these hospitals reported having EKG machines. The AHA stopped asking about EKGs by 1981 and recovery rooms, pharmacy, and EEG's by 1991.

According to Seth Goldsmith:

> With the exception of a few large municipal hospital systems, such as that of New York City, most (nonfederal general) hospitals have

TABLE 3.13
Average Yearly Rate of Change in National Health Expenditures[53]

Years	Average Percent Change per Year
1929–1935	−3.5%
1935–1940	6.6
1940–1950	12.2
1950–1955	6.9
1955–1960	8.7
1960–1965	9.2
1965–1970	12.4
1970–1975	12.2
1975–1980	13.2
1988–1989	9.5

developed in isolation from one another both clinically and managerially. But in the decade of the 1970's this fragmentation gave way, to increasing interinstitutional cooperation as we enter the 1980's. The completely freestanding hospital is rapidly becoming a thing of the past.[55]

In 1975, an estimated 24 percent of community hospitals accounting for 32 percent of their beds were in multihospital systems. A 1978 AHA survey of 5,740 community hospitals (an 83 percent response rate) showed 65 percent of hospitals shared purchasing services, up from 38 percent in 1975. Thirty-four percent shared electronic data processing, up from 21 percent in 1975. Twenty-seven percent shared laboratory services, up from 17.4 percent in 1957. Almost nineteen percent shared biomedical engineering services, up from 7.7 percent in 1955. Other shared services showed similar increases[56] (see Table 3.14).

Another measure of the hospital's increasing complexity is the growth of outpatient and emergency visits to short-term, non-federal hospitals. In 1944, outpatient visits totaled 23.7 million. In 1953, 42 million; in 1965, 92.6 million; in 1970, 124 million; and in 1979, 203.9 million. Emergency visits went from 9.4 million in 1954, to 76.6 million in 1979.[58]

1966–

The recovery from the Great Depression and then World War II saw the growth of health care expenditures. New specialties and technol-

TABLE 3.14
Community Hospitals and Beds in Multihospital Systems by Type of Ownership 1975[57]

			In Hospital Systems	
Type of Ownership	Total Hospitals	Hospitals in System	% of Hospitals	% of Beds
Voluntary	3,355	940	28%	32%
Investor-Owned	755	309	40	51
State & Local Government	1,745	156	8	22
Total	5,875	1,405	24%	32%

TABLE 3.15
Selected Services Provided by Nonprofit General Hospitals of 50–99 Beds in 1953, 1981, and 1991[59]

	Percent of Hospitals Having Service		
Service	1953	1981	1991
Post operative recovery room	17.0%	92.4%	—
Pharmacy	48.0	97.2	—
E.E.G.	3.0	51.0	—
Physical Therapy	26.0	90.1	78.4
Social Work	5.0	77.1	81.1
Occupational Therapy	3.0	21.2	54.3
Radiation Therapy	29.0	6.0	10.5

ogy increased costs. Increased costs called forth private insurance and Medicare and Medicaid. Insurance created the possibility of more technology, fueling rising costs. The growing number of elderly who use more medical care also increased total spending.

In the 1980s, hospitals grew larger and more complex. They confronted third party payers, both government and private, in a sea of regulatory constraints fostered by a concern for rising costs. This complex environment, both internal and external, resulted in hospitals creating linkages in the interests of survival.

The 1970s saw the growth of multihospital systems and alliances. Most Catholic hospitals have been associated with a particular order of sisters, but highly decentralized in their management. A number of these congregations developed larger corporate headquarters and central management.

By 1982, the Hospital Corporation of America (HCA) had operating revenues of $3.5 billion (349 hospitals); Kaiser Permanente, $2 billion (30 hospitals); Humana, $1.92 billion (91 hospitals); and American Medical International, $1.41 billion (70 hospitals). See Table 3.16.

Such large systems have political "clout," easier access to capital markets, and can attract skilled managers looking for larger responsibilities. These characteristics and the growth of managed care suggest that the expansion of systems will continue.[61] Through this process, some hospitals are achieving horizontal integration.

Hospitals are taking on new roles, including hospice programs, nursing homes, emergicenters, wellness programs, mental health crisis intervention programs, family planning, rehabilitation centers, congregate housing, and industry-related programs.[62] Through these ventures, hospitals are vertically integrating.

The rising tide of regulation began to recede with the presidency of Ronald Reagan. Local health planning agencies disappeared in some locations; in others, their role was reduced. The key to hospital construction was less the regulatory Certificate of Need than the hospital's bond rating.

The hospitals that do well in the investment arena are those that generate sufficient revenue to repay the bonds. In such an environment, the multi-institutional systems often have more capital for expansion than isolated small community hospitals.

At the College's Fiftieth Anniversary Congress on Administration in March, 1983, attendees could, in a seminar on "Health Provider Advertising: How to Do It Ethically and Legally," learn:

—to combat lawfully a competing health provider's deceptive (and competitively damaging) advertising and;
—to change as violations of the First Amendment or the federal antitrust laws, those state laws or ethical rules that unreasonably prevent a health provider from running truthful advertising.

In "Creative Alternatives for Hospital Capital Formation and Financing," participants could:

—become informed on the existence and nature of certain creative and unconventional methods of raising and utilizing hospital capital, including private capital reorganizations and private sale/leaseback reorganizations.

And in the seminar on "Competition in Health Care," administrators might learn:

—to incorporate financial planning with strategic planning especially when viewing mergers, acquisitions, restructuring or capital expansion programs.[63]

TABLE 3.16
Multihospital Systems 1981 and 1992[60]

Non-government Multi-Hospital Systems by Ownership			Number of Hospitals in These Systems		Number of Beds in These Systems	
	1981	1992	1981	1992	1981	1992
Investor-Owned	31	50	746	1,101	97,478	134,006
Catholic	113	67	516	503	137,501	118,527
Other Religious	19	14	150	95	21,771	18,563
Voluntary	93	164	465	799	94,658	180,649
Total	256	295	1,877	2,498	351,408	451,745

In 1981, 32% of all Community Hospitals (5,842 total hospitals)
In 1992, 47% of all Community Hospitals (5,292 total hospitals)

In 1981, 36% of all Community Hospital beds (983,694 total beds)
In 1992, 46% of all Community Hospital beds (920,943 total beds)

When John R. Mannix, a founding Fellow of the College, saw this seminar announcement, he said that most of these topics would be appropriate for the executive of any business. "We didn't concern ourselves with those things in 1933," he said.[64]

The hospital's complex external environment from the 1970s on has led managers to spend more time on external affairs. This encouraged the shift to the corporate form of hospital organization with a Chief Executive Officer (CEO) often focused on external affairs, long range planning and governance and a Chief Operating Officer (COO) managing the internal organization.

In 1970, there were 3.1 million HMO members.[65] By 1990, there were 33 million members of 572 HMOs. By June, 1992, HMO enrollment was reported at 42 million people, or 16.6 percent of the U.S. population.[65] (See Table 3.17.)[66] By 1990, 23 percent of people in the west were enrolled in HMO's. This underestimates the total number of people in managed care programs. Home care, hospice, ambulatory surgery, urgent care centers have all grown. The diversity of healthcare provider organizations is reflected in the change in employing organizations of College members from 1986 to 1992. See Table 3.18. Hospital employment in 1992 included 73.9 percent of the membership.

Hospitals across the country were redefining themselves as medical centers. In 1981, there was a proposal to change the College name. It required a two-thirds vote of the regents and won only 102 of 178 regents' votes (17 short). Former Chairmen Henry X. Jackson said at the time that the new name would make the ACHA the "American

TABLE 3.17
Health Maintenance Organizations and Enrollment: 1976, 1986, 1990[66]

	1976	1986	1990
All plans	174	623	575
IPA	41	384	360
Group	122	239	212
Enrollment (thousands)	5,987	25,725	33,028
IPA	390	9,932	13,741
Group	5,562	15,793	19,287
Enrollment per 1000 population			
Northeast	19.9	100.5	145.6
Midwest	15.2	116.4	126.2
South	4.3	54.4	70.5
West	96.9	190.4	232.1

TABLE 3.18
Percent of Active College Members by Employing Organization[67]

	1986	1992
Hospitals	84.8	68.9
Hospital System		5.0
Other direct providers*	3.3	11.0
Health Association/Agency	4.1	2.1
Education	6.0	1.7
Consulting		5.9
Industry and Insurance	1.2	1.0
Others**	.7	4.4
Number	13,782	16,667

HMO, long term care, ambulatory care, medical group practice.
** *Includes self-employed.*

College of Almost Anything."[68] It took another four years for the change to be approved.

Rising costs and a changing economy starting in the 1980s increased the number of Americans without health insurance. (See Table 3.19.) By 1989, almost 16 percent of Americans were without coverage. This concern led to a College member survey in 1986 on "Access to Care." Other member surveys followed. (See Table 3.20.) Some of these are about the executives' role and some about healthcare issues. A 1991 Delphi Survey conducted with Arthur Andersen & Co. of Board Chairs, CEOs, and physicians collected opinions about future trends, particularly those related to physician–hospital relations.[69] Trends expected included continued hospital closure, more managed care, and a growing attention to quality and the measurement of value. There were 160 hospital closures from 1984 to 1986 and 227 from 1987 to

TABLE 3.19
Percent of People under the Age of 65 Without Health Insurance Coverage 1980 and 1989 by Family Income[71]

Family Income ($)	1980	1989
less than 14,000	31.0	37.3
14,000–24,999	25.9	21.4
25,000–34,999	15.0	9.3
35,000–49,999	6.2	5.6
50,000 plus	3.9	3.2
Total	12.5	15.7

TABLE 3.20
Recent Selected College Member Surveys[72]

1986	Access to Care Survey
1988	Hospital Sponsored Child Care
1990	1989 Survey on Allocating Healthcare Resources (Research Series No. 1)
1989	Hospital Chief Executive Officer Role Study (Research Series No. 2)
1991	The Future of Health Care: Physician and Hospital Relations (with Arthur Andersen & Co.)
1991	Gender and Careers in Healthcare Management (Research Series No. 3)
1991	Hospital Chief Executive Officer Turnover: 1981–1990
1992	Results of the 1992 Public Policy Opinion Poll
1992	Affiliate Needs Survey
1992	Affiliate Advancement and Attrition Study
1992	Special Interest Group Studies:
	Executives in Managed Care
	Executives in Long Term Care
	Executives in Investor-owned Systems
	Physician Executives
	Nurse Executives

1989. Ninety-one percent of the respondents felt that total quality management programs would be in use by 1996.[70]

NOTES

[1] ACHA, "The Hospital Administrator . . .," 1935, The Carter Report, p. 3.

[2] Conners, Edward J. "Future of the Hospital Administrator," in American Hospital Association, *The Changing Role of the Hospital*, 1980, p. 17.

[3] Hornsby, "Standardization of Hospitals," 1913, p. 176.

[4] Toner, 1873. This census was not complete. For example, in Cleveland, Lakeside and St. Vincents Charity Hospitals were not included. (John R. Mannix interview, 1983).

[5] John R. Mannix found that 60 hospitals closed their doors and disappeared in the last 90 years in Cleveland alone (interview).

[6] Steinwald and Neuhauser, 1970. Corwin, 1946, pp. 6–7. American Hospital Association, *Hospital Statistics*, 1982; *Hospital Statistics*, 1992–1993. Bureau of the Census, *Historical Statistics of the United States*, 1975, Part 1, p. 78.

[7] Thompson and Goldin, 1975.

[8] ACHA, "The Hospital Administrator: An Analysis of his Duties . . .," 1935, p. 4.

[9] Kalisch and Kalisch, 1978, p. 350.

[10] Martin, 1926.

[11] "Standards," "National Bureau of Standardization," *Encyclopedia Britannica*, London, 1939, Vol. 21, pp. 305, 310, 311.

[12] "Hoover, Herbert." *Encyclopedia Britannica*, London, 1939, Vol. 11, pp. 732–733.

[13] John R. Mannix interview, March 1983.

[14] John R. Mannix interview. Hayes, 1938. Forbes, 1911.

[15] Report of the Committee on Simplification and Standardization of Furnishings, Supplies and Equipment," *Transactions of the American Hospital Association*, 1928, pp. 45–53 and 1937, pp. 190–195. Ochsner, 1914, 1917. Hornsby, 1913. Drew, 1918. Dickinson, 1914. Foote, 1926. Standardization continues as a national issue; witness the debate over conversion to the metric system.

[16] American College of Surgeons, 1938, p. 8.

[17] Shanahan, 1965. Martin, 1926. The American Hospital Association actively endorsed the Standardization program. Robert J. Wilson, M.D., *Transactions of the American Hospital Association*, Vol. 18, 1916, p. 295 in response to an appeal by Bowman, 1916.

[18] Brown, E. Richard, 1979, p. 155.

[19] American College of Surgeons, 1938, p. 6.

[20] Kalisch and Kalisch, 1978, p. 337, referring to Committee for the Study of Nursing Education, 1923.

[21] American College of Surgeons, 1938, p. 8.

[22] Kalisch and Kalisch, 1978, p. 10.

[23] "Germany erected the Friedrichshain [Freidrichsheim] Hospital in Berlin, generally acknowledged to be the first 'pavilion-style' hospital," ACHA, *Hospital Administration: A Life's Profession*, 1948, p. 13. See Ochsner and Sturm, 1907, pp. 23–26. This hospital was built from 1868–1874 with 624 beds. The 17 buildings of this hospital were completely separate. Other hospitals had connecting covered passages, for example, Lariboisierre Hospital in Paris, 1846, p. 466. Of the 178 U.S. hospitals reported by Toner in 1873, one hospital had 5 floors, 35 had 4 floors, 55 had 3 floors and 18 had 2 floors. The remainder either failed to respond or had one floor. Corwin, *The American Hospital*, 1946, pp. 6–7.

[24] Giedion, 1956, pp. 206–209.

[25] *Ibid.*, pp. 366–393.

[26] Dowling, 1977.

[27] Goldwater, 1929. His earlier thinking on the vertical hospital is found in his "A Plan for the Construction of Ward Buildings in Crowded Cities," 1911. This plan called for separate five-story buildings in a single, square city block.

[28] Goldwater, S. S., 1949, p. 240, Thompson and Golden, 1975, p. 196, and Chapter 6. Corwin, 1946, p. 183. Ochsner, a Chicago surgeon, was one of the early members of the American College of Surgeons. See Ochsner and Sturm, 1907. The changes in hospital architecture are well documented in the three editions of Edward F. Stevens 1918, 1921, and 1928. The 1928 edition introduces a possible multistory hospital of about 25 floors, pp. 127–137. "With the crowded conditions of our city streets, the city hospital can no longer be a spread-out affair and we must look to the air rather than to land for accommodation," pp. 132, 137. Mount Sinai Hospital in New

York is also shown as an example, p. 76. S. S. Goldwater was administrator of this hospital.

[29] "In 1928 the Columbia-Presbyterian Hospital group of buildings rose to 22 stories, at a cost exceeding $25,000,000. Similar multistoried structures were built: the Harborview Hospital in Seattle, the Charity Hospital in New Orleans, and Lakeside (University Hospital) in Cleveland." ACHA, 1948, *op. cit.*, p. 18.

[30] *Journal of the American Medical Association*, "Hospital Number," Vol. 106, No. 10, March 7, 1935, cited by Pennell *et al.*, 1939.

[31] Pennell *et al.*, 1939, p. 13.

[32] *Ibid.* p. 12.

[33] *Ibid.* p. 1.

[34] *Ibid.* p. 14.

[35] *Ibid.* p. 19.

[36] *Ibid.* pp. 22, 27.

[37] Dewey Lutes interview, April 20, 1982.

[38] ACHA, *The College Curriculum in Hospital Administration*, 1948, p. 97.

[39] The hospitals of this era were racially segregated. There were separate wards for black patients. There were over 118 black hospitals in 1931. Of these, 2 were federal, 10 state, 3 county and 7 city-owned, 38 proprietary, 40 independent voluntary, and 9 church-owned. In addition, 9 were owned by fraternal organizations. Of these, 95 were under the control of blacks. Julius Rosenwald Fund. *Negro Hospitals*, 1931, p. 8.

[40] Commission on Hospital Care, 1957, pp. 344–345.

[41] Commission on Hospital Care, 1957. U.S. Department of Health and Human Services, *Health US*, 1990, p. 180. AHA *Hospital Statistics 1992–93 Edition*, p. 7.

[42] Commission on Hospital Care, 1957.

[43] Corwin, 1946, p. 21. The Duke Endowment, 1945.

[44] U.S. Department of Health and Human Services, *Health US*, 1990, p. 184, 193. For 1929–1940 private insurance included in out-of-pocket payment, p. 193. National expenditures less research construction, health insurance administration, and government public health equals personal health expenditures, p. 254. "Other private funds" excluded from percentage distribution, p. 193. *Health Care Financing Review*, Fall 1991. *NY Times* Jan. 5, 1993, page A1, A7. "Health Care Costs Up Sharply Again" for years 1991–1994.

[45] Gabriel, 1935, p. 91.

[46] ACHA reprint from *Hospitals* of Goldwater, "The Future of Hospital Administration," 1938.

[47] U.S. Department of Health and Human Services, *op. cit.*, p. 188.

[48] USHHS, *Health US* 1990, p. 160. Lerner and Anderson, 1963, p. 220. U.S. Department of Health, Education and Welfare, 1980, pp. 186, 187.

[49] Lerner and Anderson, 1963, p. 230.

[50] *Ibid.*, p. 248.

[51] *Ibid.*, p. 288.

[52] Health Insurance Institute, 1980, p. 13.

[53] U.S. Department of Health and Human Services, *Health United States*, 1981, p. 201; *Health Care Financing Review*, Fall 1991.

[54] Block, *Hospital Trends*, circa 1957. Copies of this book were given to College affiliates in 1958. Inside the front cover was a pasted label and small mirror, "Congratulations to the American College of Hospital Administrators on its Silver Anniversary. Here is a reflection of one of those who contributed to its progress [mirror]."

[55] Goldsmith, 1981, p. 107. This book can stand as a symbol of a new era of thinking about multihospital systems in a competitive healthcare market. Hospital mergers have gone on throughout the century. F. R. Bradley, *Hospital Managment*, July 1953, p. 34.

[56] AHA, Feb. 1979. Brown and McCool, 1980, p. 479.

[57] Brown and Lewis, 1976, p. 32. Brown and McCool, 1980. Vraciu and Zuckerman, 1979.

[58] Dowling, Harry F., 1977, p. 164.

[59] Block, 1957. AHA, Hospital Statistics *1982 Edition*. AHA, *Hospital Statistics 1992–93 Edition*. Table 12A.

[60] AHA, *Data Book on Multihospital Systems 1980–1981*. Coyne and Young, 1983. AHA, Hospital Statistics *1993–94 Edition* and *Guide to the Health Care Field*, 1993.

[61] *The Internist*, American Society for Internal Medicine, Vol. 23, No. 10, Dec. 1982-Jan. 1983 issue, "Corporate Care: Threat or Challenge?"

[62] AHA, *The Changing Role of the Hospital*, 1981.

[63] ACHA, *Twenty-Sixth Congress on Administration*, 1983.

[64] John R. Mannix interview, 1983.

[65] U.S. Department of Health and Human Services, *Health United States*, 1981. Interstudy, 1982, p. 77. *AHA News*, vol. 29, no. 1, Jan. 4, 1993 p 3.

[66] USHHS *Health US*, 1990, p. 210.

[67] ACHE, *1992 Directory*, p. 1391; *1986 Directory*, p. 1169.

[68] *Modern Healthcare*, "Regents rebel, veto name change proposal," Oct. 1981, p. 77, 78.

[69] ACHE, The Future of Healthcare, 1991.

[70] *Ibid.* p. 37.

[71] USHHS, *Health US*, 1990, p. 208.

[72] See the bibliography for ACHE for full references. There have been a number of member surveys throughout the College history.

4

Superintendent to Administrator to CEO: The Role of the Healthcare Executive

In many ways the American College of Hospital Administrators is exceptional among professional societies. It rose before there was a profession, not after one had long been established. It was devoted to creating a profession, not merely advancing the professional interests of those already acknowledged as professionals. It had to develop a university without a campus, not simply to provide opportunity for leaders to read papers at annual meetings. All these it has done, and done remarkably well. The time, energy, and money so freely contributed by its members would be impossible to calculate. Its achievements can be measured in part by the present status and ability of the hospital administrator, but in whole only by the high level of medical care available in American hospitals.[1]

Kipnis, 1955

In 60 years there has been both change and consistency in the role of the administrator. This evolution is partially reflected in the modification in administrative titles. Prior to the title of "superintendent" was the title "matron," but that era predates the College. This change in forms of address was in keeping with shifts in management style and other fundamental changes in the role.

These changes were also reflected in the activities and programs of the College. The College observed these alterations through research of the administrator's role. It also mirrored these changes by restructuring its organization. Always, the College has been a force for change through its promotion of professionalism.

The 1920s and 1930s

Prior to the founding of the College, in 1927 Michael Davis described hospital administration as being "generally viewed as an inferior calling, offering a berth rather than an opportunity."[2] It was not a permanent berth either. Davis looked at 1,230 hospitals in ten states during 1920 to 1926. Of these, 43 percent had the same superintendent throughout; 35 percent had one change of superintendency; 19 percent had two changes; and 3 percent had three changes.[3] In another analysis, Davis looked at the characteristics of the senior manager in all 7,610 U.S. and Canadian hospitals in 1927. Thirty-seven percent were directed by a physician, 9 percent by a "medical director with a lay superintendent"; 20 percent by nurses; 8 percent by sisters; 10 percent by laymen; 11 percent by laywomen, with 5 percent unspecified.[4]

Robert Neff, a founding Fellow and President of the College from 1934–1935, said in his 1936 introduction to the first College survey of the hospital administrator:

> The College recognizes its obligation to study and survey the administrative field in its efforts to promote and improve the efficiency of hospital administration.
>
> The variety and complexity of the numerous relationships of the administrator—social, financial, and professional—are such as to require abilities of unusual caliber, and the facts which have been gleaned by this study naturally become interesting to those who are concerned with the relationships of the hospital administrator as a professional individual.[5]

This study was conducted by a mailed questionnaire to the administrators of approximately 6,500 hospitals listed by the American Hospital Association. About 2,200 replies were received, even fewer for specific questions. Although the research methodology used in this study was primitive when compared to later studies by the College, the information was a window to another era and defined the administrator of the 1930s.

Tables 4.1 through 4.5 reveal frequent nonresponses. In addition, total responses vary from one question to another. However, even with these statistical problems, there are some clear messages.

According to Neff, 66.9 percent of the men had university degrees as compared to 7.7 percent of the women (see Table 4.1). Two-thirds of the administrators were women. Among the men, over half were physicians; they predominated among the university men. Twelve percent of all administrators had no education beyond high school. After the M.D.s, Reverends predominated among the degree-holding

TABLE 4.1
The Academic Background of Hospital Administrators in 1935, 1992[6]

	1935		1992 ACHE Members	
	Men %	Women %	Men %	Women %
No Work beyond high school	5.1	17.6	0.2	0.3
Nursing schools	0.6	25.9		
Teachers' colleges	3.4	10.6	0.7	0.5
College or university w/o degree	10.5	20.4		
College or university with degree	66.9	7.7	9.5	7.4
College or university beyond degree	4.3	1.6	89.6	91.8
Study Abroad	2.9	2.1	—	—
Business Course	5.1	8.4	—	—
Extension courses, night school, etc.	1.2	5.7	—	—
Total	100.0	100.0	100.0	100.0
Number of Respondents	960	1,236	13,312	4,011

TABLE 4.2
The Yearly Salaries of Hospital Administrators in 1935[9]

	Men Number	Women Number
No Salary	36	77
Less than $1,000	9	39
1,000–	36	211
2,000–	76	498
3,000–	137	227
4,000–	149	61
5,000–	129 ⎫	
6,000–	119 ⎪	
7,000–	50 ⎬	25
8,000	26 ⎪	
9,000–	15 ⎪	
10,000+	23 ⎭	
Total number of respondents	805	1138

men. Twenty-six percent of the women held nursing degrees, but only 4.6 percent of the nurses were university degree holders. Among the women, the sisters were the most likely to be degree holders.

In 1935, College members were a small fraction of all hospital administrators. By 1991, they were more representative; almost 6,000

TABLE 4.3
Reasons for Entering Administration by Age and Sex, 1935[10]

Reasons for Entering Administrative Field	Men								Women								Grand Total	Grand Percent
	20s	30s	40s	50s	60s	70 & Over	Total	%	20s	30s	40s	50s	60s	70 & Over	Total	%		
Interest or Preference for Administrative Work	3	60	107	75	36	3	284	40.6	20	88	177	89	16	2	392	51.4	676	46.2
Appointed or Requested by Superiors		22	55	69	23	2	171	24.4	9	48	111	76	26	1	271	35.5	442	30.2
Financial Remuneration		7	16	17	9	1	50	7.2	3	12	9	8	2		34	4.4	84	5.8
Physical Incapacity for other Work		2	4	8	2		16	2.3			1	3	1		5	.6	21	1.4
Interest in Helping Sick	1	11	34	35	14	1	90	13.7		5	21	6	4		36	4.7	132	9.1
Carried on Work of Husband or Other Relative		2	1	3	1		7	1.0	1	1	2		2		6	.8	13	.9
Not Satisfied with Existing Conditions of Hospital Administration	1	2	10	11	5		29	4.2		1	9	3			13	1.7	42	2.8
Forced into it	1	11	10	17	7		46	6.6	2		1	3	1		7	.9	53	3.6
Totals	6	117	237	235	97	7	699	100	35	155	331	188	52	3	764	100	1463	100.0

74

TABLE 4.4
Reasons for Entering Administration by Background and Sex, 1935[11]

Reasons for Entering Administrative Field	Men						Women						Grand Total	Grand Per Cent
	M.D.	R.N.	Rev.	Non-Prof.	Total	%	M.D.	R.N.	Sister	Non-Prof.	Total	%		
Interest or Preference for Administrative Work	180	3	11	68	262	39.0	2	363	4	14	383	49.8	645	44.8
Appointed or Requested by Superiors	75		25	63	163	24.3	1	201	74	15	291	37.9	454	31.6
Financial Remuneration	31	1		19	51	7.6		28		3	31	4.1	82	5.6
Physical Incapacity for other Work	14			2	16	2.4		3	1		4	.5	20	1.3
Interest in Helping Sick	83	2	3	9	97	14.4	1	28	3	3	35	4.6	132	9.2
Carried on Work of Husband or Other Relative	2			5	7	1.0	1	2		2	5	.6	12	.8
Not Satisfied with Existing Conditions of Hospital Administration	10		4	14	28	4.2		12		2	14	1.8	42	3.0
Forced into it	44		1	3	48	7.1	2	4			6	.7	54	3.7
Totals	439	6	44	183	672	100	7	641	82	39	769	100	1441	100.0

TABLE 4.5
**Percent Reduction in Yearly Administrators'
Salary in 1935 Compared to 1929**[12]

	Percent of Respondents %
No reduction	25.3
Up to 5% reduction	1.5
−10%	24.4
−15%	13.1
−20%	12.1
−25%	7.0
−34%	8.1
−49%	4.7
−69%	3.2
−100%	0.6
Total	100.0%
Number	1433

CEO's were College members, although perhaps 40 percent of these were leading other kinds of organizations than hospitals.[7]

By 1991, 85.5 percent of college affiliates had masters' degrees, 4.7 percent doctorates, and 9 percent bachelor degrees. Of those with post-secondary degrees, 61.6 percent obtained them in hospital and health administration, 20.4 percent in business, 3.6 percent in public health and public administration, with 14.4 percent in other fields (n = 16,888).[8] By 1991, unlike 1935, there would be very little difference between men and women by degree status.

According to today's standards, 1935 salaries were very low, as shown in Table 4.2. Men received higher salaries on average than women. Well over half the women received salaries under $3,000 a year.

These figures excluded fringe benefits such as free room and board. In 1937, President Roosevelt said, "I see one-third of a nation ill-housed, ill-clad (and) ill-nourished." No doubt there was comfort in holding any job at all.[13]

For physicians, this was a time when many saw so few patients who could pay their bills that the editor of the *Journal of the American Medical Association (JAMA)* had to congratulate his readers who were willing to pay their subscription fees during such hard times.

However, as Table 4.5 shows, administrators were affected by the Depression in terms of salary cutbacks. Only 25 percent of administrators received no reduction in their salary between 1929 (before the stock market crash) and 1935.

In the 1920s, administrators of larger hospitals got together and talked about problems of construction, convalescent wards, housing for employees, and pension systems. In the 1930s, the prevalent concerns included the training of nurses, low hospital occupancy, finances, the relationship of radiologists to hospitals, the Wagner Act as it related to labor unions, the Social Security Act and national health insurance. During the war, the issues were war preparations, rationing, price and salary controls, and air raid precautions.[15]

Why did people enter the field of hospital administration? In the 1935 survey, half said they entered because of preference for administrative work. Thirty-five percent of the women were appointed or

TABLE 4.6
Membership Characteristics of the ACHE in 1944[14]

	Fellows	Members	Nominees	Total
Number	323	493	201	1,017
Men	208	195	98	501
Women	115	298	103	516
Age under 50	61	219	148	428
Age 50+	243	270	53	567
Not Given	18	4	0	22
Born in USA	230	383	154	767
Born in Canada	39	37	11	87
Other	30	39	16	20
Not Given	24	34	20	74
Education				
High school or less	25	28	14	66
Some college	175	357	127	659
College degrees	156	159	81	396
Graduate work	22	18	13	53
Degrees in Education	15	15	6	36
Not Given	14	13	4	31
Professional Status				
M.D.	81	52	14	147
R.N.	64	132	43	239
Nun	42	146	51	239
Clergyman	8	7	3	18
Laywoman	9	21	9	39
Layman	118	136	81	335
Function				
Administrator	238	356	102	696
Other (assistant, associate, staff, department head, etc.)	85	137	99	321

requested by their superiors. This was the case for nearly all the sisters. A large number of respondents admitted they did not come into the field by preference, but because of financial need (6 percent), physical incapacity for other work, or carrying on the work of husband or other relative. Seven percent of the men said they were "forced into it" as the primary reason for their position.

Twenty-three percent of respondents left private business to become hospital administrators; 21 percent came from public health and social work; 18 percent from medicine; 15 percent from nursing; and 13 percent from school teaching. Sixty-seven percent of the respondents carried out other occupations or held other positions, in addition to being administrators. It was a part-time job for most. Sixty-six percent had more than six years of hospital administration experience before assuming their present position. Sixty percent received full maintenance (room and board). This was especially true for physicians, sisters, and nurses. The higher salaried men were more likely to receive full maintenance. Only 13 percent had a written contract as the basis of their appointment. Most of the rest had verbal agreements or no agreement. The majority (88 percent) planned to continue in hospital administration. Sixty-three percent of the men and 91 percent of the women administrators were in hospitals of 100 beds or less, which accounted for 78.4 percent of the hospitals reporting. Table 4.7 shows the ratio of College Members to hospital size in 1944.

According to John R. Mannix, prior to World War II, larger hospitals were typically directed by physicians; middle size hospitals were directed by Protestant ministers or Catholic sisters; and a nurse directed the smaller hospital.[17] Physician administrators predominated in government hospitals and in proprietary hospitals. Typical administrators were in their forties.

It was an occupation with three origins: medicine for the men, nursing for the women, and a religious order for both genders. It could be a demoralizing occupation for many. The founding Fellows of the College were hardly representative of their occupation. Of the 102 Charter Fellows, 16 were women and 32 of the men were phy-

TABLE 4.7
Hospital Size of College Members, 1944[16]

Beds	Number
Under 100	181
100–199	281
200–299	170
300–499	124
Over 500	86

sicians. Many of the early founders of the College were men without one of the three primary allegiances: medicine, nursing, or a religious order. They were enthusiastically committed to a career in hospital administration; none left the field when better economic times came. However, these Fellows became representative of hospital administration in the years to come. Not only did they seek colleagueship through the College; they also used the College to encourage graduate education in health administration.

Concurrent with the collection of statistical data, the College's 1934–35 Study Committee, consisting of Fred G. Carter, M.D., Chairman, Sister M. Patricia and Asa S. Bacon, produced their report, *The Hospital Administrator: An Analysis of His Duties, Responsibilities, Relationships and Obligations.*[18] This document defined the role of the administrator, given the conditions of the day:

> ... the administrator is the executive head of the hospital, responsible to the governing board for efficient management. Such being the case, he[19] must be given complete authority in administration and he must collaborate with the medical staff in order that the patient may be restored to health as quickly, safely and pleasantly as possible.[20]

This wording recognizes the hospital's "three-legged stool": board, administrator, and medical staff. To accomplish administrative objectives, the document advised administrators to involve themselves in formulating a body of rules: a constitution and bylaws. Such rules should not be too detailed, the document noted. However, "they may and should be supplemented by more detailed rules for the guidance of hospital employees."

Coordination of effort may be accomplished to a large extent by detailed regulations which are commonly referred to as standing orders. These are issued by the administrator and by establishing fixed routine, wherever possible, they greatly facilitate the work of the hospital.

> Organization charts indicating the division of labor and lines of authority clarify the functions of the various departments of the hospital and help to prevent overlapping and the resulting friction which usually develops out of failure on the part of department heads properly to appreciate the limits of their respective functions. The organization record (book of job descriptions) is valuable as a supplement to the organization chart. In this the duties and authority of each worker are put into written form and little is left to his imagination so far as his place in the organization is concerned.[21]

These words were clear reflections of the classical school of management theory, a philosophy which existed prior to the development of the human relations school and later studies of the "informal organization."[22]

The document continued:

> The administrator selects all department heads. In order to perform his duties it will be necessary for the administrator to delegate part of his responsibility . . . depending largely on the size of the hospital. But even though duties are delegated, the administrator is ultimately responsible.
>
> In the smaller hospital the relations between executive and employee and between employees are very simple; directions are for the most part verbal and relations in general quite elementary.
>
> [In larger hospitals] it is perfectly natural to organize all of those performing closely related duties into groups or departments in order to facilitate the administration of the affairs of the institution.[23]

Today, it is hard to envision a time when hospitals were so small and uncomplicated that departmental organization was unnecessary. Similarly, it is difficult to imagine a hospital where all tasks were so clearly defined as to leave little to the worker's imagination.

"The administrator fixes hospital fees and rates which are to be charged . . . and instructs the business office to see that such charges are made, entered in the patient's account and collected,"[24] the document stated. Prior to health insurance, less rate regulation existed. It was a simpler world. "The accounting office assists the administrator in preparation of the budget for presentation to the governing board," noted the report. This was an objective more than a fact; many hospitals did not use budgets until Medicare regulations required them to do so in the late 1960s.

> Legal decisions in practically all states of the union have thrown on the governing board of the hospital responsibility for seeing that the patient has proper care and the administrator, as the representative of this body, must assume that responsibility.[25]
>
> Ordinarily the administrator acts as a liaison officer between the medical staff and the governing board, but in some hospitals there are joint conference committees consisting of board members and staff members which meet with administrators to discuss and solve the purely medical problems of hospital administration. The danger in this type of organization is that the joint conference committee will overstep the bounds of propriety by enlarging the scope of its activities to include more than the purely medical phases of hospital administration. A more desirable arrangement is created through the appointment by the staff or its executive officer of a medical advisory

committee of the staff to confer with the administrator on matters of staff interest. . . . The administrator relays the wishes of the staff as expressed through the committee to the governing board, and he may, if it seems desirable, in the case of highly technical matters ask the members of such advisory committee to assist him in his representations to the governing board. Incidentally, staff members should not be asked to assume the anomalous, dual role of board member and staff member because this arrangement is incompatible with sound principles of organization.[26]

This proposal, consistent with classical organization theory, was rejected in time. Evidence accumulated that good rapport between board and medical staff contributed to higher quality of care.[27] Instead of later human relations theories, there was the following comment:

The administrator should be interested in the social activities of the personnel, particularly of those living in the institution. His interest should not be in the nature of interference but rather he should encourage social intercourse when off duty and render all assistance possible in promoting recreation and amusement when called on to do so.[28]

The qualifications of the administrator were summarized as requiring "infinite tact, diplomacy, patience and tolerance for the views and opinions of others," as well as firmness tempered with consideration for the weaknesses of others.

He must be an organizer, a community leader, have a sense of seriousness in his work, be absolutely honorable and just, a judge of human nature, industrious, of broad education, neat and tidy appearance, an educator, a good buyer, of a mechanical turn of mind, an ability to work with others, familiarity with laws affecting the hospital, and he should constantly seek comments and constructive criticism.

Of the 18 listed qualifications, number nine stated, "He must have administrative ability, the degree varying directly with the size of the hospital. In the very large hospital he will be almost entirely an administrator but in the smaller one he will actually do much of the work with fewer subordinates on whom he will depend."[29]

With this list of qualifications, the report concluded, "This survey describes the niche into which the American College of Hospital Administrators feels that its members may or should strive to fit themselves in a general way."[30]

The Transition of the 1940s and Later

In 1935, only a small percentage of administrators were members of the College. This had changed by 1944, when Dean Conley analyzed the coded questionnaires from 1,107 administrator members. From these questionnaires, he prepared "a statistical survey based on the 1944 Directory of Membership" for the Central Committee on Institutes of the College (see Table 4.6).[31]

The analysis was carried out by transcribing the questionnaire data onto punch cards. A statistical tabulating service was used to do the analysis that the "already overloaded headquarters staff" of the College was unable to complete. The result—methodologically speaking—was a major improvement over the 1935 survey.

In 1944, there were slightly more women affiliates than men. However, Fellows were twice as likely to be men than women.[32] Table 4.8 demonstrates the age and gender of College members in 1944. Although Fellows were older on average, male members were younger. Of members age 30–39, 104 of 125 were men; of members over 60 years old, 74 were men and 149 women. The nurse and physician members were somewhat older on average than the lay members. There was a decrease in the number of nurses entering hospital administration.[33]

The level of education of members in 1944 was higher than for the entire field in 1935. Laymen were the largest single group of members; sisters and nurses tied for second place; and physicians were third. Over two-thirds of the members were administrators, with the remainder being mostly associate and assistant administrators.

Most of the College members represented hospitals over 200 beds in size, even when most hospitals were under 100 beds.

The College membership of 1944 reflected the transition away from nurse and physician administrators to younger lay administrators.[35]

TABLE 4.8
Age and Gender of College Members, 1944, 1991 Active Affiliates[34]

Age	Men		Women	
	1944	1991	1944	1991
Under 30	3	295	0	328
30–39	104	3684	21	1580
40–49	163	6245	137	1358
50–59	148	2443	198	517
60+	74	811	149	233
Not given	9	—	15	—

The College represented larger general hospitals that offered more services. Of the 1,107 hospitals represented, 573 had outpatient departments; 703 had nursing schools; 531 had interns; and 381 had resident training programs.[36] College members continued to be unrepresentative of the larger body of hospital administrators. Signs of the future were clearly written in these figures.

At the start of World War II, military hospitals were usually managed by physicians. However, as the war progressed and the need for such hospitals grew, an increasing number were managed by non-physician male administrators. The College encouraged these administrators to join the College if they planned to continue in the field, and many did. Thus, the war helped change the profession of hospital administration.[37]

When Arthur Bachmeyer was President of the College in 1940–41, he predicted that there would be increased interest in hospital administration at the end of World War II. In order to estimate the size of this demand, the College sent questionnaires to Medical Service Corps administrators and received about 1500–2000 replies expressing interest in training and civilian careers. According to Dean Conley, this survey added fuel to the post war development of hospital administration courses.[38]

Since World War II, career officers in all branches of the military service have been actively involved in the College. Before the 1967 reorganization, Major General James McGibony represented the military on the Board of Regents. Today, the uniformed services are represented by a member of the Board of Governors and have the status of a "district." All the services recognize College involvement. In the Air Force, pay and rank are affected by College status.[39]

In 1948, the College published *Hospital Administration: A Life's Profession* in response to frequent requests of the College, "principally for vocational guidance purposes and more specifically for men and women deciding on a life's work."[40] The book noted:

> The increasing number of hospital trustees, administrators and others, seeking persons whose background and training qualify them for positions leading to a career in hospital administration.[41]
>
> A sound case can be made for the professional status of the hospital administrator . . . Hospital administration is a unique and highly complex activity. Involving as it does problems of finance, hospital care of the sick and injured, institutional management, interrelations of professional groups, as well as cutting across the fields of political economy, sociology, psychology, and technology, it encompasses many of the disciplines and principles of several distinct professional areas. Moreover [the administrator] must be skilled in effective human relations with an emphasis on such personal attitudes as diplomacy and

sympathetic understanding. Further the administrator must possess the somewhat abstract quality known as sound judgment.[42]

In 1948, annual administrative salaries were $7,500 a year and up, including maintenance (room and board). Some administrators of large institutions were "receiving $15,000 upwards with the privilege of engaging in consultant work." In moderately sized institutions, nonresident positions were paying a salary of $7,500 a year. Starting salaries were around $5,000 plus maintenance.[43]

The ACHA document went on to describe the ten graduate programs in hospital administration. For the first time, graduate education was proposed by the College as the primary entry point for a career in hospital administration, thus heralding a new era. By the 1950s, there were an estimated 10,000 hospital administration positions in American hospitals. By 1955, about 2,594 of these positions were held by affiliates of the College.[44] In the 1960s, the weight of College membership had shifted to masters'-degree program graduates. The mid-fifties saw the proportionate decline of the physician administrator.[45]

As part of his work on the Joint Commission on Education of the ACHA and AHA in 1948, Charles E. Prall surveyed hospital administrators on the major problems they confronted.[46] See Table 4.9.

This started a series of such surveys in 1961 (Levey and McCarthy),[47] 1963 (Dolson),[48] 1978 (Carper),[49] and 1990 (Agho and Cyphert).[50] Business and financial management has gone from 5th to first in the list of problems. Quality of medical care has held a steady middle place. Legal issues have remained low. The correlations shown in Table 4.10 show the most similarity between 1948 and 1963, and 1963 and 1978.[51]

After the initiation of Medicare, hospitals continued to grow in size, complexity, and costs. In 1968, Richard Stull said that one of the "major unsolved problems bedeviling the practice of truly effective administration in hospitals today . . . is our failure to secure competent supportive staff skills and to develop a middle level management of qualified and specialized individuals."[53]

The 1970s saw the proportion of College members who were employed in nonhospital settings reach 20 percent and remain at that level throughout the decade.[54] This figure reflected the diversity of health care organizations in this era of regulation and environmental complexity. By 1981, Stuart Wesbury estimated that only 60 percent of the graduates of masters' programs were employed in hospitals,[55] with the remaining 40 percent employed in a wide variety of health-related organizations.

TABLE 4.9
Comparison of the Rankings for the 1948, 1961, 1963, 1978, and 1990 Studies[52]

Problem Area	Rank Order				
	1948	1961	1963	1978	1990
Working with medical staff	1	7	4	4	2
Personnel management	2	2	3	3	3
Departmental functioning	3	4	1	1	6
Providing quality medical care	4	3	5	6	4
Business and financial management	5	1	2	2	1
Community relations	6	6	6	9	7
Physical plant and equipment	7	8	8	8	5
Dealing with the governing board	8	10	7	5	9
Affiliation with other institutions	9	5	9	7	10
Legal aspects and litigation	10	9	10	10	8

TABLE 4.10
Spearman Rank-Order Correlations for the 1948, 1961, 1963, 1978, and 1990 Problem Area Rankings[52]

	1948	1961	1963	1978	1990
1948	1.000	—	—	—	—
1961	0.539	1.000	—	—	—
1963	0.842**	0.697*	1.000	—	—
1978	0.697*	0.588*	0.891**	1.000	—
1990	0.770**	0.594*	0.697*	0.539	1.000

* $p < 0.05$, one-tail test.
** $p < 0.01$, one-tail test.

As of December 31, 1983, the College had 17,499 affiliates. This number included 81 Honorary Fellows, 642 Life Fellows, 1,758 Fellows, 348 Life Members, 6,079 Members, 5,413 Nominees, and 3,178 Student Associates.[56] This was the largest number of affiliates in the College's history.

Of the 12,471 active affiliates, 82 percent worked in hospitals and hospital systems; 3 percent in other direct providers; 8 percent in health agencies and associations; 5 percent in education and consulting; 1 percent in industry and insurance; and 1 percent in other settings.[57] Of those working in hospitals, 63 percent were chief executive officers or chief operating officers. Of those working in other organizations, 47 percent were chief executive officers.[58]

A 1983 staff study completed by James B. Gantenberg showed that in 1982, there were 202 physicians identified as hospital chief executive officers as compared to 813 in 1972. For registered nurses, 54 were identified as CEOs in 1982 as compared to 294 in 1972.

Table 4.11 shows the percentage of women affiliates of the College in November, 1982. At that time, women were returning to hospital administration, after a decline in the 1960s that accompanied a general decrease in the number of women in Catholic religious orders.[59]

Forty-five percent of student affiliates were women. In 1981, 51 percent of students in graduate programs in health administration were women, up from 9 percent in 1969.[60] This growth in the percentage of women in graduate schools could also be found in law and medicine.

Only 8.54 percent of Members were women. Fellows were 11.9 percent women, reflecting the earlier cohort of administrators when there were more women.

The two retired categories of Life Member and Life Fellow reflected several factors: the higher percentage of women in administration in the earlier years of the College; the longevity of women; and the lesser likelihood of women advancing from Member to Fellow because they served as administrators of smaller hospitals.

In 1990, the College in collaboration with the Graduate Program in Hospital and Health Administration of the University of Iowa conducted a national study of the careers of female and male College affiliates.[62] In order to control for length of time in the field, three cohorts were created. Those entering the field in 1971–1975, entering between 1976–1980, and entering between 1981–1985. (Members of

TABLE 4.11
Percent of Women by College Status, November 1982, Jan. 1991[61]

	% Female	
	1982	**1991**
Student	44.7	62.1
Faculty Associate	NA	26.1
Candidate for Nomineeship	NA	54.9
Nominee	16.2	36.0
Member	8.5	14.1
Fellow	11.2	8.5
Honorary Fellow	13.5	NA
Life Member	36.2	18.6
Life Fellow	27.0	NA

Life Members and Life Fellows are retired.

religious orders were excluded.)[63] As Table 4.12 shows, women were less likely to have become CEO's. Length of time in the field increases the likelihood of becoming a CEO.[64] In Cohort I, 61 percent of males and 37 percent of females earned more than $75,000. In Cohort II, 38 percent of males and 20 percent of females earned over $75,000. (Both are statistically significant differences.) For Cohort III, 15 percent of males and 9% of females earned over $75,000 (not significant). Women were more likely to report having a mentor,[65] but less likely to socialize with other executives outside of work.[66] Men were more likely to be married and married to their first spouse.[67] Women were more likely to have a spouse with graduate education.[68] Women were more likely to say that their spouse's career and child rearing were obstacles to their careers.[69] Men were much more likely to aspire to become a CEO,[70] and more likely to move to do so.[71]

The College, in collaboration with the AHA and Heidrick and Struggles, Inc., has studied hospital CEO turnover from 1981–1990.[73] (See Table 4.13.) Adjusted turnover rose in the middle 1980's to over 18 percent, and then declined. Based on surveys in 1989 and 1990, 65 percent of turnover was voluntary (career moves, 31 percent; personal events like retirement, 15 percent; job dissatisfaction, 15 percent; and other, 4 percent). The 35 percent involuntary turnover was due to disagreements (14%) and reorganization (11%), with 10 percent of unknown cause. High turnover hospitals are more likely to be smaller, part of multihospital systems, investor-owned, in the south or west, in large cities, non-teaching, low occupancy, and low operating margins.[74]

TABLE 4.12
1990 Survey of Current Position, Females and Males by Cohort of Entry into the Field[72]

	Cohort I 1971–75		Cohort II 1976–80		Cohort III 1981–85	
	Female	Male	Female	Male	Female	Male
CEO	17	37**	9	24**	7	17*
COO/Associate	32	37	22	29	18	28
Vice President	36	14	40	32	35	34
Department Head/Staff	14	8	22	11	29	17
Other	1	4	7	4	11	4
Total	100%	100%	100%	100%	100%	100%
n	106	120	139	119	137	113
No answer			3	1	3	2

* Chi Square significant $p < .01$
** Chi Square significant $p < .001$

Table 4.13
Turnover in General Hospital CEO's, 1981–1990[75]

Year	Adjusted CEO Turnovers	Number of Short Term Hospitals
1981	13.7	5,687
1982	14.0	5,678
1983	12.8	5,672
1984	15.4	5,665
1985	15.9	5,651
1986	16.9	5,626
1987	17.5	5,583
1988	18.4	5,526
1989	16.2	5,454
1990	12.8	5,398
1991	16.7	—

Minority Relations

In an address to the American Hospital Association in 1968, Whitney Young spoke to the General Assembly, stating that he did not see many black faces in the audience. He urged the encouragement of young African Americans into the profession of hospital administration.

One result of this speech was the creation of a Task Force on Minorities within the ACHA. In 1968, there were about 50 black members of the College. Many of them were instrumental in founding the National Association of Health Services Executives (NAHSE) in 1968.[76] Dr. Albert W. Dent was the first black Fellow of the College and President of Dillard University from 1941 to 1969. There is now an ACHE scholarship in his name.

Another black Fellow of the College, Charles E. Burbridge, was the first graduate of the doctoral degree program at Iowa, and thus, the first person to be awarded a doctorate in hospital administration. From 1971 to 1980, he was Executive Director of Freedman's Hospital, Washington, D.C.[77]

In 1947, the AHA held its annual meeting in St. Louis. Charles Burbridge's hotel reservation was not honored because of his race. Dean Conley, George Bugbee and Edwin Crosby visited the St. Louis Convention Bureau, asserting that there would never be another AHA convention in St. Louis unless blacks were accepted at the city's hotels.[78] Thus, the college and the AHA took early public positions against segregation.

A Code of Ethics

Unlike the professions of medicine, law, dentistry, and nursing, there is no code of ethics for managers in general. Unlike graduates of medical schools who traditionally have risen to take the Hippocratic oath or its equivalent when receiving their degrees, graduates of business schools initiate their careers unrestrained by such professional standards.[79]

The College, however, from its earliest days, maintained its concern for a code of ethics for hospital administration. As early as 1934, it was noted that:

> In the Fellowship Pledge of the American College of Hospital Administrators this sentiment stands out in bold relief:
>
> > Especially do I pledge myself to honest administration within my own hospital, to consider ever primary to my own welfare that of my institution.
>
> The Fellows of the College in faithfully keeping this their pledge, will make an immense contribution to hospital administration not only in their own institutions but, by their precept and example, to every hospital on this continent.[80]

Table 4.14 summarizes key developments in the College's ongoing concern with a code of ethics. In 1938, the College Executive Committee appointed a special committee chaired by Dr. G. Harvey Agnew, secretary-treasurer of the Canadian Hospital Council, Toronto, to develop a code of ethics. "The drafting proved to be long and painful."[81]

"After the College committee had struggled with the code for some time, it was decided that an administrator's code could not logically be separated from a code applying to all hospital workers so a Joint ACHA and AHA Committee was established," said Dr. Agnew, Chairman, one of a large number of able Canadians active in the early College.

Since the subject matter was ethics, the views of the various religious hospital associations were considered, even though there was no representation from these associations. However, care was taken to see that major religions had influential members on the drafting committee. Not until June, 1941, did the Code receive final approval by both ACHA and AHA and was published. According to Kipnis, this was a further step in the professional development of hospital administration.[82]

One reason for the delay in the development of the Code was the College's requirement that the administrator/affiliate's hospital be approved by the American College of Surgeons (the forerunner of approval by the Joint Commission of the Accreditation of Hospitals, now the Joint Commission on the Accreditation of Healthcare Organiza-

TABLE 4.14
The Code of Ethics Chronology[83]

1938	The College Executive Committee appoints a special committee chaired by Dr. G. Harvey Agnew to develop a code of ethics.
1939	The Joint ACHE-AHA Committee established to develop a code of ethics.
June 1941	The Code of Ethics approved by both the AHA and ACHE. Published by the AHA.
Feb. 1942	Code published in ACHE *News*.
1947	Joint Committee revises code approved by AHA + ACHE.
1956	New Joint Committee appointed Dr. A. P. Merrill, Chairman.
1957	Revised Code accepted by both organizations.
1958	Revised Code published.
1963	New Joint Committee chaired by Jack A. L. Hahn, revises the Code. Approved in June by the College, and in November by the AHA Trustees.
1964	New Code published.
1970	The ACHE publishes its own code, adopted Sept. 14, 1970.
1973	Special Committee on Ethics of the College revises the Code. Approved by the Council of Regents August 20, 1973.
1974	The Board of Trustees of the AHA accepts their "Guidelines on Ethical Conduct and Relationships for Health Care Institutions."
1980	The College republishes their 1973 Code and the 1974 AHA Guidelines. The AHA revises and updates its Code.[84]
1985	College develops Public Policy statement on Ethics.
1987	New Code of Ethics published. Review of Grievance Procedure.
Nov. 1987	AHA Guidelines on Ethical Conduct for Health Care Institutions Approved.
Feb. 1990	First Ethical Policy Statement, "Impaired Health Care Executive".
Mar. 1992	Second Ethical Policy Statement, "Responsibility to Employees."
Aug. 1992	Code of Ethics revised. (As amended by the Council of Regents, July 28, 1992).[85]

tions (JCAHO)), and be registered with the AHA. This resulted in a controversy with the Catholic Hospital Association (CHA), because Catholic hospitals were "registered" with the CHA rather than the AHA. Reverend Griffin wrote to College President Bachmeyer that he could not serve on the Code of Ethics Committee (he was Vice President of the CHA) "because of the strained relations between our organizations due to the refusal of your board to recognize the Catholic Hospital Association." The problem was aggravated by the fact that sisters constituted a large percentage of the potential College membership. The

College revised its position and deleted the ACS and AHA requirements for candidates for admission.

By 1942, sisters were 13 percent of the Fellows; 29 percent of Members; and 20 percent of Associate Members. Rev. Griffin was included as a member of the Joint Committee.[86]

Other members of the committee included Asa S. Bacon, Superintendent of the Presbyterian Hospital, Chicago, a President of the AHA, and its Treasurer for years. Not only was he well-remembered by John Mannix,[87] the American Hospital Association's outstanding library is named in his honor.

In addition, there were S. S. Goldwater, M.D., Commissioner of Health for the City of New York, and one of the leading men of his day; the Right Reverend Monsignor M. F. Griffin; James A. Hamilton; Malcolm T. MacEachern, M.D.; and Ada Belle McCleery.[88] Ex-officio members included A. C. Bachmeyer, M.D.; B. W. Black, M.D.; B. W. Caldwell, M.D.; Fred G. Carter, M.D.; and Gerhard Hartman, Ph.D. The preface stated: "A Code of Ethics is the crystallization of the principles underlying civilization"—an elegant ecumenical summary.[89]

With ongoing revisions, the Code of Ethics became more generalized. The changes reflected shifts in the field. According to the Code, "the hospital is to render care to the sick and injured as its primary responsibility. Financial concerns and other interests should be of secondary consideration. The duty of the hospital is also to advance scientific knowledge and the education of all participating in the work, and to take an active part in the promotion of general health." This was at once an obvious and profound statement of the central values of the hospital field. "Trustees have the duty to determine policies and provide equipment and facilities consistent with community needs."[90] This statement was made before regional health planning legislation appeared in 1966, long before the Hill–Burton Act of 1946.

"They must also see that proper professional standards are maintained for the care of the sick." This was before the *Darling* versus *Charleston Hospital* decision which gave legal force to this view in 1965. In addition, "no member of the board should profit by his connection with the hospital." The voluntary hospital was the focus; the Code was inappropriate for proprietary hospitals.

The Code requested that administrators assure "that the medical staff be properly organized"[91] for medical records to be complete and adequate. Adequate medical records were concerns of the American College of Surgeons and Malcolm MacEachern since 1918. They remain a concern of the JCAHO to this day. "There should be no solicitation for patients by a hospital or any person connected with it."[92]

The Federal Trade Commission and the rise of marketing as a legitimate activity for hospitals have obviously changed this position. Relationship to other hospitals "should bear to each other a spirit of friendly cooperation and interest. When possible, efforts should be directed to not duplicate unnecessarily the facilities of competing institutions."[93] However, competition between hospitals received open acceptance in the late 1970s. "Hospitals should refrain from participating in contracts with companies, organizations, municipalities, governments or other bodies at rates which are obviously unfair to other hospitals in the community."[94] In taking this stand against capitation contracts or lower than average contracted group rates, the College reversed an earlier decision not to take such positions.[95] This policy continued in the 1947 and 1958 Codes, but disappeared from the 1973 Code of Ethics.

During the presidency of Dean Conley (1941–1966), the College was not particularly active in using the Code as a basis for disciplining unethical behavior. This was due both to the difficulties of sorting fact from hearsay evidence and the desire for fairness.

One reason for the separation of the AHA and ACHE codes in 1967 was the unwillingness of the AHA to adjudicate ethics violations. The ACHE went on to develop and publish a definitive grievance procedure. In the early days, the basic Code was summarized as: "If you can stand to have that story printed on the front page of your local paper it's probably o.k." At that time, unethical behavior included personal aggrandizement, proselytizing employees of other neighborhood hospitals, and actively seeking to displace a colleague.

Teas or open houses for nurses of other hospitals as a recruitment technique were considered unethical. Administrators were criticized if they used the shotgun approach to send out large numbers of resumes.

As of 1983, the ACHE Ethics Committee focused on much more critical ethical violations such as kickbacks, stealing, sexual harassment, or misappropriation of funds. This is not to imply that the ethics of hospital administrators had deteriorated.

Gone were the days when the trustees of one city's hospital took home 5 percent of hospital revenues or when an administrator in another city kept a 45-caliber revolver in his desk drawer.[96]

HMOs were bitterly opposed by many physicians, not only in this country, but also in England where a company (through a friendly society) would seek the lowest bid from a doctor to provide medical care. In an era before the Flexner reforms made doctors scarce, there were doctors willing to bid low prices and provide minimal care.[97] With respect to employees and interns:

Anyone who has broken a contract with another hospital or who has left service in another hospital on short notice should not be accepted without adequate evidence that such action was justified.

All hospitals operated by a church organization and for all patients who are members thereof, it is expected that the Moral Code of that denomination be observed.[98]

By 1980, this had become: "Health care institutions, wherever possible, and consistent with ethical commitments of the institution, should ensure respect and consideration for reasonable accommodation of the individual religious and social beliefs and customs of patients, employees, physicians and others."[99] In earlier decades, the ethnic and religious focus of many hospitals was more narrowly defined. In more recent years, this has been replaced with a more ecumenical view.

The Joint Committee of the AHA and the ACHE continued its work publishing revisions in 1947, 1957 and 1963. The 1956 Committee was chaired by Dr. A. P. Merrill, superintendent of St. Barnabas Hospital for Chronic Diseases in New York City. Representing the AHA were Dr. Frank R. Bradley, Director of Barnes Hospitals, St. Louis, and Joseph G. Norby, a Milwaukee hospital consultant. Robert Cunningham was editor of *Modern Hospital* and Bradley and Norby were both former leaders of the AHA and ACHA. Representing the ACHA were Dr. Edwin L. Harmon, Director of Grasslands Hospital, Valhalla, New York, and Donald M. Rosenberger, Director of the Portland Maine Medical Center.[100]

The College revised this Code in 1973, a version that remained in effect through 1983. The AHA revised its Code under the title, "Guidelines on Ethical Conduct and Relationships for Health Care Institutions" in 1974, and again in 1980.

The 1973, the Code of Ethics of the College focused specifically on the administrator:[101] "Health services administration must meet two primary accountabilities—one as a member of the College, and the other in activities performed as an institutional executive."[102]

The Preamble[103] served as a strong statement of the executive's role:

An expected condition of affiliation with the American College of Hospital Administrators is that the individual's behavior will be ethical as a way of life in the conduct of personal and business affairs.

Inherent in any human dealings are the possibilities of unethical behavior in a variety of forms. The environment of health institutions and related programs presents complex and unique settings of human relationships, replete with potentials for behavior in conflict with desired ethical standards and projects consequences contrary to a favorable public image.

Table 4.15 highlights some of the differences between the 1973 and the 1992 Code of Ethics.[104] The 1973 Code is explicit about adhering to the AHA Guidelines, while the 1992 one is not. The 1973 Code is explicit about respect for religious practices, while the 1992 Code does not mention this. The 1973 Code calls for accountability

TABLE 4.15
Selected Changes in the ACHE Code of Ethics 1973 and 1992[105]

1973	1992
Expected adherence to AHA Guidelines on Ethical Conduct for Healthcare Institutions.	Implied adherence to AHA Guidelines on Ethical Conduct for Healthcare Institutions.
"Respect for social and religious practices and customs of patients, employees."	"Respect the customs and practices of patients."
"Health services administration must meet two primary accountabilities— one as a member of the College and the other in activities performed as an institutional executive."	"I. Responsibilities to the Profession of Health Care Management II. Obligations to Patients or Others Served, to the Organization and to Employees"
"Cooperate with other entities to promote accessibility and the conduct of quality health programs"	"Conduct both competitive and cooperative activities in ways that improve community health care services."
Reports to the public should include factual information and interpret clearly institutional status, accomplishments, and objectives.	Provide prospective consumers with adequate and accurate information.
"Effectiveness in administrative performance depends upon mutual respect and harmonious relationships between the hospital administration and the governing body."	—
No mention of employees.	No mention of governing body or medical staff.
—	An affiliate of the College has a duty to communicate violations of this Code to the ACHE Ethics committee.
No supplement Principles for Students.	Statement of Principles for Students.

to the College and employing organizations, while 1992's refers to the profession, patients and others served, to the organization, and to employees. Employees were not mentioned in 1973. In 1992, the Code allows both cooperation and competition. It refers to "consumers" and is explicit about avoiding discrimination. The 1992 Code does not mention specifically the governing board or medical staff. In 1973, there was no explicit duty to report ethical violations to the College. The principles for students are new.

Grievances reviewed by the Ethics Committee
Beginning in 1975, reports of the College ethics committee were made to the membership.[106] Table 4.16 summarizes the decisions made by this committee from 1980 to 1992. Most cases are dismissed with no cause. A few have not been acted upon because the affiliate had resigned or was suspended for nonpayment of dues. Actions vary from censure to probation to suspension to expulsion (severance).

The growing interest in health care management ethics is reflected in a number of publications, including a book of case problems published by the college on this topic,[108] a text, and a regular column in *Healthcare Executive* magazine.[109]

APPENDIX
*American College of Healthcare
Executives Code of Ethics*

Preface

The Code of Ethics is administered by the Ethics Committee, which is appointed by the Board of Governors upon nomination by the Chairman. It is composed of nine Fellows of the College, each of whom serves a three-year term on a staggered basis, with three members retiring each year.

The Ethics Committee shall:

• Review and evaluate annually the Code of Ethics, and make any necessary recommendations for updating the Code.
• Review and recommend action to the Board of Governors on allegations brought forth regarding breaches of the Code of Ethics.
• Refine the Code of Ethics to specific applications and to relate the Code to several membership classifications as compared to the Code for hospitals as institutions.

As amended by the Council of Regents at its annual meeting on July 28, 1992.

TABLE 4.16
Number of Grievances Considered and Actions by the Committee on Ethics[107] 1980–1992

Year	Invalid Complaint	Dismissed	In Abeyance Due to Affiliate Resignation or Suspension	Censure	Probation	Suspension	Severance Expulsion
1980–82		9		2			5
1982–83		3					2
84		2					1
85		3		2			
86							1
87	1	1					
88	1	1	2			1	
89	4		1				
90	2	3		1	1		
91	1	2					
1991–92	2	3		1			

- Prepare a report of observations, accomplishments, and recommendations to the Board of Governors at the annual reporting session, and such other periodic reports as required.

The Ethics Committee invokes the Code of Ethics under authority of the ACHE Bylaws, Article II, Affiliation, Section 11 (b), Termination of Affiliation, as follows:

> Affiliation may be terminated by action of the Board of Governors as a result of violation of the Code of Ethics, nonconformity with the Bylaws or Regulations Governing Admission, Advancement and Recertification or conduct unbecoming an affiliate, as determined by the Board of Governors. No such termination of affiliation shall be effected without affording a reasonable opportunity for the affiliate to consider the charges and to appear in his or her own defense before the Board of Governors or its designated hearing committee, as outlined in the "Grievance Procedure," Appendix I of the College's Code of Ethics.

Preamble

The purpose of the Code of Ethics of the American College of Healthcare Executives is to serve as a guide to conduct for affiliates. It contains standards of ethical behavior for healthcare executives in their professional relationships. These relationships include members of the healthcare executive's organization and other organizations. Also included are patients or others served, colleagues, the community and society as a whole. The Code of Ethics also incorporates standards of ethical behavior governing personal behavior, particularly when that conduct directly relates to the role and identity of the healthcare executive.

The fundamental objectives of the healthcare management profession are to enhance overall quality of life, dignity and well-being of every individual needing healthcare services; and to create a more equitable, accessible, effective and efficient healthcare system.

Healthcare executives have an obligation to act in ways that will merit the trust, confidence and respect of healthcare professionals and the general public. To do so, healthcare executives must lead lives that embody an exemplary system of values and ethics.

In fulfilling their commitments and obligations to patients or others served, healthcare executives function as moral agents. Since every management decision affects the health and well-being of both individuals and communities, healthcare executives must evaluate the possible outcomes of their decisions and accept full responsibility for the consequences. In organizations that deliver healthcare services, they must safeguard and foster the rights, interests and prerogatives of patients or others served. The role of moral agent requires that health-care executives speak out and take actions necessary to promote such rights, interests and prerogatives if they are threatened.

I. The Healthcare Executive's Responsibilities to the Profession of Healthcare Management

The healthcare executive shall:

A. Uphold the values, ethics and mission of the healthcare management profession;

B. Conduct all personal and professional activities with honesty, integrity, respect, fairness and good faith in a manner that will reflect well upon the profession;

C. Comply with all laws in the jurisdictions in which the healthcare executive is located, or conducts professional or personal activities;

D. Maintain competence and proficiency in healthcare management by implementing a personal program of assessment and continuing professional education;

E. Avoid the exploitation of professional relationships for personal gain;

F. Use this code to further the interests of the profession and not for selfish reasons;

G. Respect professional confidences;

H. Enhance the dignity and image of the healthcare management profession through positive public information programs;

I. Refrain from participating in any endorsement or publicity that demeans the credibility and dignity of the healthcare management profession; and

J. Refrain from using the College's credential or affiliation with the College to promote or endorse external commercial products or services.

II. The Healthcare Executive's Obligations to Patients or Others Served, to the Organization and to Employees

A. Commitments to patients or others served

The healthcare executive shall:

1. Assure the existence of a process to evaluate the quality of care or service rendered;

2. Avoid exploitation of relationships for personal advantage;

3. Avoid practicing or facilitating discrimination and institute safeguards to prevent discriminatory organizational practices;

4. Assure the existence of a process that will advise patients or others served of the rights, opportunities, responsibilities and risks regarding available healthcare services;
5. Provide a process that assures the autonomy and self-determination of patients or others served; and
6. Assure the existence of procedures that will safeguard the confidentiality and privacy of patients or others served.

B. Commitments to the organization
The healthcare executive shall:
1. Provide healthcare services consistent with available resources and assure the existence of a resource allocation process that considers ethical ramifications;
2. Conduct both competitive and cooperative activities in ways that improve community healthcare services;
3. Lead the organization in the use and improvement of standards of management and sound business practices;
4. Respect the customs and practices of patients or others served, consistent with the organization's philosophy; and
5. Be truthful in all forms of professional and organizational communication and avoid information that is false, misleading, and deceptive or information that would create unreasonable expectations.

C. Responsibilities to employees
Healthcare executives have an ethical and professional obligation to employees of the organizations they manage that encompass but are not limited to:
1. Creating a working environment conducive for underscoring employee ethical conduct and behavior.
2. Assuring that individuals may freely express ethical concerns and providing mechanisms for discussing and addressing such concerns.
3. Assuring a working environment that is free from harassment, sexual and other; coercion of any kind, especially to perform illegal or unethical acts; and discrimination on the basis of race, creed, color, sex, ethnic origin, age or disability.
4. Assuring a working environment that is conducive to proper utilization of employees' skills and abilities.
5. Paying particular attention to the employee's work environment and job safety.

6. Establishing appropriate grievance and appeals mechanisms.

III. Conflicts of Interest

A conflict of interest may be only a matter of degree, but exists when the healthcare executive:

A. Is in a position to benefit directly or indirectly by using authority or inside information, or allows a friend, relative or associate to benefit from such authority or information.

B. Uses authority or information to make a decision to intentionally affect the organization in an adverse manner.

The healthcare executive shall:

A. Conduct all personal and professional relationships in such a way that all those affected are assured that management decisions are made in the best interests of the organization and the individuals served by it;

B. Disclose to the appropriate authority any direct or indirect financial or personal interests that might pose potential conflicts of interest;

C. Accept no gifts or benefits offered with the expectation of influencing a management decision; and

D. Inform the appropriate authority and other involved parties of potential conflicts of interest related to appointments or elections to boards or committees inside or outside the healthcare executive's organization.

IV. The Healthcare Executive's Responsibilities to Community and Society

The healthcare executive shall:

A. Work to identify and meet the healthcare needs of the community;

B. Work to assure that all people have reasonable access to healthcare services;

C. Participate in public dialogue on healthcare policy issues and advocate solutions that will improve health status and promote quality healthcare;

D. Consider the short-term and long-term impact of management decisions on both the community and on society; and

E. Provide prospective consumers with adequate and accurate information, enabling them to make enlightened judgments and decisions regarding services.

V. The Healthcare Executive's Duty to Report Violations of the Code

An affiliate of the College who has reasonable grounds to

believe that another affiliate has violated this Code has a duty to communicate such facts to the Ethics Committee.

Appendix I
American College of Healthcare Executives Grievance Procedure

1. To be processed, a complaint must be filed in writing to the Ethics Committee of the College within three years of the date of discovery of the alleged incident; and, the Committee has the responsibility to look into incidents brought to its attention regardless of the informality of the information, provided the information can be documented or supported or may be a matter of public record. The three-year period within which a complaint must be filed shall temporarily cease to run during intervals when the affiliate is in inactive or suspended status, or when the affiliate resigns from the College.

2. The committee chairman initially will determine whether the complaint falls within the purview of the Ethics Committee and whether immediate investigation is necessary. However, all letters of complaint that are filed with the Ethics Committee will appear on the agenda of the next committee meeting. The Ethics Committee shall have the final discretion to determine whether a complaint falls within the purview of the Ethics Committee.

3. If a grievance is initiated:
   a. Specifics of the complaint will be sent to the respondent by certified mail. Committee staff will inform the respondent that the grievance procedure has been initiated and will ask the respondent to cooperate with the Regent investigating the complaint. The respondent may respond directly to the Ethics Committee.
   b. The Ethics Committee shall refer the matter to the appropriate Regent who is best able to investigate the alleged infraction. The Regent shall make inquiry into the matter, and in the process the respondent shall be given an opportunity to be heard.
   c. Upon completion of the inquiry, the Regent shall present a complete report and recommended disposition of the matter in writing to the Ethics Committee. Absent unusual circumstances, the Regent is allowed 60 days to complete his or her report and recommended disposition and provide them to the Committee.

4. Upon the Committee's receipt of the Regent's report and recommended disposition, the Committee shall review them and make its written recommendation to the Board of Governors

as to what action shall be taken. A Copy of the Committee's recommended decision along with the Regent's report and recommended disposition to the Board will be mailed to the respondent by certified mail.

5. Within 30 days of the receipt of the Ethics Committee's recommended decision, the respondent may file a written appeal of the recommended decision with the Board of Governors. The written appeal must be received by the Board of Governors within 30 days after the recommended decision of the Ethics Committee is received by the respondent. The Board of Governors shall not take action on the Ethics Committee's recommended decision until the 30-day appeal period has elapsed. If no appeal to the Board of Governors is filed, the Board shall review the recommended decision and determine action to be taken.

6. If an appeal to the Board of Governors is timely filed, the College chairman shall appoint an ad hoc committee to hear the matter. This ad hoc committee shall consist of three Fellows from the region of the respondent's area of employment at the time of the alleged infraction of the Code of Ethics. Adequate notice of the formation of this committee, notice of the hearing date, with an opportunity for representation, shall be mailed to the respondent. At least 30 days' notice of the hearing date shall be given to all parties concerned. Reasonable requests for postponement shall be given consideration.

7. This ad hoc committee shall give the respondent adequate opportunity to present his or her case and to be represented if so desired. At the close of the hearing, the ad hoc committee shall write a detailed report with recommendations to the Board of Governors.

8. The Board of Governors shall decide what action to take after reviewing the report of the ad hoc committee. The Board shall provide the respondent with a copy of its decision. The decision of the Board of Governors shall be final. The Board of Governors shall have the authority to accept or reject any of the findings or recommended decisions of the Regent, the Ethics Committee or the ad hoc committee and to order whatever level of discipline it feels is justified.

9. At the level of the grievance procedure, the Committee and the Board of Governors shall have the sole discretion to notify or contact the complainant relating to the grievance procedure.

Appendix II

Once the grievance procedure has been initiated, the Ethics Committee may take any of the following actions based upon its findings:

1. Determine the grievance complaint to be invalid.
2. Dismiss the grievance complaint.
3. Recommend censure.
4. Recommend probation.
5. Recommend suspension.
6. Recommend expulsion. . . .

[Because of its length, Appendix III, the AHA "Guidelines on Ethical Conduct and Relationships for Health Care Institutions," is not reprinted here.]

Appendix IV
American College of Healthcare Executives
Statement of Principles for Students
(Supplement to the ACHE Code of Ethics)

"The life of the health administrator is dedicated to the achievement of the highest possible level of performance in the competent and humane delivery of health services, and in education and research conducted in the interest of healthcare."

Council of Regents, ACHE

Students of health administration have the opportunity to participate in the building of a worthy, purposeful, and progressive profession. This opportunity, however, is not without obligation, for the viability of the profession will rest on the integrity as well as the capability of its members. It is necessary, therefore, that the individual's behavior be ethical as a way of life in the conduct of personal and academic affairs. In pursuing this objective the student shall:

1. Conduct self at all times in a dignified, exemplary manner.
2. Abide by the procedures, rules, and regulations of the educational institution.
3. Respect the guidelines prescribed by each professor in the preparation of academic assignments.
4. Be objective, understanding, and fair in academic performance and relationships.
5. Strive toward academic excellence, improvement of administrative skills and expansion of other professional knowledge.
6. Encourage and assist colleagues in the pursuit of academic excellence, improvement of administrative skills, and expansion of other professional knowledge.
7. Encourage, aid, and teach others in the principles and practices of health services administration.

8. Not denigrate the work of colleagues.

9. Neither engage in, assist in, nor condone cheating, plagiarism, or other such activities.

10. Foster and support sound programs of education and research to assure the proper direction of the profession.

11. Contribute interest, support, and leadership toward the overall improvement of the community, with special emphasis on delivery of healthcare, health education, and related objectives.

12. Respect and protect the rights, privileges, and beliefs of others.

NOTES

[1] Kipnis, 1955, p. 123.

[2] Davis, Michael, 1927, p. 27.

[3] *Ibid.*, pp. 17–18. Based on data from AMA hospital directories for these years.

[4] *Ibid.*, p. 8. Titles as listed in the 1927 *AMA Directory*.

[5] ACHA, "A Survey of the Hospital Administrator," 1936. (Robert Neff, "General Statement.")

[6] ACHA, "A Survey of the Hospital Administrator," 1936, p. 5. ACHE *1992 Directory*, p. 1386. There was very little difference between genders in 1992.

[7] ACHE, *1992 Directory*, p. 1386.

[8] *Ibid.*, p. 1387.

[9] ACHA, "A Survey of the Hospital Administrator," 1936, p. 8.

[10] *Ibid.*, p. 27.

[11] *Ibid.*

[12] *Ibid.*, p. 64. In March 1933, President Roosevelt requested an Economy Act that would reduce government employee salaries by up to 15 percent and cut veterans' pensions. Morris, 1953, p. 342. Also see Faxon, N., 1959, p. 13.

[13] Morris, 1953, p. 355.

[14] ACHA, "A Statistical Survey Based on the 1944 Directory of Membership," 1944, Part I. Tables 1–6.

[15] Society of Medical Administrators, 1967.

[16] ACHA, "A Statistical Survey Based on the 1944 Directory of Membership," 1944. Tables 9, 10. Of these, 771 were general hospitals, 12 mental, 13 tuberculosis, and 46 other types of hospitals.

[17] John R. Mannix interview, 1982.

[18] ACHA, *The Hospital Administrator: An Analysis of His Duties, Responsibilities, Relationships, and Obligations,* 1935. Carter was president of the ACHA in 1935–1936. Asa Bacon was a Charter Fellow; they also give credit to Dr. MacEachern and Dr. T. R. Ponton.

[19] "The male pronoun is used throughout this study as an editorial convenience only." *Ibid.*, p. 3, footnote.

[20] *Ibid.*, p. 7.

[21] *Ibid.*, pp. 7–8.

[22] About 10 miles away from the College offices, at the Hawthorne plant of the General Electric Company, Elton Mayo, Fritz Roethlisberger and their colleagues were finishing the "Hawthorne studies," which would change this perspective completely. By the 1950s, the College ran conferences on human relations across the country. Roethlisberger and Dickson, 1939.

[23] ACHA, 1935, *op. cit.*, pp. 8, 9.

[24] *Ibid.*, p. 11.

[25] *Ibid.*, p. 12. This was written 30 years before "Darling vs. Charleston Community Hospital," 211 N.E. 2nd 53 (1965) and the U.S. Supreme Court's refusal to hear an appeal of this case, *cert. denied*, 383 U.S. 946 (1966).

[26] *Ibid.*, p. 13. The quote continues, "The preservation of the liaison characteristics of the administrator's position will be found to be highly desirable at all times. Deviations from this conception of the administrator's place in the organization lead to trouble sooner or later. The organization of the proprietary hospital represents a somewhat different problem which need not enter into present considerations."

[27] Shortell *et al.*, 1976, p. 103.

[28] ACHA, 1935, *op. cit.*, p. 9.

[29] *Ibid.*, pp. 19–20.

[30] *Ibid.*, p. 24.

[31] ACHA, "A Statistical Survey Based on the 1944 Directory of Membership," 1944.

[32] The number of female affiliates of the College increased due in part to the number of nuns who joined after Father Schwitilla lifted "the bans" on ACHA interaction. Father Schwitilla opposed the College at its onset. Gerhard Hartman, personal communication, 1983. Kipnis, pp. 65–66. The number of female affiliates fell during the 1960s due to the declining number of women in Catholic religious orders and the substitution of administrators who were nuns with lay male administrators. W. Richard Kirk interview, 1983.

[33] ACHA, *Minute Book*, Vol. 1, August 19, 1944.

[34] ACHA, "A Statistical Survey Based on the 1944 Directory of Membership," 1944, Part II. Table 1. ACHE, *1992 Directory*, p. 1385.

[35] ACHA "A Statistical Survey Based on the 1944 Directory of Membership," 1944, op. cit. Part IV. Table 8.

[36] *Ibid.*, Part III. Table 3.

[37] Personal communication. Oscar Weissman, M.D., and Robert Griggs, M.D., 1983. The College continued to welcome military hospital administrators. "The Value to Medical Service Corps Officers of Affiliation with the American College of Hospital Administrators," *U.S. Airforce Medical Service Digest*, Vol. 10, February 1959, p. 27.

[38] Dean Conley interview, April 21, 1983.

[39] W. Richard Kirk interview, March 14, 1983.

[40] ACHA, *Hospital Administration: A Life's Profession*, 1948. "Foreword" by Dean Conley, executive secretary. This work relies heavily on Rappleye (1922), Davis, Michael M. (1929), and the ACHA reports of 1934–35 (Dr. Fred Carter) and 1937 (Dr. Alphonse Schwitalla), and gives thanks to Drs. Arthur C. Bachmeyer, Malcolm MacEachern, Claude Munger, Charles Prall,

and John Gorrell. In the same year the College also published a more popular document *At the Helm of the Hospital: The Story of a New Profession*, 1948, as part of a fundraising project for the College.

[41] ACHA, *Hospital Administration: A Life's Profession*, 1948, p. 7. The committee members responsible for this report were Howard Bishop (Charter Fellow, Chairman 1937–38), Robert Bishop, M.D. (Chairman 1943–44), Arden Hardgrove (Fellow and administrator of Norton Memorial Infirmary, Louisville, 1938–1958), and Edgar C. Hayhow, Ph.D. (Chairman 1947–48).

[42] *Ibid.*, pp. 41–42.

[43] *Ibid.*, p. 51.

[44] Kipnis, pp. 121, 129. There were an additional 42 College members working outside of the United States and Canada as of January 1, 1955.

[45] Katzive, "The Vanishing Medical Hospital Administrator," *Hospital Topics*, Vol. 43, Feb. 1965, p. 41. This was a topic of discussion at the Society of Medical Administrators (1967) at their 1953, 1954, and 1956 meetings. The 1960s saw the near disappearance of the physician chairmen of the AHA and ACHA.

[46] Prall, *Problems of Hospital Administration*, 1948, p. 43.

[47] Levey and McCarthy, 1962.

[48] Dolson, 1965.

[49] Carper, 1982.

[50] Agho and Cyphert, 1992 (22.6 percent response rate).

[51] *Ibid.*, p. 134.

[52] *Ibid.*

[53] Stull, "Management of the American Hospital," pp. 61–76 in Hague, 1968.

[54] ACHA, Wesbury, April 1981.

[55] *Ibid.*, p. 5.

[56] ACHA, "Affiliate Reconciliation Report from January 1, 1982 to December 31, 1982." Data run December 31, 1982. Honorary Fellows, Life Fellows, and Life Members do not pay dues. Student Associates have special reduced fees.

[57] ACHA, internal report, "Table of Organizations in which the ACHA Affiliates are Employed," January 11, 1983.

[58] ACHA, Nov. 1982 data, computer printout. N = 9,824 for hospitals; 3,076 for other organizations.

[59] W. Richard Kirk interview March 14, 1983.

[60] Stephen Shortell, personal communication, 1983.

[61] ACHA, Dec. 7, 1982, computer printout. Prepared by Peter Weil, Ph.D. ACHE *1992 Directory*, Fig. 1A, p. 1382.

[62] ACHE, "Gender and Careers in Healthcare Management," 1991. Research Series No. 3.

[63] *Ibid.*, p. 1

[64] *Ibid.*, p. 3

[65] *Ibid.*, p. 12

[66] *Ibid.*, p. 23

[67] *Ibid.*, p. 26, 27

[68] *Ibid.*, p. 27

[69] *Ibid.*, p. 30

[70] *Ibid.*, p. 35

[71] *Ibid.*, p. 71

[72] *Ibid.*, p. 3

[73] ACHE, "Hospital Chief Executive Officer Turnover 1981–1990," 1991.

[74] *Ibid.*, p. 8

[75] AHA data tapes used here have been adjusted for incorrect reporting and interim positions. Hospitals are short term, general medical and surgical, and non-federal. ACHE "Hospital Chief Executive Officer Turnover 1981–1990," p. 7, "Hospital CEO Turnover Rates for 1991" ACHE March 16, 1992, mimeo.

[76] Interview, W. Richard Kirk.

[77] *Ibid.* and ACHA, *1981 Directory.* Lewis Weeks interview with Gerhard Hartman, 1982, p. 24. Gerhard Hartman received his doctorate in business administration from the University of Chicago in 1942, with a concentration in hospital administration. His doctoral dissertation, "Hospital Malpractice Insurance," was published in *The Journal of Business* of the University of Chicago, Vol. 16, No. 4, Part 2, Oct. 1943 and specially reprinted by the ACHA. With respect to the Iowa doctoral program in hospital administration, see Hartman and Wever, 1965, and Hartman and Levey, 1962.

[78] Interview, W. Richard Kirk.

[79] Friedlander, 1977.

[80] *Bulletin of the American College of Hospital Administrators*, Vol. 1, No. 1, 1934–1935, quoting Bert W. Caldwell, M.D., executive secretary of the AHA.

[81] Kipnis, p. 53.

[82] *Ibid.*

[83] Kipnis, pp. 53, 65–66. AHCA, *Code of Ethics*, 1941, 1947, 1958, 1964, 1970, 1973, 1980, 1987, 1992.

[84] AHA, "Ethical Conduct and Relationships for Health Care Institutions," 1981.

[85] ACHE, *1991–1992 Annual Report and Reference Guide.*

[86] *Kipnis*, pp. 65–66.

[87] John R. Mannix interview, 1982.

[88] AHA and ACHA, *Code of Hospital Ethics*, November 21, 1941.

[89] *Ibid.*, p. 3.

[90] *Ibid.*

[91] *Ibid.*, p. 4.

[92] *Ibid.*, p. 6.

[93] *Ibid.*, p. 7.

[94] ACHA and AHA, *Code of Ethics*, Dec. 1947, paragraph 9.

[95] Kipnis, pp. 16–17. Policy issues were left to the AHA.

[96] John Mannix personal communication, 1982.

[97] In 1908, "The Forresters of Reading offered physicians a per capital sum of three cents a week, while Philadelphia lodges paid only two cents," p. 123, in Burrow, 1977.

[98] ACHA and AHA, *Code of Ethics*, Dec. 1947, paragraph 10, 11.

[99] ACHA, *Code of Ethics,* approved Aug. 10, 1974, and AHA *Guidelines on Ethical Conduct and Relationships for Health Care Institutions,* approved April 1, 1974. Published in a brochure by ACHA, copyright, 1980, p. 11.

[100] "AHA, ACHA Approve Revised Ethical Codes," *Hospitals JAHA,* Vol. 31, Oct. 16, 1957, pp. 124, 126, 127.

[101] ACHA *Code of Ethics,* 1974.

[102] *Ibid.,* p. 3.

[103] *Ibid.,* pp. 2–3.

[104] ACHE *Code of Ethics* approved July 28, 1992, printed in ACHE *1991–1992 Annual Report and Reference Guide,* pp. 45–48.

[105] *Code of Ethics,* 1973 and 1992, cited above.

[106] *ACHA News,* Vol. 36, No. 10, Nov. 1975.

[107] 1980–1982 information from *ACHA News,* Vol. 45, No. 8, August 1982, p. 5. Other years from "ACHE Council of Regents Agenda Materials." Annual Reports of the Ethics Committee yearly.

[108] ACHE, "Council of Regents Agenda Materials," July 28, 1992. Annual Meeting Report No. 8. Ethics Committee 1991–1992 Annual Report.

[109] Darr, *Ethics for Health Services Managers.* Volume 4: Case Studies in Health Administration. ACHE, 1985.

5

The Education of the Healthcare Executive

No hospital can do a really good job whose superintendent is not vigorous, well-informed, sympathetic, unselfish and an enemy of make-believe.

If you were asked what you considered the most important single quality in a hospital administrator, what would you say? If this question were put to me I would answer sympathy or compassion.

Dr. S. S. Goldwater, Honorary Fellow[1]

EARLY TRAINING PROGRAMS

At the end of his 1929 book, *Hospital Administration: A Career,* Michael M. Davis, Ph.D. presented a brief history of U.S. education in hospital administration:

> Up to the present time (1929) the outstanding educational resource of the hospital field has been those individual hospital superintendents who have been interested not only in their own institutions, but in hospital administration as a profession, and who have made their hospitals centers for training of younger men and women by personal apprenticeship.

This occurred especially at the Massachusetts General Hospital, Johns Hopkins Hospital, Mount Sinai Hospitals in New York and Cleveland, and Grace Hospital in Detroit.[2]

This early personal apprenticeship training resulted in genealogies of administrators training the next generation. One such genealogy, starting at the Massachusetts General Hospital, is shown in Table 5.1. Prior to the 1930s, this was the only ongoing source of education

109

TABLE 5.1
One Partial Educational Genealogy of Apprentice-trained Hospital

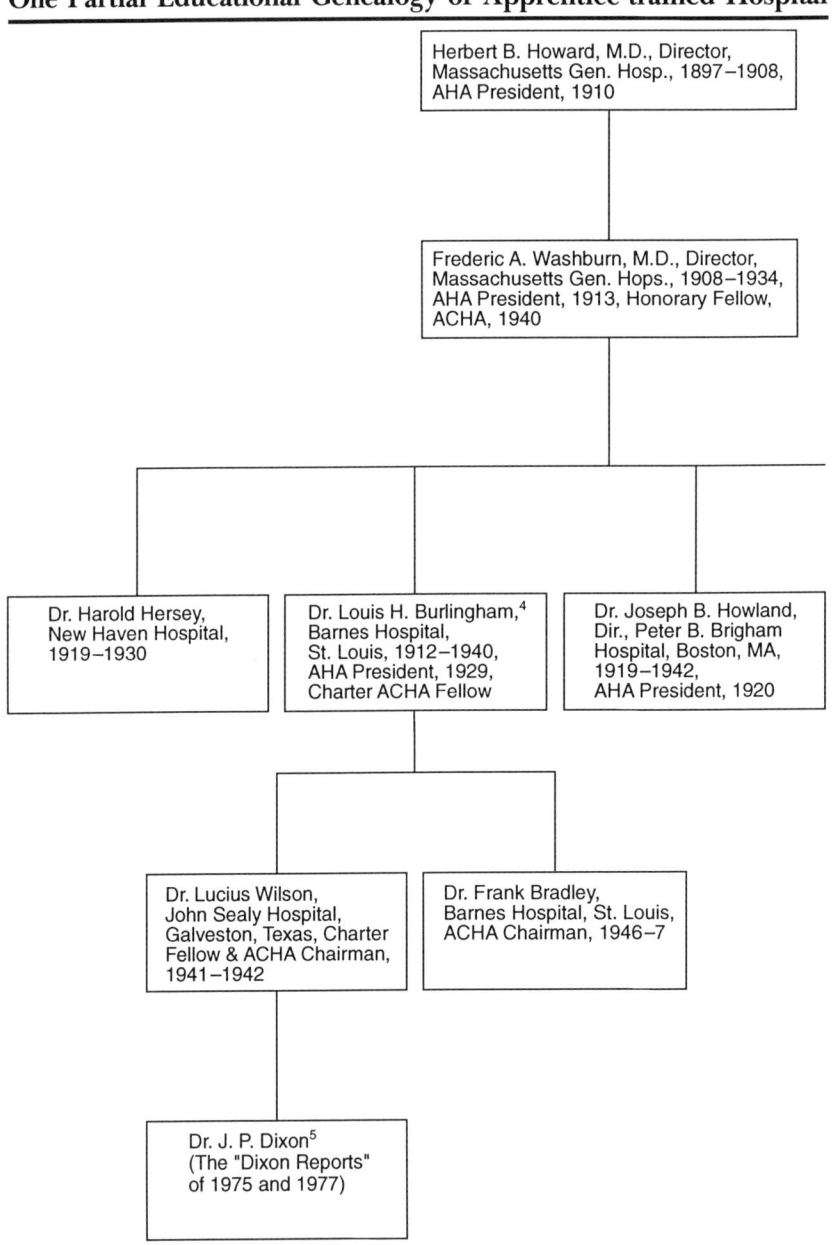

Herbert B. Howard, M.D., Director, Massachusetts Gen. Hosp., 1897–1908, AHA President, 1910

Frederic A. Washburn, M.D., Director, Massachusetts Gen. Hops., 1908–1934, AHA President, 1913, Honorary Fellow, ACHA, 1940

Dr. Harold Hersey, New Haven Hospital, 1919–1930

Dr. Louis H. Burlingham,[4] Barnes Hospital, St. Louis, 1912–1940, AHA President, 1929, Charter ACHA Fellow

Dr. Joseph B. Howland, Dir., Peter B. Brigham Hospital, Boston, MA, 1919–1942, AHA President, 1920

Dr. Lucius Wilson, John Sealy Hospital, Galveston, Texas, Charter Fellow & ACHA Chairman, 1941–1942

Dr. Frank Bradley, Barnes Hospital, St. Louis, ACHA Chairman, 1946–7

Dr. J. P. Dixon[5] (The "Dixon Reports" of 1975 and 1977)

Administrators: Five Generations Shown: "The Begats"[3]

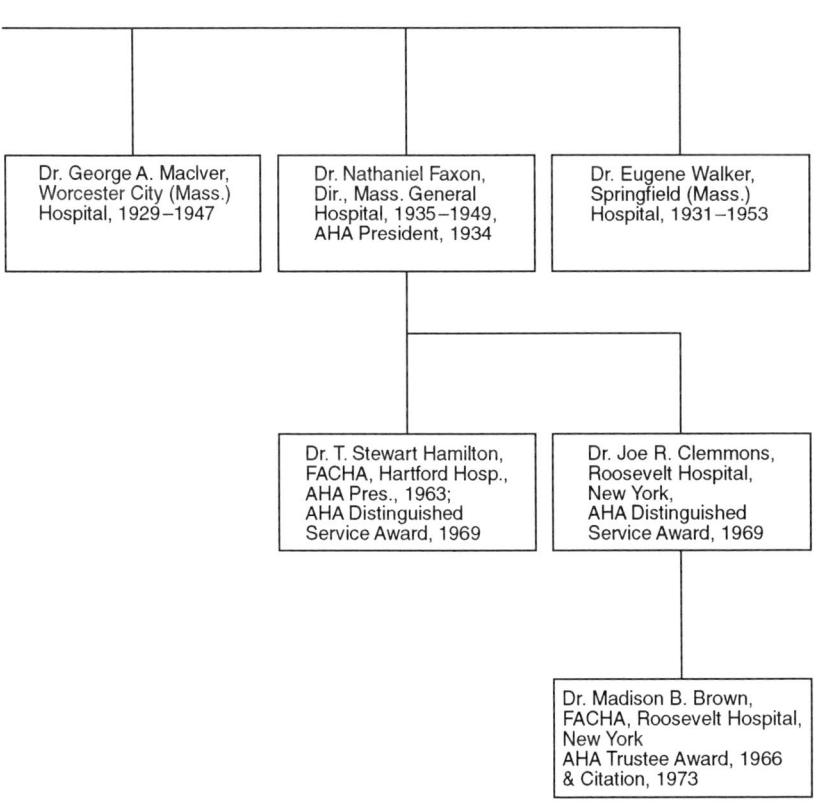

Dr. George A. MacIver,
Worcester City (Mass.)
Hospital, 1929–1947

Dr. Nathaniel Faxon,
Dir., Mass. General
Hospital, 1935–1949,
AHA President, 1934

Dr. Eugene Walker,
Springfield (Mass.)
Hospital, 1931–1953

Dr. T. Stewart Hamilton,
FACHA, Hartford Hosp.,
AHA Pres., 1963;
AHA Distinguished
Service Award, 1969

Dr. Joe R. Clemmons,
Roosevelt Hospital,
New York,
AHA Distinguished
Service Award, 1969

Dr. Madison B. Brown,
FACHA, Roosevelt Hospital,
New York
AHA Trustee Award, 1966
& Citation, 1973

in hospital administration. Yet only a small fraction of all administrators took advantage of it.

In 1911, Drs. Washburn and Howland described an informal training course in hospital administration for nurses at the Massachusetts General Hospital[6] (see Table 5.2). In 1916, Annie Goodrich, RN, a faculty member of the Department of Nursing and Health, Teachers College, Columbia University, spoke at the American Hospital Association annual meeting of the need to train superintendents of small hospitals:

> One can conceive of no greater piece of constructive and enduringly valuable work for this Association (AHA), no greater contribution toward a rapid standardization of hospitals—than the raising of a fund sufficient to establish at least one school of hospital or institutional administration and to command the services of the most highly experienced administrator in the field for its director, with an adequate staff of lecturers and instructors.[7]

In 1919, Arthur C. Bachmeyer, M.D., described a proposed curriculum in hospital administration at the University of Cincinnati in the College of Medicine with courses in the College of Commerce. Although this proposal was unsuccessful, Bachmeyer was prepared to endorse the idea of a graduate program in hospital administration when he moved to the University of Chicago.[9]

In addition, a number of universities gave courses in hospital administration. New York University, for example, gave classes on "Hospital and Institutional Management" and "Community Relations of Hospitals." However, these were discontinued in 1928–1929 for financial reasons. Columbia Teachers College, New York; Temple University in Philadelphia; McGill University, Montreal; University of Iowa, Iowa City; the Illinois Training School for Nurses in Chicago; Peabody College in Nashville; and Michigan State College, East Lansing, also gave classes in hospital management. The Harvard School of Public Health offered a course in 1927, but it was discontinued for lack of students. The University of Western Canada gave a nine-month course leading to a certificate, but not a degree.[10]

The first degree-granting program in hospital administration with a "more or less complete curricula" was at Marquette University in Milwaukee. In 1927, two students, both sisters, were given degrees. Undergraduate, two-week graduate, and summer courses were planned. But by 1928, this program had failed.[11]

The idea for this course came from Father Moulinier, the guiding force behind the Catholic Hospital Association,[12] and a member of the 1922 Rockefeller Commission on the Training for Hospital Execu-

TABLE 5.2
Landmark Reports on Education for Hospital Administration

The Age of Apprenticeship or No Training

1911: F. A. Washburn, M.D. and W. B. Howland, M.D.	"The Training of Hospital Administrators" *Transactions of the American Hospital Association*
1916: Annie Goodrich, R.N.	"How shall the superintendents of small hospitals be trained?" *Transactions of the American Hospital Association*
1919: A. C. Bachmeyer, M.D.	"A Course in Hospital Administration" *Transactions of the American Hospital Association*
1922: Willard Rappelye	*Report of the Rockefeller Committee on the Training for Hospital Executives: Principles of Hospital Administration and Training of Hospital Executives*

The Heroic Age: 1929–1945[8]

| 1929: Michael M. Davis | *Hospital Administration: A Career.* New York, NY: privately published. |
| 1937: Committee on Educational Policies of the ACHA | *University Training for Hospital Administration Career.* A Report by the Committee on Educational Policies of the American College of Hospital Administrators. Committee on Educational Policies, Chicago, IL: ACHA |

The Age of the Practitioner: 1945–1965[8]

| 1948: "The Prall Report: | *The College Curriculum in Hospital Administration.* The Joint Commission on Education of the ACHA and AHA, Charles E. Prall, Director. Chicago, IL: Physicians Record Company. |
| 1954: "The Olsen Report" | *University Education for Administration in Hospitals.* Commission on University Education in Hospital Administration, Herluf V. Olsen, Director. Washington, D.C.: American Council on Education. |

The Age of the New Man, 1966–1980[8]

| 1967 | Hospital Administration. JACHA, Special issue on Education, Fall, 1967 |
| 1969: T. E. Chester | *Graduate Education for Hospital Administration in the United States: Trends.* Chicago, IL: ACHA, 1969, p. 31 |

TABLE 5.2
Continued

1975, 1977: "The Dixon Reports"	Commission on Education for Health Administration Vol. I, 1975 Vol. II, 1975 Vol. III, 1977. A Future Agenda. Ann Arbor, MI: Health Administration Press.
1978	*The Report of the Task Force on the Report of the Commission on Education for Health Administration.* Chicago, IL: ACHA, 1978.
The Age of Lifelong Learning 1980–	
1981: ACHA	*Enhancing Executive Competence*
1984: ACHA	Report of the Task Force on Beginning and Early Career Development
1984: ACHE (revised 1987)	Guidelines for Postgraduate Fellowships and Management Development Programs in Health Services Administration
1984	First Directory of Postgraduate Fellowships and Management Development Programs in Health Services Administration.
1992: ACHE, AUPHA	Report of the Task Force on Beginning and Early Career Development.

tives.[13] Father Moulinier and Father Fox set up the degree granting program at Marquette in September, 1924, with courses following the Rockefeller Commission recommendations. The course was, according to Shanahan, "an outgrowth of the great movement for the progressive betterment of hospitals that is taking place in the country."

The school was also "a natural outgrowth of the movement for hospital standardization." Malcolm MacEachern and S. S. Goldwater were among the guest lecturers. Just why this program ended is not clear, but it was probably because of lack of funds.[14]

In 1929, Michael Davis proposed a two-year graduate degree curriculum in hospital administration. In the first nine months, the student would have six hours of accounting; five hours of statistics and methods of presentation; six hours on organization and management; six hours on economics and social sciences; three hours on history and status of hospitals, clinics, and the health professions; eight hours of practical observation; and six hours of seminar. In the second year, the student would have 24 hours of practical work; seven hours of seminar related to the student's thesis; six hours of business policy; and three hours of public health and labor relations.[15] Thus, Davis focused on management skills more than nursing or medical skills.

The final report of the Commission on the Costs of Medical Care in October, 1932, stated:

> Hospitals and clinics are not only medical institutions, they are also social and business enterprises, sometimes very large ones. It is important, therefore, that they be directed by administrators who are trained for their responsibilities and can understand and integrate the various professional, economic, and social factors involved. Definite opportunities should be provided in universities or in institutes of hospital administration connected with universities, for the theoretical and practical training of such administrators. The administration of hospitals and medical centers should be developed as a career which will attract high-grade students.[16]

Davis had the opportunity to put his thoughts into action when he started the world's first successful master's degree program in hospital administration within the business school of the University of Chicago.[17] This course was formally decided upon on February 14, 1934. Looking back on his work, Davis said:

> By 1933, I had experience as an administrator, a teacher and a consultant. . . . This experience had led me to several conclusions, including the very firm one to the effect that hospitals would be much better off if their administrators had training for the job.
> . . . most administrators were absorbed in institutional detail and lacked broad basic objectives toward which administration should be headed. The trustees who employed them did not in most instances expect their executive officers to be more than housekeepers.

The considerable sum of money required to set up a research institute was unavailable. The Rosenwald Fund provided from $5,000 to $7,000 for three years to start the Chicago program. It was placed in the business school for purely practical reasons and relied heavily on existing courses.[18]

In 1937, the Rosenwald funds which supported the University of Chicago program were coming to an end. Michael Davis, Dean William Spencer, and Gerhard Hartman visited Robert Hutchins, President of the University of Chicago, and asked for his blessing and strategic support to seek Commonwealth Fund financing. In Hartman's words:

> When we came, he was sitting at a work table in his shirt sleeves. He said to the Dean, "Bill, what's up?" The Dean told him why we were there. Hutchins said, "Oh, yes." Then the commentary was made on why the HA program should be carried forward. I won't repeat the

precise profanity he used except that he called the field just G__ d___ technocracy, that is just the antithesis of what a university should represent and that it would go forward over his dead body.

The Dean, of course, was used to working with him, but I was just innocent enough so that I spoke up and said: "As an individual enrolled, may I say that it is respectable academically." Then, I indicated some of the faculty. When I named (the economist) Jacob Viner, he asked, "Did you study with him?" "That's my major," I said. He asked, "with Frank too?" "Yes, Professor Knight (another noted economist) is a man I'm working with day and night. I am not obligated to take the courses, but they are the men from whom I learn." I threw in the names of Ruth Emerson and Louis Wirth. I said, "I would like to respectfully suggest that it be given another three-year test interval with sufficient interim reporting to you so that you know what is really happening." He smiled and said, "So be it." That was it.[19]

What would have happened to graduate education in hospital administration if Hutchins had actually closed the Chicago program in 1937?

Gerhard Hartman reviewed the experience of this program from 1934 to 1937 in an article published when he was Executive Secretary of the ACHE.[20] This program was, after the first three years, supported by The Commonwealth Fund and later by the Kellogg Foundation.[21] Open to students with a bachelor's degree, it was a joint project of the Business School and the University of Chicago Clinics. Applicants were interviewed by either Davis or Bachmeyer.[22]

The link between the College and the University of Chicago was a close one. Michael Davis was elected the first Honorary Fellow in 1935. Gerhard Hartman earned his doctorate degree at Chicago, was an instructor in that course, and Executive Secretary of the College from 1937 to 1941.

Bachmeyer was the second head of the Chicago program, active in its inception, Charter Fellow, and President of the College in 1940–1941. Davis was also Medical Director for the Julius Rosenwald Fund of Chicago at this time, and Director of the Chicago program for a year.[23]

Many aspects of the Davis curriculum became prototypes for future degree programs. But 25 years would pass before master's degree programs were able to educate sufficient numbers to meet the need projected by the 1948 Prall Report.[24]

Both the College membership and the Chicago program epitomized the future of the profession. They were not representative of the field as a whole during the first years of the College.

The College Institutes: 1933–1964

From its inception, the College was concerned with improving the education of hospital executives. In the first 25 years of the College, one of its largest undertakings was its short educational programs. These programs lasted up to two weeks. Usually held in conjunction with a university and often cosponsored by other associations, they were refresher courses for professionals actually involved in administration at the time.[25]

The first College-sponsored program was September 18–October 6, 1933. It was the Chicago Institute for Hospital Administrators under the auspices of the University of Chicago, the American Hospital Association, the American Medical Association, the American College of Surgeons, and the Chicago Hospital Association. One hundred ninety-six administrators attended.[26] In 1947, the 15th Chicago Institute continued with the same sponsoring organizations and 123 attendees. From that date, to the 23rd program in 1955, the institute was sponsored by the University of Chicago and the College alone. There were also five one week Chicago Advanced Institutes from 1950 to 1954 (see Table 5.3).

Starting in 1948, similar regional institutes were conducted. By far the largest attendance over the years was at the Chicago Institute (2,738 total participants in 23 Institutes), followed by the Minnesota Institute (1,006 total participants in 15 Institutes).

For example, the 13th Chicago Institute, in September, 1945, covered topics including operating fundamentals of organizations, nursing education, hospital planning and construction, maintenance of the physical plant, volunteer services, food services, public relations, laundry and linen, analysis of financial statements, purchasing, fund raising, medical records, and public health. A large part of the two-week course was taken up with visits to Chicago hospitals. The faculty included Drs. Claude Munger, Malcolm MacEachern, Robin Buerki and Charles Wilinsky.[27]

Perhaps this high attendance at Chicago helps explain why the approach of the Chicago master's degree program became so widespread. In 1959, of 16 programs that were members of the AUPHA, nine had directors who were program graduates. Of these, five were graduates of the Chicago program.[28]

Almost all of these Institutes were held under the auspices of universities and colleges, bringing the College and the participants into contact with some of America's most notable educational institutions.

The College also sponsored other short courses and meetings: ten Fellows' seminars from 1944 to 1954 lasting four days at universities throughout the country (255 total attendance); four Members' con-

TABLE 5.3
The Institutes for Hospital Administration, 1933 to 1955[29]

		Total Attendance
23 Chicago Institutes[30]		
1933–1955 (2 weeks)	University of Chicago	(2738)
5 Chicago Advanced Institutes		
1950–1954 (1 week)	University of Chicago	(242)
6 Midwest Institutes	University of Colorado, Boulder and	(335)
1941–1954 (1 week)	Denver, Colorado, Womens College	
15 Minnesota Institutes		
1939–1955 (1 week)	University of Minnesota	(1006)
6 New England Institutes		
1940–1953 (10 days)	Harvard, Brown, Lasalle, Yale	(443)
6 New York Institutes	Columbia, Cornell, Francis Delafield	(528)
1939–1954 (2 weeks)	Hospital	
1 Southeastern Institute		
1952 (1 week)	University of Tennessee	(105)
9 Southern Institutes	Duke, Tennessee, Rollins, Medical	(635)
1939–1954 (1 week)	College of Virginia, and others.	
4 Southwestern Institutes		
1941–1953 (1 week)	Southern Methodist, Baylor, Houston	(308)
6 Western Institutes		
1938–1954 (10 days)	Stanford	(491)
3 Canadian Institutes	University of Western Ontario,	(273)
1947–1951 (1 week)	Queens	
2 Inter American Institutes	San Juan, Lima, and Mexico City,	(169)
1940, 1944 (2–3 weeks)	University of Puerto Rico	

ferences from 1945 to 1949 (196 total attendees); and 17 conferences on human relations from 1951 to 1955 throughout North America lasting two days each (885 total attendees). From 1949 to 1957, there were eight two-day meetings on graduate education for hospital administrators focusing primarily on residency preceptor training (431 total attendees). There were also three four-day educational conferences for hospital administrators in 1955 (273 attendees).[31]

Thus, in 22 years, the College sponsored short courses with a total attendance of 9,313. No doubt, many administrators came to more than one Institute, but the College's presence was widespread. In the absence of degree programs, the Institutes were a major source of education in hospital administration.

The Institutes continued into 1964, when the 11th Western, 10th Midwest, 32nd Chicago, 9th Southeast and 7th Southwest Institutes were held. Also held then were the 3rd Canadian, 2nd Northwest, 15th Chicago, 2nd Midwest and 1st Southeast Advanced Institutes. There were also Regional Member meetings and the 18th Fellows' Seminar.[32]

By April 1961, total registration at all College sponsored programs from 1933–1961 had reached the 15,000 mark.[33] However, by 1963, the Institutes had declined in attendance.[34] Perhaps they had fulfilled their role. In June, 1964, the Board of Regents accepted a new educational approach.[35] There were to be annual Assemblies in each of the eight College districts plus the Fellows' Seminar.[36] The first of these Assemblies was held at the University of California at Berkeley, June 21–25, 1965.[37] By 1968, in addition to the Regional Assemblies, seminars on executive skills were given across the country.[38]

The annual Congress on Administration of the College started in 1958. Ray Brown (1913–1974), a member of the Board of Regents at that time, chaired the committee to organize the first Congress. The AHA provided a contribution of $5,000 to start it. According to Bernard Lachner, Ray Brown was "probably the best known hospital administrator of his era and his time. He represented what you and I dream about, fantasize and work a lifetime to emulate. He was a man of his profession!" Lachner went on to describe Ray Brown as "a tough, warm, chainsmoking, card playing, Southern roughneck."[39]

The Congresses brought together leading thinkers on administration to share ideas. The 1961 Congress included as speakers: Melville Dalton and Warren Bennis on administration; Raymond A. Bauer on motivational research; Donald Pelz on controls; and James D. Thompson on organizational conflict.[40]

A 1967 national survey of 250 hospital administrators by Kenneth Matzick attempted to evaluate continuing education in the field of hospital administration. Administrators reported that their most valuable source of continuing education was through interaction with fellow administrators, followed by hospital journals, continuing education courses, interactions with others, and other journals.[41] According to Matzick, the respondent administrators' first choice for responsibility to develop a more formalized approach to continuing education was the ACHA.[42] In terms of overall value, the ACHA Fellows' Seminar was ranked highest out of eight educational categories.[43]

By 1966, the College provided eight regional "ACHA Assemblies on Hospital Administration," the Congress on Administration, and the ACHA Fellows' Seminar. In 1967, the American Hospital Association sponsored several Institutes on special topics. Several universities also provided management development courses, and there were a number of government-sponsored institutes.

The annual Congress on Administration continues as the major educational activity of the College, drawing 3,600 attendees in 1983 and 4,300 in 1993. In the 1980s, "Executive Briefings" typically consisted of six speakers, each presenting a different topic. College seminars focused on particular topics. The briefings and seminars were two or two-and-one-half days in length, and were held from four to twelve times a year at various sites throughout the country. Fees were charged; non-affiliates of the College attended, but at slightly higher fees.[44] Audio cassette tapes of speeches were produced and marketed.[45] All of the activities were managed by the Division of Education.

By 1993, the College was meeting the diverse learning needs of healthcare executives through a wide variety of educational programs, including conferences, institutes, and seminars. Conferences were two-day programs characterized by large attendance and leading speakers on a variety of health care management topics. The three conferences the College presented in 1993 included the Healthcare Management Ethics Conference, a program that helped raise awareness of issues related to responsible and ethical decision making, and the Eastern and Western conferences, regional programs that offered major addresses, educational seminars, skill-assessment programs, membership activities, and career-planning presentations.

The College also offered three institutes, which were characterized by workshop formats, smaller attendance, and in-depth coverage of a single topic. The College's 1993 institutes included the three-day Partnership Institute for teams of board chairs, CEOs, and medical staff presidents; the five-day Healthcare Executive Leadership Development Institute, a skill-assessment and enhancement program for senior-level executives; and the three-day Healthcare Executive Public Policy Institute, which provided an intensive look at the health care polymaking process.

In addition to conferences and institutes, the College held 135 offerings of 23 different seminars. Among the College's offerings were a special Canadian seminar that addressed issues of interest to Canadian health care executives and a special program exclusively for Fellows of the College. Other ACHE seminars focused on a variety of topics, including health care reform, integrated delivery networks, community collaboration, managed care, and hospital-affiliated group practices. Presented in a classroom, the seminars provided an opportunity for one-on-one interaction with faculty. College seminars were often held at programs called "Clusters," which allowed participants to take a number of highly rated seminars at one location in a single five-day period.

THE COLLEGE PROMOTES GRADUATE EDUCATION IN HOSPITAL ADMINISTRATION

The Committee on Educational Policies: 1936–1937

On October 1, 1935, the "Committee on the Training of Hospital Administrators" or "Committee on Educational Policies," chaired by Dr. MacEachern, met to set the basic goals of the College's educational program, "goals which have since been developed and greatly expanded, but which still remain the core of the College activity."[46]

Dr. Fred Carter (ACHA Chairman 1935–36) stated that education was divided into two areas: improving the ability of administrators already in the field and training those who wanted to enter the field. Kipnis noted, "The committee agreed with Dr. MacEachern that the College should assume responsibility for placing the training of hospital administrators on the same basis as the training of physicians."[47] Reverend Alphonse M. Schwitalla, S.J., Ph.D., Dean of the St. Louis University School of Medicine and Editor of *Hospital Progress*, said:

> The hospital administrator of the future should be an executive who can advise his board and act as a policymaker and coordinator. Such an administrator could not be trained by taking a couple of (short) courses in hospital administration after securing a Bachelor's degree in some other field of specialization.[48]

A subcommittee consisting of Father Schwitalla, Dr. Bachmeyer, and Dr. Benjamin Black, superintendent of Alameda County Hospital, was appointed to develop a proposal for university curriculum which would lead to a degree in hospital administration.[49] The result of this committee's work was presented for the approval of the Committee on Educational Policies in 1936 and 1937, and published in 1937:[50]

> The validity of the concept of hospital administration as a separate and independent career has not yet passed beyond the point of controversy.
>
> The American College of Hospital Administrators has carefully weighed the arguments for and against recognition of hospital

administration as a separate and independent career. As a result of these deliberations, it has announced its policy that hospital administration is validly to be considered as a special profession and secondly, that concerning present hospital executives, this profession demands some form of specialized preparation.[51]

This Committee went on to recommend that "the hospital administrator should have at least a Master's degree" and that such a degree "seems not only highly desirable but, in view of the present status in health development, practically indispensable."

They also advocated that bachelor's degree preparation include prerequisites and that a fourth of the undergraduate curriculum be devoted specifically to hospital administration. Because the College survey had found that 46 percent of current administrators were nurses and 28 percent were physicians, the Committee recommended two separate educational tracks for these groups. The Committee stated:

> . . . the American College of Hospital Administrators is in no sense interested in discouraging doctors of medicine or graduate nurses entering the field of hospital administration; quite the contrary is the case. The College is merely interested in seeing to it that before a doctor of medicine or a registered nurse be designated a hospital administrator, he or she should have at least a rudimentary acquaintanceship with certain basic, professional and specialized aspects of the profession of hospital administration.

The bachelor's degree program in hospital administration was to lead to master's degree training that would include English and preferably German; philosophy, including psychology; history; science, preferably biology; accounting; finance; statistics; business management; industrial organization; personnel administration; sociology (community organization, social problems, public welfare and social service in hospital administration); socio-legal economic history (economic history, principles of economics and law); and hospital administration (hospital statistics, medical and nursing essentials, financial administration in hospitals, hospital staff organization and legal problems).

The fifth year would be taken up by an internship leading to a certificate. The sixth year, and possibly a seventh, would be committed to academic work for a master's degree in administration and organization, management, finance administration, or community relations. Half of these courses would be specifically related to the hospital field.[52]

For physicians who had completed their internships, it was proposed that there be one year of basic professional courses related to administration; a year of administrative internship leading to a certificate; and then one to two years of academic study leading to a master's degree in hospital administration. For nurses, there would be three years of nursing education; two years of general education; two years of professional courses related to hospital administration; and then a year of internship followed by one or two years of graduate study leading to a master's degree in hospital administration.

In the concluding section of this report, the Committee responded to some concerns they had received.

What would be the effect of these substantial educational requirements on "the tenure of position" of present executives? Would they precipitate rifts among hospital executives, creating two classes of hospital administrators—those with extensive education and those who worked their way up through the "school of hard knocks?"[53] The Committee responded that this problem occurred in other areas, including medicine, dentistry, nursing, and law, whenever professionals had attempted to elevate standards. "During the period of transition both groups must coexist side by side," concluded the Committee.[54]

On October 19, 1937, MacEachern sent a letter to College members inviting their comments on the report.[55] At Dr. MacEachern's urging, the College published a number of these replies.

Philip Vollmer, Superintendent of Fairview Park Hospital, Cleveland, bridged four centuries of ideas from the learned gentlemen members of a professional College to the present by justifying a liberal arts education on the grounds of creativity and self-understanding in the following reply:

> It is apparent that no profession today or of the future can be worthy of the name unless its representatives are men and women possessing a cultural background. . . . but surely the creative professional man or woman must first understand through the medium of history, language, literature and philosophy, his world and himself, and from this proceed to concentration on the achievements and techniques of his chosen profession.[56]

Harvey Agnew, M.D., Secretary, Department of Hospital Service, Canadian Medical Association, was concerned about the future of physician administrators:

> On the question of relative superiority of medical, lay or nursing administrators, I have always refrained from taking any active part. It has been my conviction that each one of these three types of administrators can fill a definite place in our general plan of hospital work, that each brings to the position of administrator a distinct viewpoint not shared as fully by the others and that hospital administration is

such a complex and varied undertaking that at best an administrator can expect to have but a portion of the qualifications required.[57]

Agnew interpreted the report as suggesting that "a mere handful of medical graduates scattered over the field as administrators would be adequate" and "that the Committee looks upon hospital administration primarily as a business." The result of the lengthy training proposed for physician administrators would be to drive them out of this field, he believed. If there were mostly non-medical administrators, "the problem of cooperation with the AMA and ACS and other medical bodies would be intensified." He wrote:

> . . . it would be fatal if the medical profession and the hospitals became separated, or worked at cross purposes. This would be quite probable if the primary viewpoint of the hospital administrators became that of hospital economics and efficiency of organization rather than of the care of the patient.

E. Muriel Anscombe, Administrator of the Jewish Hospital, St. Louis, wrote:

> I am wondering if it might not be a good plan to supplement this report with one showing the turnover in administrative positions to give a true picture of the opportunities in this occupation.
> Social unrest as well as economic loss result from the overcrowding of any profession. Do you think that such a situation might develop in the field of hospital administration?[58]

Asa Bacon, Superintendent of The Presbyterian Hospital, Chicago, stated:

> I am sure it will need quite a campaign of education to make boards of managers (trustees) see the necessity of engaging trained people as administrators.
> The Committee on Educational Policies has done well not to demand "slavish adherence to any program of preparation" but rather to point the way for a general understanding of what is needed.

Amy Daniels, Administrator, Wing Memorial Hospital, Palmer, Massachusetts, added:

> I trust . . . that you will also promote or provide facilities for hospital administrators who are occupying positions of responsibility to further their education and gain additional knowledge of hospital administration. I feel that (the College's) plan of regional institutes

is an excellent one and will raise the standards of hospital administration.[59]

Sister M. Olivia, Dean, School of Nursing, The Catholic University of America, Washington, D.C., thought the first five years for the nurse administrator were "not feasible. Would it not be more desirable to construct a course for hospital administrators regardless of previous general or professional education?" she asked. This, of course, was the direction education took.

S. B. Crawford, an Assistant Superintendent, Maryland General Hospital, who "though having several years of college, is not a graduate," added:

> We are practical administrators, rather than college theorists. The result is reflected in the character of our service and in the financial statement at the end of the year. Without endowments and with a 46% free service, we show a credit balance at the end of our fiscal year. I personally am heartily in favor of a college education, but I do not feel that a qualified administrator should be refused admission, now or in the future, simply because he lacks "a sheepskin."[60]

Two physicians wrote to express their fears that "medical men as administrators will become a thing of the past."[61]

> Probably 60% of the hospitals in the country are not of sufficient size to warrant the expenditure of employing an executive who has had this theoretical and practical training.[62]

This ambitious proposal to not only restructure undergraduate training, but also to initiate graduate education, was developed at a time when there was only one degree program in existence, graduating a handful of students annually. No wonder these proposals failed to define the educational future. However, they elicited widespread agreement that university education was essential for hospital administration, and laid the groundwork for the College report of 1948.

In 1948, Harvey Agnew, M.D., reviewed the worldwide state of training in hospital administration:

> Tremendous progress has been made in the United States during the past few years. In this the American Hospital Association and the American College of Surgeons have made invaluable pioneer contributions, but the greatest stimulus to this movement during the past few years has been the American College of Hospital Administrators.[63]

Not only were there the College cosponsored Institutes, the master's degree and evening seminar at the University of Chicago, there were longer courses too:

There is a four-year combined apprenticeship and university course at Antioch College. The University of Pittsburgh has a three to four-year course for graduate nurses leading to a Bachelor of Science degree. Yale is considering a graduate course. The University of St. Louis (where Father Schwintilla taught) has a four-year course patterned after the ambitious curriculum report (1937) of the American College of Hospital Administrators.[64]

In 1943, the Committee on Educational Policies was chaired by Dr. Bachmeyer.[65] The scope of this committee's activities included: determination of policies for the development of institutes and reading courses; promotion of organized courses in universities for new entrants; development of educational programs for Nominees and Members seeking advancement in the College; creation of two or three-day conferences for Fellows; and the promotion of scholarships for students.[66]

The second master's degree program in hospital administration was started at Northwestern University in Chicago in 1943, under the directorship of Malcolm MacEachern.

The Growth of the Graduate Programs: 1945–1965

In 1945, the W. K. Kellogg Foundation funded the Joint Commission on Education of the AHA and ACHA, chaired by Charles E. Prall,[67] an Honorary Fellow of the College.

According to Prall,[68] "The Joint Commission on Education was the culmination of about 10 years of striving to upgrade the hospital superintendency. Certain leading spirits in the American College of Hospital Administrators had a pretty clear idea of what they would like to see happen at long range." The ultimate objective "was to make over hospital administration in such ways as to permit it a place among the professions."[69] Prall found that of 232 persons becoming administrators in larger voluntary hospitals, 18 percent came from occupations unrelated to health administration. Only 36 percent came to that position with experience as an assistant administrator or as an administrator of a smaller hospital, suggesting a limited amount of on-the-job learning.[70] The commission felt that a good supply of college graduates in hospital administration would change this situation.[71]

After three-and-a-half years of work, it produced its final report.[72] The first section of this two-part document consisted of personal interviews with 100 hospital administrators.[73] The second portion recommended a course and curriculum for training hospital administrators: *The College Curriculum in Hospital Administration.*[74]

This report focused primarily on graduate education, harkening back to the ideas of Michael Davis. There was no mention of undergraduate programs *per se*, ignoring this part of the Schwitalla report of 1937.[75]

The Prall Report built its curriculum proposals upon its study of problems facing hospital administrators. It was therefore more practical and less academic, especially when compared to later studies.[76] The major impact of this report was to foster the growth of new graduate programs.

Concurrent with the Prall Commission, the Kellogg Foundation supported the creation of eight new university-based hospital administration graduate programs, all but one in schools of public health.[77] Like the original program at Chicago, these programs provided a year of internship and "curricula structured to give the student basic administrative skills with a strong emphasis on business management and the broad responsibility of the hospital in the field of public health."[78]

In the summer of 1947, the College reviewed the status of the ten existing degree programs in hospital administration.[79] According to this review, there were four established courses and six newer ones. Chicago graduated 13 students in that year (three of these students were physicians). Columbia University, where C. W. Munger, M.D., was serving as Professor of Hospital Administration, graduated 22 students (six physicians).

The Northwestern University program, established in September, 1943, and directed by MacEachern, graduated students at the bachelor's and master's degree level. The Duke University Medical School and Hospital program, which opened in 1930, had by 1983 provided 29 students with 24-month apprenticeships. Duke's master's degree program started in 1962. Washington University, St. Louis, was the only program located in a medical school.

The new University of Minnesota program was directed by James A. Hamilton and included Ray Amberg on the faculty. The new Yale program admitted its first class in 1947. Members of the Department of Public Health (Ira V. Hiscock, Sc.D., Chairman) included Professor Albert Snoke, M.D., Director of Grace New Haven Hospital, and Clement Clay, M.D. The new program at the University of Iowa was jointly directed by Gerhard Hartman, Superintendent of University Hospitals, and Dean E. T. Peterson of the Graduate College. St. Louis University had an undergraduate program in hospital administration since 1936. Between that time and 1947, six students had graduated.[83] The University of Toronto School of Hygiene offered a new program under the direction of Harvey Agnew, M.D., and Leonard Bradley, M.D., Associate Professor.[84]

The total number of degree graduates in the summer of 1947 was 48 at the master's level and one at the bachelor's level.[85] Many of these professors had close links to the College. A. C. Bachmeyer, Ray Brown, Claude Munger and James Hamilton were all College Chairmen. MacEachern and Agnew were Honorary Charter Fellows; Michael Davis an Honorary Fellow; and Hartman was the second executive of the College.

The 1950s and 1960s saw a steady growth of new graduate degree programs. These are listed by date in Table 5.4.

Since then there has continued to be a growth in baccalaureate, masters, doctorate, and other education programs. Table 5.5 lists newer colleges and universities which have student affiliates of the College.

The Association of University Programs in Hospital Administration

The Joint Commission on Education of the AHA and the ACHE was "of marked assistance to various established (graduate) programs and aided in the establishment of new programs." Both Prall's Joint Commission and the new programs were supported by the W. K. Kellogg Foundation. Under the Joint Commission's guidance, "directors and faculty of the various courses were brought together for seminars and discussion of common problems."

The first of these meetings was held at Purdue University in the fall of 1945. After preliminary discussion in 1948, an organizational meeting to develop the constitution and bylaws for the new organization was held in New York City December 17–19, 1948, under the Chairmanship of Arthur C. Bachmeyer, with Ray Brown as Chairman of the committee. At the next meeting, in Chicago in May, 1949, the constitution was approved in principle. A decision was made to issue a standing invitation to the Kellogg Foundation and the ACHA to meet with the association. Thus, the Association of University Programs in Hospital Administration (AUPHA) was born as a nonprofit corporation in Illinois in 1950.[86]

Between December, 1949, and October, 1954, eight meetings were held by the College in cooperation with the AUPHA and program faculty.[87] "Dean Conley almost never missed a meeting" of AUPHA and he "made it a point to visit every one of the programs in hospital administration and to encourage students therein in their chosen profession with the admonition that they were professional people and if they had not the recognition at the time it would soon be forthcoming."[88]

TABLE 5.4

Graduate Programs in Hospital and Health Administration in the United States and Canada as of January 1, 1971 by Starting Date with Early Founding Director[80]

Decade	Program	Starting Date	Early Founding Directors
1930s	University of Chicago	1934	Dr. Michael M. Davis, '34–'35
			Dr. Arthur Bachmeyer, '35–'51*
			Ray Brown,* George Bugbee*
1940s	Northwestern University	1943	Dr. Malcolm MacEachern, '43–'56*
			Dr. Charles Letourneau, M.D.
	Columbia University	1945	John Gorrell, M.D.*
			E. Dwight Barnett, M.D.
			Ray E. Trussell, M.D.
	University of Minnesota	1946	James A. Hamilton*
	Washington University	1946	Dr. Frank R. Bradley*
	University of Toronto	1947	Dr. G. Harvey Agnew*
	Yale University	1947	Dr. Clement C. Clay, '47–'50,
			George Buis*
	University of California Berkeley	1948	Richard J. Stull*
	St. Louis University	1948	Rev. John S. Flanagan, S.J.*
1948	Founding of AUPHA		
1950s	University of Iowa	1950	Dr. Gerhard Hartman*
	University of Pittsburgh	1950	
	Baylor University (U.S. Army)	1951	
	Cornell University	1955	
	University of Michigan	1955	
	University de Montreal	1956	
	Virginia Commonwealth University	1956	
	Xavier University	1958	
	George Washington University	1959	
1960s	University of California, Los Angeles	1960	
	Duke University[81] (1930)	1962	
	University of Florida	1964	
	University of Ottawa	1964	
	Georgia State University	1965	
	Trinity University	1965	
	University of Alabama	1966	
	University of Missouri, Columbia	1966	
	University of Puerto Rico	1966	
	University of Alberta	1968	
	University of Colorado	1968	
	Temple University	1968	
	City University of New York	1969	
	Ohio State University	1969	
	Tulane University	1969	
	University of Pennsylvania	1970	

*Presidents of AUPHA from 1948–1973.

TABLE 5.5
Additional Degree Programs with ACHE Student Chapters in 1993[82]

Alfred University
Appalachian State University
Arizona State University
Arkansas State University
University of Arkansas—Little Rock
Auburn University
Baruch College/Mt. Sinai School of Medicine
Bellarmine College
Boston University
Bowling Green State University
Brigham Young University
University of British Columbia
California State University—Fresno
California State—Los Angeles
California State—Northridge
California State
University of Cincinnati
Cleveland State University
Concordia College
University of Dallas
University of Detroit Mercy
Eastern Michigan University
Fairleigh Dickinson University
Florida Atlantic University
University of North Florida Medicine/ Health Sciences
University of Florida
Governor's State University
Hofstra University
University of Houston—Clear Lake
Howard University
Idaho State University
University of Illinois Urbana—Champaign
Indiana University—Indianapolis
Indiana University—Northwest Campus
Iona College
James Madison University
Johns Hopkins University
University of Kansas—Lawrence
University of Kentucky
LaSalle University

Loma Linda University
Long Island University
Marshall University
University of Mary Hardin-Baylor
University of Maryland University College
Maryville University
Medical University of South Carolina
Meharry Medical College
Memphis State University
Mercer/Atlanta University
Metropolitan State University of Denver
University of Miami
University of New Hampshire
New York University
State University of New York at Buffalo
University of North Carolina—Chapel Hill
University of Oklahoma—Oklahoma City
University of Oklahoma—Tulsa
Oregon State University
University of Osteopathic Medicine and Health Sciences
Pennsylvania State University
Quinnipaic College
Rush University
Rutgers University
San Diego State University
University of Scranton
Seton Hall University
Simmons College
University of South Carolina
University of South Dakota
University of South Florida
University of Southern California—Los Angeles
University of Southern California—Sacramento
Southern Illinois University—Carbondale
Southwest Texas State University
Stonehill College
Suffolk University
University of Texas—Medical Branch at Galveston

TABLE 5.5
Continued

University of Texas—Southwestern Medical Center—Dallas	Western Kentucky University
	Wichita State University
Texas Technical University	Widener University
Texas Women's University	Wilberforce University
Union College	Winthrop College
University of Washington—Seattle	University of Wisconsin—Madison
Weber State University	University of Wisconsin—Milwaukee

In 1950, the AUPHA requested that the ACHA's Board of Regents accredit programs in hospital administration. However, it took until 1968 to organize program accreditation.[89] Since then graduate programs have been accredited by the Accrediting Commission on Education for Health Services Administration (ACEHSA). It has six corporate members, ACHE, American College of Medical Practice Executives, AHA, American Public Health Association, AUPHA, and a joint Canadian seat held by the Canadian Hospital Association and the Canadian College of Health Service Executives. As of 1993, the Canadian seat was held by the Canadian College of Health Service Executives. There are also two public members. The Association of Mental Health Administrators and the American College of Health Care Administrators (long-term care) hold consulting memberships. As of 1990, there were 57 accredited graduate programs and 64 in 1993. There is no formal accreditation program for baccalaureate education.[90]

By November, 1961, there were 3,120 graduates from the 16 graduate programs in hospital administration. In addition, there were 240 administrative residents who would graduate in 1962 for a total of 3,360 graduates.[91]

Of the 3,120 graduates, 37 percent were administrators; 24 percent assistant administrators; 8 percent administrative assistants; 5.5 percent other health field organizations; 7 percent in the armed forces; and the remainder in other positions (department heads, teaching clinic managers, consulting, medical practice and others).[92]

By 1970–1971, there were 33 member programs of AUPHA with 1,666 enrolled students.[93] In the early 1970s, the AUPHA changed its name to the Association of University Programs in Health Administration to reflect the diverse interests of faculty and the varied positions taken by program graduates.[94] By 1978, the AUPHA had become "an international consortium of 120 universities in 19 nations."[95] By 1982, the AUPHA consortium had grown to 153 educational programs in 144 colleges and universities and has continued at this level since then.[96]

The Administrative Internship

In the 1930s, the administrative internship could exist independently of a degree program,[97] evolving easily out of the earlier administration apprenticeships. In 1939, Claude Munger, M.D., described the important components of such a program.[98] Because the internship was often the path of direct entry into the field, he felt it necessary to define the traits of a good administrator:

> Hospitals need administrators who are humanitarians, energetic men and women able to meet people and assume leadership. Hospital administration holds no place for the educated sophisticate, the petty martinet, or, above all, the man who wants an easy job. Quiet persistence, tact, a judicial attitude, good appearance, a sense of humor, and the ability to speak and to write about hospitals' work are valuable attributes. Those who have failed in other fields and who seem likely to repeat the process in hospital work must be avoided.

With respect to the administrative internship:

> It is preferable that the student live in the institution.[99]
> The student should have a desk in the administrator's outer office during the first two months.
> A helpful means of giving the intern a grasp of the administrator's work is to assign him to open and read the mail that comes to the administrator's office.
> The student should make and record several case studies of individual patients, with an interpretation of the reasons for the various procedures and with an evaluation of the efficiency with which the various phases of the work for that patient are executed.
> Lay persons who expect to administer hospitals must be permitted to witness as many surgical operations and like procedures as seem necessary to give them a clear knowledge of these procedures and of the administrator's relation to them.
> In the seventh to tenth months the student should work on special problems such as:
> - a system for key issuance and control
> - devising and putting into operation in a storeroom a system of perpetual inventory.[100]

Master's degree programs grew in the 1940s, '50s and '60s. Programs often consisted of one academic year and one year of administrative internship. Hospital administration programs also developed linkages with particular administrators who accepted students. Sometimes, these administrators were chosen because of their status as program graduates, their reputation as administrators, or their willingness to provide good learning experiences for students. If these administrators found students able, they would often be helpful in launching early careers.

By 1946, some of the programs sought College help in placing interns and students. Aware that to be a Nominee they must satisfactorily complete courses in hospital administration approved by the College, many students inquired whether certain internships would be acceptable to the College.[101]

The Board of Regents agreed to set up a subcommittee of the Educational Policies Committee to implement an internship approval program. Claude Munger, Chairman of the College in 1946, addressed the College as follows:

> It is my strong belief that the College should accept leadership in establishing an approval program for administrative apprenticeships, in somewhat the same manner as the American Medical Association maintains an approval program of hospitals desiring to offer medical internships. I urgently recommend that the College undertake such a project forthwith. Thought should be given also to the possibilities of initiating in the College an approval program for the hospital administration courses themselves. We already hear of plans of questionable soundness for the initiation of courses under various auspices.[102]

Dr. Prall believed that the responsibility for choosing an internship belonged to the university course director. Dean Conley, however, took the opposite view. College files on its members could be a unique source of information about possible preceptors. All the existing course directors were Fellows or Members of the College, as were 900 chief administrators. Conley believed no developed internship program could exist without College cooperation. Because membership in the College "was rapidly becoming essential to a successful career in hospital administration, few students would be so reckless as to accept an internship unsatisfactory to the College."[103]

As a result of College prodding, the Joint Commission organized a conference in January, 1947, at Columbia University to discuss the criteria for a good internship. Later that year they published *The Administrative Internship in the Hospital*,[104] recommending that half the internship year be spent rotating through hospital departments.

After the end of the Joint Commission's work in June, 1948, the College continued to propose guidelines for administrative residency, as it came to be known in 1953.[105] From 1949 to 1954, the College sponsored eight two-day conferences for preceptors.[106]

The College's residency guidelines were republished until 1965. After this date, with the growth of the two-year academic programs, the residency disappeared from many programs.[107] However, by 1982, with an abundance of program graduates, the residency/fellowship returned.[108]

The Olsen Report: 1954

In 1952, the W. K. Kellogg Foundation made a grant to the AUPHA to establish a Commission on University Education in Hospital Administration. Its report was published in 1954.[109] The Commission was chaired by James A. Hamilton (Chairman of the College 1939–1940), and directed by Herluf V. Olsen,[110] an Honorary Fellow of the College.

A major component of the work of this commission was taken on by the College: the mailing and analysis of 6,000 questionnaires to administrators to survey present and future needs of hospital administrators.[111]

The Commission reviewed the existing 13 graduate programs and discussed issues related to research, faculty qualifications, admissions policies, teaching methods, and program costs.[112] As a result of the College survey, the report estimated that 602 hospital administrative positions would become available annually and that several additional programs should be established.[113]

The Commission recommended that the age of admission to the graduate programs be between 21 and 27 years of age.[114] From 1934 to 1952, of 1,224 graduates, the average age of admission to the programs was above 30 years of age.[115] As the programs accepted younger students, they also helped to extend the administrator's years in middle management.

The Commission also recommended that candidates to the graduate programs have two semesters of accounting as well as one semester of statistics in administration, principles of administration, personnel administration, finance, marketing, business law, and general business conditions.

Students should go directly from this undergraduate training into the graduate program, the Commission believed. Residency training should continue without exceptions for experience. Teaching in the graduate programs should be by seminar and, therefore, class size should be from 10 to 15 students. Research should be part of the program. Faculty should be at least two full-time equivalents.[116]

Although not an explicit recommendation, the report also stated:

> In the opinion of this commission the graduate curricula, teaching methods and materials, and personnel of the schools of business administration most nearly approximate those considered most de-

sirable for the program that the commission is proposing, with its emphasis on management and administration.[117]

The debate over this controversial suggestion nearly destroyed the AUPHA, whose members split in their preference for a business school of health-based educational programs.[118]

1966–1983

The College's continued interest in graduate education was reflected by the special issue of *Hospital Administration* devoted to this topic in 1967. In 1969, Professor Theodore (Teddy) Chester of the University of Manchester, England, wrote a report on *Graduate Education for Hospital Administration in the United States*, which the College published without officially endorsing its content. Although Chester found the U.S. programs in a rapid state of growth, he nevertheless concluded that the 400 students expected to graduate in 1968 were not an adequate number.

In his 1969 report, Chester stated:

> It seems to me possible to divide the development of (the graduate) programs since their inception into three distinct periods: "The age of the pioneers," "the age of the practitioners," and "the age of the new man," the latter of which is just emerging. The "heroic age" can be said to have begun in 1929 with the Michael Davis book. This period, which came to an end around 1945, was characterized by the pioneering efforts and the outstanding personalities of Dr. Arthur C. Bachmeyer and Dr. Malcolm T. MacEachern.
>
> During the subsequent period—from 1945 to 1965—students graduating from (the first) two programs became the disciples of their masters; they spread their words and their writings over the face of the United States. A substantial number of them became themselves program directors. Generally speaking, they saw as the main goal of the newly founded schools training for the practice of hospital administration. They did not bother too much about generalized theory or fundamental research, but relied on . . . their own practical experience and achievements as a major source of their teaching material.

These programs consisted of one academic year, plus the residency and a thesis. "Program faculty lived at best in uneasy coexistence with the other members of the university," concluded Chester.[119] In recent years, Chester saw the picture change:

> The age of the new man has begun to dawn. More and younger men are coming forward, some already as program directors, who them-

selves have a very respectable academic background, including doctorates, and who are not only anxious to put the whole teaching program on a sound theoretical basis but also to prove to all their colleagues in the university that their academic respectability is without blemish. It seems to me that it is largely against this background that the recent trend to increase the time allocated to academic studies, while decreasing practical training, has to be seen.[120]

When the Cornell program started in 1958, it was a two-year academic program based in their Sloan School of Management.[121] In the 1960s, the Chicago program also changed to a two-year academic program and other programs followed.[122]

This occurred for several reasons, including faculty members' beliefs that the required knowledge could not be conveyed in one academic year and because students were now more committed to this specific field—and so they would accept the increased preparatory demands to join the profession. Finally, the College's efforts probably contributed indirectly since it supported the development of graduate health administration programs.

By the 1970s, three-year, two-degree programs appeared, offering coordinated public health and business administration degrees (Columbia, Yale).[123]

A two-year academic program effectively doubled the size of the on-campus student body, thereby building the economic foundation for a larger academic faculty for these programs. As these programs developed major funded research efforts, they were also able to support more full-time faculty.[124] Jon Jaeger, FACHE, writing in 1972, said:

> Since its inception 50 years ago, education for hospital administration has undergone an amazing transformation. Originally a highly pragmatic, situationally oriented instruction format, course curricula by successive stages have now become increasingly theoretical with increasing reliance upon empirical rather than intuitive decision methods. And while the advantages attributed to older approaches are still wistfully remembered, the forces that have brought about the current orientation are rooted in the basic changes occurring in our twentieth century society.[125]

Full-time faculty tend toward a more academic, scholarly research focus. They bring a different perspective than the program founders who often had substantial administrative experience and held leading positions in the College. At the present time, relatively few faculty play leading roles in the College. This division between teaching and practice parallels similar trends in medicine, law, business, engineering, and other professions.

The close link between the early master's program faculty and the College required no adjustment of College admission requirements to apply to full-time faculty. Just prior to 1960, a modification was made in the College admissions criteria:

> Candidates who are duly appointed faculty members of an approved course in hospital administration at the time of their election to the College, and have completed satisfactorily an approved course in hospital administration, or have had the required years of experience in a responsible administrative position in a hospital . . . have the same eligibility . . . as persons actively engaged in hospital administration.[126]

As faculty were drawn increasingly from scholarly academic disciplines, proportionately fewer could qualify for College membership.[127] Even with the growth of full-time faculty, many practicing hospital managers maintained close relationships with the master's programs as residency preceptors. The College had a direct impact on education through its published standards for acceptable residency training. As more programs moved to two academic years, the linkage between academia and practice became less pronounced.[128]

The Commission on Education for Health Administration: 1972–1977

Funded by the W. K. Kellogg Foundation, the Commission on Education for Health Administration was chaired by James P. Dixon, M.D., President of Antioch College, and had Charles Austin of the Xavier University Graduate Program in Hospital and Health Administration as its Staff Director.[129] The commission worked from 1972 to 1974, publishing two volumes in 1975, and a third in 1977.[130]

They found that fewer than 25 percent of executive positions were filled by people with education in health administration. They recommended diversity in academic approaches to meet these needs.[131] The Commission's 30 percent sample of 2,402, 1972–1973 graduates of the health administration programs (2,100 master's degree, 170 baccalaureate, and 132 associate degree graduates), showed that 57 percent went into hospital administration; 13 percent into government agencies; 7 percent into health planning; 4 percent into ambulatory care; 3 percent into voluntary health agencies; 4 percent into long-term care and mental health administration; 1 percent into third party agencies; 4 percent to become university faculty; and 7 percent to further education.[132] This demonstrated the diversity of organizations and positions that became available after 1966. The program graduates felt the programs were strongest in administrative theory, and weakest in financial management, systems analysis and electronic data processing.[133] In the master's degree programs, 61 percent of the faculty held doctorate degrees and the average number of full-time faculty was 5.7. Thirteen percent of master's program students were minorities.[134]

The College appointed a task force to study the report of this commission, chaired by R. Zach Thomas, Jr.[135] This task force and the College leadership viewed the Dixon report as "developed largely by educators and for educators," ignoring the role of both the practitioner and the College in education. It led to a discussion about how the College might broaden its admission and advancement criteria to fit the developing specialized areas in healthcare administration.[136]

The College task force pointed out that the Dixon commission defined healthcare administration very broadly, to include hospital administration (17–18,000 practitioners); nursing home administration (16–20,000 practitioners); public health agency administration (5–6,000); voluntary health agencies (10,000); comprehensive health planning (500–1,000); and clinic management (1,000).[137]

Although the commission found that only one-fourth of these managers had education in health administration, the College task force pointed out that this was hardly the case for hospitals for which the supply of program graduates was abundant and perhaps even excessive.

The task force recommended that "universities should give serious attention to developing an appropriate alignment between programs of professional education and employment opportunities for graduates."[138] Explicitly taking an administrative practitioner perspective,[139] the task force urged that the graduate program faculty "translate the realities of administrative practice into educational endeavors."

> Opportunities and incentives for faculty development should be geared less to scholarly endeavor in the academic tradition and more to pursuits enabling educators to keep abreast of advances in the professional practice of health administration.[140]

The College task force stressed a major point:

> The professional society creates an orientation and an environment conducive to the lifelong learning which undergirds development of administrative competence and leadership. Beyond this the profes-

sional society is cognizant of the educational needs of the practitioners, and is in an advantageous position to design structured educational programs responsive to these needs.[141]

Reflecting the growing specialization in the field, the task force
finally recommended that the College expand its educational functions "through the development of specialized examinations in major
areas of health administration."[142]

The Multi-Institutional System: 1979–Present

In 1975, the Dixon Report viewed healthcare as "fragmented, plu-
ralistic and disorganized," a trend they felt would continue in the future.[143] But could the rise of multi-institution systems be a response
to this fragmentation? According to John Griffith, FACHE, half of
the two billion dollars third parties spent in Michigan in 1982 was paid
to only five large healthcare providers.[144] Career paths in these large
organizations will call for increased specialization by healthcare managers in such areas as finance, engineering, law, nursing and medicine.[145]

At the same time, program faculty have become increasingly specialized. Many of these faculty would not be able to manage a hospital
the way faculty of the "heroic age" of the 30s and 40s could.

Enhancing Executive Competence, 1981–

This ACHE report became the basis for the College's program of self-
assessment and continuing education. It was the product of the College's Self-Assessment Project Committee, chaired by James D. Harvey.
This committee presided over four specialist panels. Governance and
Control (David S. Ramsey), Environmental Relations (L. Russell Jor-
don), Resource Acquisition and Management (Russell B. Williams) and
Service Delivery (Robert H. Brandow).[146] Table 5.6 lists their task domains. In each area, task knowledge and skill statements are listed.
For example, under Comprehensive Systems of Patient Services, tasks
include: "protects the confidentiality of information concerning patients" and "enforces institutional policies and operating procedures."

Knowledge statements include "ethical, legal and religious mores
relative to patients' rights and well being" and "major environmental
forces in the healthcare field." Skills include "motivating others," "conducting meetings," "delegating."[147]

In 1979, the College received a grant from the Kellogg Foundation to develop a general management assessment appropriate for use
by College members. From 1982–1988 there were 18 different man-

TABLE 5.6
Task Delineation, Enhancing Executive Competence, 1981[148]

Governance and Control
  Strategy Planning and Policy
  Board/Medical Staff/Administrative/Accountability Relations
  Preservation of Assets
Resource Acquisition and Management
  Financial Management
  Human Resources Management
  Plant and Facility Management
  Systems Management
Service Delivery
  Comprehensive Systems of Patient Services
  Quality Assessment and Assurance
  Professional Relations
Environmental Relations
  Community/Public Relations
  Governmental Relations/Regulations
  Hospital and Health Inter-organizational Relations
Generic Areas
  Marketing
  Planning
  Education
  Research
  Law and Ethics

Each section above lists task statements, knowledge of and skills in.

agement areas. These were consolidated to 11 with the 1989 revision.[149]

The *General Management Assessment* is a loose leaf notebook that can be used by the affiliate to define their own important management areas, assess their competence in these areas, and design their own continuing education, including seminars to attend at the annual Congress. These management areas are governance and organization, finance, human resources, marketing, planning, operations management, quality assessment/improvement, organizational arrangements and relationships, external relations, professional relations, and profession/law and ethics. After defining these areas, the next section allows the affiliate to clarify career goals and objectives and relate these to the eleven management areas. The next section contains 175 multiple choice questions related to one-paragraph descriptions of realistic management problems. After scoring their own assessments, managers are able to compare their performance with others at similar positions and organizations. The summary scores combined with self-assessed areas of importance becomes the basis for a continuing education plan. A bibliography is included. College seminars and Congress seminars are linked to the eleven areas.

Another self-assessment program of the College is the *Administrative Communication Techniques* (ACT) exercise originally developed in 1983 and revised in 1991. It is currently used by about 200 affiliates per year.[150] This self-assessment consists of an in-basket exercise and a writing assessment based on a hospital setting, a cast of characters and six scenarios. The member takes the role of the CEO who has been away from the hospital for a week and is confronted with an in-basket and the resultant need for four written responses. Four hours are the expected completion time.

The Ambulatory Care Administration/Medical Group Management Simulations of 1986 are jointly used by ACHE and the American College of Medical Practice Executives. Seven problems are followed by choices. A special marker is used to bring out the consequences of choice. There is a companion multiple choice exam with a scanable code sheet. The Simulation is used by about 150 College affiliates and about 100 American College of Medical Practice Executives affiliates yearly.[151]

The College also worked with AUPHA on executive competence. A joint ACHE and AUPHA Task Force report on beginning and early career development in 1992, reviewed the changes of the 1980s.

> "Applications to graduate programs in health services administration declined steadily from 1980 to 1989 before starting an upward trend. The programs increasingly serve "nontraditional" learners, individuals who are more than 25 years old and working full time. They have career patterns distinct from those of typical health administration graduates of an earlier era who entered their programs directly from undergraduate studies and who rarely worked even part-time before graduating."[152]

This report noted the growth in mid-career students with clinical or other training with prior work experience. The report expects that the majority of master's degree students will be part-time. There will be bright opportunities in long term care, managed care and medical group management.[153]

The task force recommended that students develop career plans and should seek positions with apprentice stage attributes. Careerists should develop long term personal career planning which includes assessment of skills, a continuing education plan and College affiliation. As careerists gain experience, they should take on a mentoring role to newer entrants. This report clearly accepts the concept of lifelong learning.

The 1970s saw the greatest separation of academia and the College. The 1980s saw the development of new ways to build bridges. A new faculty category of affiliation was created.[154] Student Associates were started. Arrangements to allow faculty to spend time in health care organizations were undertaken. Faculty editorial boards and book publishing created new links.

Other initiatives included the student competition, which at first invited student teams from accredited masters programs in health administration to participate in a computer simulation "game." Developed by faculty at Georgia State University, the game offered programs the opportunity to play consecutive rounds. The top three programs' participants were then invited to come to the Congress on Administration to finish the game. Later, this competition was replaced by Hill-Rom Company's sponsored essay writing contest—one at the master's and one at the baccalaureate level. These links culminated with James Hepner, Ph.D., the program director at Washington University becoming College chair in 1991–1992.

Finally, the College in the 1980s began to play a more active role in supporting health services research. New initiatives included (1) becoming an institutional sponsor of the newly formed Association for Health Services Research; (2) sponsoring a $500 annual best paper award for the Academy of Management's Health Administration Section and (3) providing a $5,000 Health Management Research Award to encourage faculty from accredited health administration programs to conduct research to enhance managerial effectiveness and career opportunities in health services administration.

The College invites faculty to teach both in short courses and in the annual Congress seminars.[155] One way the College and academia have merged is through the background of each of the College's chief executive officers. Gerhard Hartman, Ph.D. (1937–1941), was concurrently a faculty member at the University of Chicago. Dean Conley (1942–1965) was, prior to working for the College, Business Manager of the University of Minnesota Health Service from 1935–1941. Richard J. Stull (1965–1979) was the founding Director of the program at the University of California, Berkeley. Stuart A. Wesbury, Jr., Ph.D. (1979–1991), was Director of the Graduate Program in Health Services Management at the University of Missouri—Columbia, from 1972 to 1978.[156] Thomas C. Dolan, Ph.D. (1991–) was on the faculty of the Graduate Program in Health Services Management at the University of Missouri—Columbia and was Director of the Saint Louis University Center for Health Services Education and Research from 1979 to 1986.[157]

The College was started in the era of "the begats" or apprenticeship education. It was closely linked to the development of graduate education in hospital administration. By the 1970s, university education in health management was almost universal. The 1970s saw the specialization of faculty and their separation from the College. The 1980s brought both groups closer together and the College embarked on creative approaches to systematic lifelong learning for its associates.

NOTES

[1] Goldwater, quoted on the first page of the *Bulletin of the ACHA*, Vol. 1, No. 1, 1934 or 1935.

[2] Davis, Michael, 1929, p. 90.

[3] Society of Medical Administrators, 1967. AHA *Guide Issue 1982*, p. B4–5. Kipnis. All the listed hospital administrators are physicians and members of the Society of Medical Administrators. The author trained in part with Silas Wass, who in turn was trained by Madison Brown, and could therefore be considered a seventh generation in this genealogy. Johns Hopkins provided apprentice training for the following physician presidents of the AHA: Henry Hurd, 1912; Winford Smith, 1916; George O'Hanlon, 1922; Lewis Sexton, 1931; Edwin L. Crosby, 1953; and Russell Nelson, 1960. The Montreal General Hospital educated Basil MacLean in 1942, Donald Smelzer in 1945, Peter Ward in 1946, and Albert Snoke in 1957. All these physicians were members of the Society of Medical Administrators. Madison Brown, M.D., personal communication, April 8, 1983. ACHA *1981 Directory.* "The Begats," Sidney Lee, personal communication. Madison Brown, 1984, p. x.

[4] Dr. L. H. Burlinghams' name is misspelled in the 1981 list of ACHA Charter Fellows, *1981 Directory*, but is correct in Kipnis, 1955.

[5] Commission on Education for Health Administration 1975, 1977.

[6] Washburn and Howland, 1911.

[7] Goodrich, 1916, p. 361.

[8] Chester, 1969. His terms describe the teachers and program faculty of these times.

[9] Bachmeyer, 1919.

[10] Davis, Michael, 1929, pp. 90–93

[11] *Ibid.*

[12] Shanahan, 1965, p. 60.

[13] Rappleye, 1922. The importance of this study was recognized at the time. "Committee on Training of Hospital Executives Issues Momentous Report," *Modern Hospitals*, Vol. 19, No. 1, July 1922, pp. 1–6.

[14] Shanahan, 1965, pp. 60–61.

[15] Davis, Michael, 1929. This was not the first such list. The 1922 Rappleye report listed curriculum content, and Dr. Goldwater in Sept. 1920 listed the content areas for the administrator's self-education.

[16] Committee on the Costs of Medical Care. *Final Report*, 1932, cited by Ray Brown, p. 1, in Ray Brown (editor), 1959.

[17] *Michael M. Davis, A Tribute*, 1972.

[18] Davis, Michael, "Development of the First Graduate Program in Hospital Administration," pp. 6–21, in Ray Brown, 1959. Davis, Michael, 1938 (ACHA reprint). Davis, Michael, "Studies in Hospital Administration at the University of Chicago," *Hospitals*, March 1936.

[19] Lewis Weeks interview with Gerhard Hartman, Ph.D., 1982, pp. 12–13.

[20] Hartman, "Graduate Education in Hospital Administration," 1938.

[21] *ACHA News*, Jan. 1938, p. 11. "Kellogg didn't become interested until Andrew Pattullo, who was, I think, in the last class I taught with Bachmeyer [at the University of Chicago], left to join Graham Davis and Emory Morris in his [administrative] residency or fellowship at Kellogg." Lewis Weeks interview with Gerhard Hartman, Ph.D., 1982, p. 13. Because Kellogg funded the first wave of new hospital administration programs after World War II, this is one way the Chicago program influenced education in hospital administration.

[22] Hartman, *op. cit.*, 1938.

[23] Wren, 1980, p. 34

[24] ACHA, *The College Curriculum in Hospital Administration*, 1948, projected a yearly need for 230 new administrators and not less than 160, pp. 77–83.

[25] ACHA, MacEachern, "Institutes for Hospital Administrators," Sept. 13, 1937.

[26] Kipnis, 1955, pp. 139–142. Malcolm MacEachern organized and directed that Institute, according to George Bugbee (personal communication, 1983).

[27] "Program of the 13th Chicago Institute for Hospital Administrators, September 17–28, 1945." Cosponsored by the ACHA, AHA, ACS, AMA, University of Chicago, and the Chicago Hospital Council and held at International House of the University of Chicago. The course content largely follows that outlined by MacEachern, *op. cit.*, 1937.

[28] Everett A. Johnson, "A Review of the Several Graduate Programs in Hospital Administration," in Brown, Ray E., 1959. Charles Prall, p. 31 in Brown, Ray E., 1959. The University of Chicago program "served as a model of how such programs can be structured by a university," George Bugbee, p. vii in Brown, Ray E., 1959.

[29] Kipnis, 1955, pp. 139–142. The latest date reported by Kipnis is 1955.

[30] The 1933 Chicago Institute was the first year of participation in this program by the College, Kipnis, 1955, note p. 139.

[31] Kipnis, 1955, pp. 139–142.

[32] *ACHA News*, April 1964, Vol. 28, No. 4.

[33] *ACHA News*, April 1961, Vol. 25, No. 4.

[34] ACHA, 1964 *Annual Report*, pp. 8–9.

[35] *ACHA News*, April 1964, Vol. 28, No. 4.

[36] *ACHA News*, March-April 1965, Vol. 29, Nos. 3, 4.

[37] *ACHA News*, May 1965, Vol. 29, No. 5.

[38] *ACHA News*, Feb.-March 1968, Vol. 32, No. 2.

[39] Lachner, Foreword to the ACHA's commemorative edition of Brown, Ray E., *Judgment in Administration*, 1982.

[40] *ACHA News*, Jan. 1961, Vol. 25, No. 1.

[41] Matzick, 1967, p. 33.

[42] *Ibid.*, p. 38.

[43] *Ibid.*, p. 67.

44 ACHA, *Professional Continuing Education Catalog*, March through Dec., 1982. *Professional Development Catalog*, Jan. through Dec. 1983.

45 ACHA, *Educational Audio Cassette Catalog, 1982/83*. There is also a publications catalog (circa 1982).

46 Kipnis, 1955, p. 27.

47 *Ibid.*

48 Kipnis, pp. 27–28.

49 *Ibid.*, p. 28.

50 Parts 1–4 presented Feb. 17, 1936. Parts 5 and 6 presented Sept. 28, 1936. Summary, Conclusions, Principles and Recommendations were presented to the Committee on Educational Policies on Feb. 15, 1937. The whole document was published with a Foreword by Father Schwitilla in 1937. Thus, it became known as the "Schwitilla report" and titled *University Training for Hospital Administration Careers, a report by the Committee on Educational Policies of the ACHA*, Malcolm T. MacEachern, M.D., chairman, 1937. The other members of this committee were Father Schwitilla; Robert Bishop, M.D.; Robert E. Neff; Nathaniel W. Faxon, M.D. (director of the Massachusetts General Hospital); Joseph C. Doane, M.D.; and Michael M. Davis, Ph.D.

51 ACHA, *University Training for Hospital Administration Careers*, 1937.

52 *Ibid.*, pp. 9–11.

53 S. B. Crawford, assistant superintendent, Maryland General Hospital. *ACHA News*, Jan. 1938, pp. 8–9.

54 ACHA, *University Training for Hospital Administration Careers*, 1937, p. 15.

55 "Opinions Here and There," *ACHA News*, Jan. 1938, p. 4.

56 *Ibid.*, pp. 4–5.

57 *Ibid.*, pp. 5–6.

58 *Ibid.*, p. 6.

59 *Ibid.*, p. 8.

60 *Ibid.*, p. 9. "In the minds of many present-day administrators there is some anxiety lest this rapidly spreading realization of the value of adequate training for administration should undermine their own personal position. For those individuals who just drifted into administration years ago when little beyond personal acceptability was required, adequate contact with the achievements of today can be maintained by attending Institutes, not once but repeatedly . . ." G. Harvey Agnew, M.D., president of the American Hospital Association, "Training in Hospital Administration," *Hospitals*, July 1939.

61 *Ibid.*, pp. 9–10. A. F. Anderson, M.D., superintendent, Royal Alexandra Hospital, Edmonton, Alberta, and A. K. Haywood, M.D., general superintendent, The Vancouver General Hospital, British Columbia.

62 *Ibid.*, p. 11. Worth L. Howard, administrator, The City Hospital of Akron, Akron, Ohio.

63 Agnew, "Training in Hospital Administration," *ACHA News*, March, 1940, pp. 2–4. Agnew says in Great Britain the Corporation of Certified Secretaries (incorporated in 1923) gives examinations for administrators of hospitals and other organizations leading to Association and Fellowship (F.C.C.S.). In addition, the British Incorporated Association of Hospital

Officers has recently developed examinations leading to association and fellowship (F.H.O.A.). However, these British developments seem to have had no effect on developments in North America.

[64] *Ibid.*, p. 3.

[65] The other members of the committee were Benjamin Black, M.D.; Robin Buerki, M.D.; Claude Munger, M.D.; James A. Hamilton; Malcolm T. MacEachern, M.D.; Ada Belle McCleery; and Lucius R. Wilson, M.D. Consultants to the committee were Robert Elsasser, Edward Fitzpatrick, H. V. Olsen, and L. C. White.

[66] "Report of the Committee on Educational Policies of the American College of Hospital Administrators," *ACHA News*, Nov. 1943, p. 3.

[67] W. K. Kellogg Foundation, 1955. The grant was $94,700. Kipnis, 1955, p. 90.

[68] Prall was a former dean of education at the University of Pittsburgh, 1934–38; field coordinator, American Council on Education, 1939–44; and later dean, School of Education, Woman's College, University of North Carolina, 1949–58. ACHA, *1960 Directory*, p. 323.

[69] Charles E. Prall, "A Review of the Report of the Joint Commission on Education for Hospital Administration," pp. 29–31 in Brown, Ray E., 1959.

[70] ACHA, "Joint Commission on Education for Hospital Administration," ("The Prall Report") 1948, pp. 75–80. This was based on a mailed questionnaire to new administrators between 1945 and 1946 from hospitals listed in the American Hospital Directory of the AHA. The sample was confined to 1,700 hospitals of between 75 and 600 beds, but it excluded federal and Catholic hospitals.

[71] Prall in Brown, Ray E. *op. cit.*, 1959, p. 30. The Joint Commission members were R. H. Bishop, Jr., M.D. (chairman); Frank R. Bradley; Arthur Bachmeyer; R. C. Buerki; George Bugbee; J. R. Clemmons, M.D.; Dean Conley; Edwin Crosby, M.D.; James A. Hamilton; Edgar C. Hayhow; Malcolm MacEachern; Ada Belle McCleery; Claude Munger; Sister M. Patricia; J. Gilbert Turner, M.D.; and staff Charles E. Prall and Paul B. Gillen. ACHA, "The Prall Report," 1948.

[72] Wren, 1980. p. 34.

[73] Prall, *Problems of Hospital Administration*, 1948.

[74] ACHA, *The College Curriculum in Hospital Administration*, 1948.

[75] None of these previous studies are cited by Prall. Wren, 1980, p. 35.

[76] ACHA, *op. cit.*, 1948, pp. 25–56.

[77] W. K. Kellogg Foundation, 1955. These programs were Columbia, Johns Hopkins (not a hospital administration program, specifically), Yale, Washington University of St. Louis, Minnesota, Toronto, Chile, and Sao Paulo, Brazil.

[78] *Ibid.*, p. 108.

[79] *ACHA News*, June-July 1947, pp. 2–7.

[80] The two sources for this table are Ray E. Brown, "Health Services Management Preparation, pp. 18–29 (Table 1, p. 26), in *Education for Health Services Administration at the University of Michigan, Proceedings of the Workshops*, 1972, and Sophie V. Zimmerman, "A Historical Summary of the Graduate Programs in Hospital Administration," pp. 184–190, in Brown,

Ray E., *Graduate Education for Hospital Administration*, 1959. Founding dates and listing of programs are from Brown, 1972, Table 1. He included only programs in existence then. Therefore he excluded Northwestern, which was not graduating students in 1971. The founding directors are from Zimmerman, which is why they stop at 1956. This list stopped when the source material ran out, rather than continued to include or exclude particular programs. A history of these programs, singly or collectively, has yet to be written. AUPHA presidents from AUPHA, 1973. Zimmerman, op. cit., also lists the Medical College of Virginia, starting in 1950, and Emory University, starting in 1956. These programs are not listed by Ray Brown in 1972. Zimmerman says the U.C. Berkeley program started in 1947, Pittsburgh in 1948, Army-Baylor in 1950. Olsen lists early courses (p. 12). His starting dates agree with R. Brown for Berkeley and Pittsburgh. He does not list Baylor, but does list Johns Hopkins, 1947, Ernest L. Stebbins, M.D., director. *University Education for Administration in Hospitals*, 1954.

[81] The Duke University program was established in 1930. It was a certificate program up to 1962 when it began offering the MHA degree. "Bulletin of Duke University program in Health Administration 1973–1974," Durham, Duke University, 1974. Andrew Pattullo, "Foundations and Their Role in the Development of Graduate Education in Hospital Administration," in Brown, Ray E., 1959.

[82] Sources: ACHE *1991–1992 Annual Report and Reference Guide*, p. 26, and AUPHA *Health Services Administration Education 1991–1993*. Of programs listed in Table 5.4, the following did not have ACHE student chapters in 1992: Columbia University, University of Toronto, University of Alberta, and University of Pennsylvania. Columbia University is the only program listed in Table 5.4 that was not a 1992 AUPHA member.

[83] Sister Mary Giovani of St. Joseph, Minnesota, received the first degree in 1940. *Ibid.*, p. 5.

[84] "HM Salutes Frank R. Bradley, M.D.", *Hospital Management*, Vol. 85, April 1958, p. 34.

[85] *Ibid*. Wren, 1980, greatly overestimates the number of graduates in 1948, p. 36. In 1948 Dean Conley reported 76 program graduates, rising to 165 graduates in 1952, Conley. 1953.

[86] James W. Stephan, "The Development of the Association of University Programs in Hospital Administration," in Brown, Ray E., 1959, pp. 68–70. AUPHA *Minute Book 1945–1961*. AUPHA Library, Arlington, Virginia. Attendees at the Dec. 17, 1948, organizational meeting included Dr. John Gorrell (Columbia), Dr. Malcolm MacEachern and Laura Jackson (Northwestern), James Hamilton and James Stephan (Minnesota), Frank Bradley and Clement Clay (Yale).

[87] James W. Stephan, *op. cit.*, p. 71. Kipnis, 1955, p. 141.

[88] "Hospital Management Salutes Dean Conley," *Hospital Management*, Vol. 101, March 1966, p. 53.

[89] Kipnis, 1955, pp. 102–104.

[90] AUPHA, *Health Services Administration Education 1991–1993*, pp. 15–16.

[91] Gerhard Hartman *et al.,* "The Impact of Graduate Programs in Hospital Administration," 1962, Table 1.

[92] Hartman, Levey, and McCarthy, 1962, pp. 54–57.

[93] Brown, Ray E., in *Education for Health Services Administration at the University of Michigan, Proceedings of the Workshops,* 1972, p. 27.

[94] ACHA, Wesbury, April 1981, pp. 4–5.

[95] Quatrano, 1978. Foreword, Gary Filerman, p. vii.

[96] AUPHA, 1982, p. iii.

[97] This was the case at Duke. *ACHA News,* June-July, 1947, p. 4.

[98] W. Munger, 1939, reprinted in Bachmeyer and Hartman, 1943, pp. 123–132.

[99] This was the preferred and typical approach for medical interns at the time.

[100] W. Munger, *op. cit.*

[101] Kipnis, 1955, p. 92.

[102] *Ibid.,* p. 93.

[103] *Ibid.,* p. 95.

[104] ACHA, *The Administrative Internship in the Hospital,* 1947, with Gillen and Prall. *The Hospital Administrative Internship: A Conference Report,* joint commission, 1947.

[105] ACHA, *The Administrative Residency in the Hospital,* 1953, 1954, and 1956. *The Hospital Administrative Residency,* 1965.

[106] Kipnis, 1955, p. 141.

[107] Gary L. Filerman, "Toward a reexamination of education for health administration," in Stimson and Taylor, 1973, p. 68.

[108] Of the 22 graduates of the class of 1982 of the master's program in hospital administration of the University of Michigan, 10 (45 percent) went into administrative residency or fellowship positions, *The Eclectic,* Vol. 25, No. 1, Jan. 1983, "Class 1982."

[109] *University Education for Administration in Hospitals.* Washington, D.C., American Council on Education, 1954, Kipnis, p. 106. Wren, 1980, pp. 36–38.

[110] Olsen was dean, Amos Tuck School of Business Administration, Dartmouth College, 1937–51, and professor, 1926–60. He was a member of the ACHA book award committee in 1959–60. ACHA *1960 Directory* 1960, pp. 304–305.

[111] Kipnis, 1955, pp. 106–107.

[112] The Commission members were James A. Hamilton (chairman); Milo Anderson (hospital administrator, Ohio State University Health Center); Donald G. Borg (trustee); Francis J. Brown (American Council on Education); Ray E. Brown; James P. Dixon, M.D. (Commissioner of Public Health, Philadelphia); John E. Gorrell, M.D. (former assistant director of the hospital administration program at Columbia); J. Steele Gow (trustee); and Leon N. Hickernell (director, Vancouver General Hospital), *University Education for Administration in Hospitals,* 1954. Also, Charles E. Prall, "A Review of the Report of the Joint Commission on Education for Hospital Administration," pp. 29–42, in Brown, Ray E., 1959.

[113] *University Education For Administration in Hospitals,* 1954, pp. 122–123.

[114] *Ibid.,* p. 156.

[115] *Ibid.*, p. 179.

[116] *Ibid.*, pp. 156–165. Olsen accepted the residency and because of this said, "If the program of study in hospital administration is limited to one graduate academic year, than none of that year should be devoted to making up deficiencies in these basic foundation courses [proposed for preadmission requirements]." Charles E. Prall, p. 46, in Brown, Ray E., 1959.

[117] *University Education For Administration in Hospitals*, 1954, p. 89.

[118] James W. Stephan, p. 71, in Brown, Ray E., 1959. Wren, 1980, pp. 36–39.

[119] ACHA, Chester, 1969, pp. 10–11.

[120] *Ibid.*, p. 12.

[121] Wren, 1980, p. 39.

[122] Bugbee, 1967.

[123] AUPHA, 1979, p. 84.

[124] The University of Michigan program, directed by Walter McNerney, in 1960 had developed a large research staff resulting in the two-volume report, McNerney *et al.*, 1962.

[125] Jaeger, 1972, pp. 1–2.

[126] ACHA, *1960 Directory*, p. 13

[127] "ACHA regulations, up to the early 1960s, prevented faculty from advancing to Fellowship or Membership. As a result, many of these individuals dropped their affiliation with the College and still have not rejoined, in spite of changes that permit advancement opportunities. Their position is understandable because the College denied their attempts to advance at the time they were prepared to do so." ACHA, Wesbury, April 1981, p. 5.

[128] *Ibid.*, p. 4.

[129] Of the 16 members of the Commission, only three are listed as College members in the *1981 Directory:* Lloyd Detwiller, Lawrence Hill, and Joseph B. Mann. Of these three, the first two had spent a major part of their careers in hospital administration education. Dixon was a member of the Olsen Report Commission in 1947, former Commissioner of Public Health of Philadelphia, and a member of the Society of Medical Administrators.

[130] The reports of the Commission on Education for Health Administration are Vol. I and Vol. II, published in 1975, and *Vol. III, A Future Agenda*, 1977, and *Summary of the Report of the Commission on Education for Health Administration*, 1974. Wren, 1980, pp. 39–42.

[131] Report of the Commission on Education for Health Administration, Vol. I, 1975, p. 43.

[132] *Ibid.*, p. 58.

[133] *Ibid.*, p. 66.

[134] *Ibid.*, pp. 76, 78.

[135] The other members included Everett Fox, Aladino Gavazzi, L. Russell Jordan, Stephan Morris, William N. Wallace, and David Youngdall. ACHA, "The Report of the Task Force on the Report of the Commission on Education for Health Administration," 1978, and "Report of the Joint Meeting of the ACHA Board of Governors Task Force on the Report of the Commission on Education for Health Administration," Aug. 10, 1977.

[136] ACHA, "The Report of the Task Force on the Report of the Commission on Education for Health Administration: Compilation of Reactions of Officers and Governors," May 4, 1977, pp. 15, esp. p. 14.

[137] ACHA, *The Report of the Task Force on the Report of the Commission on Education for Health Administration*, 1978, p. 14.

[138] *Ibid.*, p. 15.

[139] *Ibid.*, p. vi.

[140] *Ibid.*, p. 20.

[141] *Ibid.*, p. 27.

[142] *Ibid.*, p. 30.

[143] *Report of the Commission . . .*, Vol. I, 1975, *op. cit.*, p. 122.

[144] John Griffith, personal communication, Dec. 1982.

[145] Howard Zuckerman, personal communication, Dec. 1982.

[146] ACHA, *Enhancing Executive Competence*, 1981, p. 81.

[147] *Ibid.*, pp. 57–58.

[148] *Ibid.*, pp. 44–71.

[149] Interview with Cynthia Hahn and Arthur Strobeck, Nov. 1992. ACHE, General Management Assessment program, 1989, developed in cooperation with Professional Examination Service, New York City.

[150] Interview with Cynthia Hahn, Nov. 1992. Administrative Communication Techniques workshop folder has no date, but Hahn reports this revision is of 1991.

[151] ACHE, American College of Medical Group Administrators, *Health Executive Professional Assessment: A System for Professional Development*. Two sections, 1986. Cynthia Hahn interview, 1992.

[152] ACHE, AUPHA "Report of the Task Force on Beginning and Early Career Development," 1992, p. 5.

[153] *Ibid.* p. 9.

[154] ACHE, *1991–1992 Annual Report and Reference Guide*, pp. 39, 43.

[155] Of the 67 faculty at the 1983 Congress on Administration, 6 were academics and 40 were from consulting and similar fields. These consulting firms can provide useful information to practitioners when, increasingly, academics have focused on scholarly work of less immediate interest. Of the 67 faculty, 7 were College Fellows, one was an Honorary Fellow, and 9 were College Members; ACHA, *Twenty-Sixth Congress on Administration*, March 1983. The 31st Congress, 1988, lists 75 seminars with 115 speakers. Of these, 20 were College Fellows and 8 were listed as academics; ACHE, *Congress on Administration: 31 Years of Educational Excellence*, Feb. 1988.

[156] ACHE, *1981 Directory*.

[157] ACHE, *1992 Directory*, p. 272.

6

Evaluating Excellence

Undoubtedly the American College of Hospital Administrators, by its emphasis upon higher standards for administrators, will be of inestimable assistance in elevating the status of this field and already it has had a very appreciable effect.

G. Harvey Agnew, M.D. 1939[1]
Honorary Charter Fellow, ACHA

If the College was to elevate the standard of hospital administration, it had to establish a standard of competency for hospital administrators which would be reflected in the qualifications for Fellowship in the College.[2] These qualifications would undoubtedly change with time. They would be based on professional evaluation, as distinct from simple economic measures, such as employment and salary. And, they would be distinct from the predilections of trustees who, in 1933, had to be educated as to the need for professionally qualified administrators.

New Beginnings: 1933–1945

The first qualification was the personal selection of Dewey Lutes and a few of his Chicago administrator friends, Maurice Dubin of Mt. Sinai; Ernest Erickson of Augustana; and Charles A. Wordell of St. Luke's.[3]

On their second meeting at Ravenswood Hospital, this group invited an additional 48 administrators to form the nucleus of the organization.[4] At the Chicago meeting on February 13, 1933, Maurice Dubin outlined a constitution and bylaws providing for three classes of membership: Member, Fellow, and Honorary Fellow.[5] On February 14, 1933, the officers were authorized to develop temporary standards for membership.[6]

Later, in Milwaukee, on September 10, 1933, in conjunction with the annual AHA meeting, a secret Credentials Committee of five was

appointed to pass on proposed names for membership.[7] The anony-
mous chairman of this committee was Malcolm MacEachern.[8] He was
the real power there. "No other individual knew so many administrators personally, nor was acquainted with the actual administrative conditions of so many hospitals," wrote Kipnis. This committee approved
70 names for Charter Fellowship and 11 for Honorary Fellowship. In
February, 1934, an additional 44 names were approved for admission
as Charter Fellows and four for Charter Honorary Membership.[9] As
Kipnis notes, membership classifications were a bit confusing in those
days.[10]

This early effort created the Charter Fellows and Charter Honorary Fellows.[11] In the second year, the first Members were elected
along with other administrators who were appointed directly to
Fellowship[12] and Honorary Fellowship. Because of the tradition of the
American College of Surgeons, the ACHE was able to reach consensus
on the criteria for Fellowship within the first two years of its existence.
Table 6.1 summarizes professional criteria and levels involved in the
evaluation of excellence as of 1982.

Position. At the September 23, 1934, meeting of the Board of Regents, it was proposed that eligibility for admission be expanded from
"administrators" to those "whose major interest lies in hospital administration." This proposal was defeated. Another proposal to make executive secretaries of hospital associations eligible was similarly voted
down. The general feeling was that membership should be limited to
active hospital administrators. Others active in the health care field,
whose work merited recognition by the College, would be eligible to
election as Honorary Fellows.[13]

This specific focus on the hospital administrator was a critically
important decision for the College. It set the conditions which would
result in the creation of other specialized associations.[14] By 1967, the
College began to admit non-hospital administrators.[15] From the start,
Fellows of the College would not lose their standing if they went on
to manage another type of organization during a later phase of their
careers.

Through 1941, administrators of hospitals under 25 beds were
not considered eligible. In addition, the administrator's hospital required approval by the American College of Surgeons (accreditation)
and registration through the American Hospital Association.

In 1941, the College dropped requirements that the hospital be
accredited and registered.[16] By the 1950s, such a large proportion of
hospitals (over 95%) was accredited, that it was no longer an issue.

The College decided to admit associate administrators and assistant administrators, but not specialized department heads.

TABLE 6.1
1982 Professional Criteria for Evaluating Excellence Criteria for College Nomineeship (N), Membership (M) and Fellowship (F)[17]

Criteria	Level at Which Requirement Must be Met in 1982*
I. *Position in Administration*	
Position in organization hierarchy:	
Administrator, assistant, etc.	N, M, F
Type of organization	N, M, F
Hospital	
Minimal hospital size	
Accreditation, registration	
Other healthcare organizations	
Country: Canada, USA	
Hospital administration faculty	
II. *Experience and Longevity*	
Years spent in hospital administration education:	
Residency and administrative positions	N, M, F
Years of longevity of College affiliation	M, F
III. *Education*	
Level of Education, general and professional:	
Education in Hospital Administration	N, M, F
Attendance at continuing education programs:	
Independent continuing self education	M, F
IV. *Reputation held by College Affiliates*	
Ethical Conduct	N, M, F
Leadership Activities	M, F
Recommendations and References	N, M, F
V. *Examination*	
Oral, Written	M
VI. *Fellowship projects*	F
Case Reports	
College Thesis	

Experience. In the original constitution, Members were to have five years of experience in "an acceptable institution." Members in good standing for three years might advance to Fellowship by "application and qualification."[18] Age was not used as a criterion, although it was indirectly involved in the experience standard.

Education. At the start, Members were to have "adequate academic education," although they were not required to have a college degree.[19] Elaboration of these standards would come at a later time.

Reputation and Recommendation. Malcolm MacEachern's opinion was important at the beginning of the College. Ethical conduct was considered important. Dewey Lutes remembers the early expulsion of a College member for unethical conduct.[20] By 1973, this process was to become a formalized grievance procedure. As time progressed, the College adjusted and in some instances, completely altered the original membership criteria. Table 6.2 outlines the chronology of these changes. At the start of the College, the Constitution read:

> Application for Membership or Fellowship may be made voluntarily or by invitation. Before the application is considered by the Credentials Committee, all Members and Fellows within the same state as that of the applicant will be asked to render an opinion regarding his or her administrative ability and other qualities. In this respect you are reminded that friendship should not obscure your vision.
>
> Bear in mind that Fellows and Members share the responsibility for maintaining an organization of Dignity and Quality. The Credentials Committee suggests that the present Members and Fellows survey the administrative field in their state and propose the names of those who in their judgment meet the requirements for membership.[21]

Examination. A written examination for advancement from Nomineeship to Membership began in 1951[22] (see Table 6.3 for a partial copy of the 1952 College exam).

Case Reports or Thesis. In 1933, it was proposed that all members submit a yearly thesis on hospital administration. By 1934, this was changed from annually to periodically. By 1938, the thesis had become a one-time requirement for Fellowship, although advancement to Fellowship was possible without it until 1940.[23]

The difficulty of each of these criteria could vary. In 1936, the College had 191 Fellows, 184 Members, and 33 Junior Members. In 1940, there were 334 Fellows, 395 Members, and 161 Associate Members (formerly Junior Members and later to be designated Nominees). By then, some of the Fellows had concluded that it was simply too easy to achieve Fellowship. They felt that the Junior Membership was diluted by "personnel directors, directors of nurses, administrative and executive assistants, chiefs of clinics, chief accountants, superintendents of surgery, purchasing agents, etc."[49] The individuals had gained admittance as Junior Members by having three years experience in responsible hospital positions and by indicating that they desired to prepare themselves for careers in hospital administration. In addition, they had been recommended by a Fellow and had passed an examination.[50]

TABLE 6.2
Changes in College Membership Criteria

1933–1934	Admission to Fellowship by invitation[24]
1934–1935	First admission to Membership by invitation; Membership to be limited to active hospital administrators
1935	Admission by application begins
1938–	Junior Members (Nominees) admitted for the first time.[25]
1940	End of direct admission to Fellowship. From now on the thesis or equivalent will be required for Fellowship.
1941	Strict requirement that the administrator's hospital be accredited was dropped.
1944	Educational Psychologist Consultant hired, for expert advice on examination, content, and evaluation.
1947	Nominee category created replacing Junior Membership, requiring a baccalaureate degree, or the equivalent.
1950–1953	Professional Examination Service employed for exam construction.
1950	Master's degree proposed (but not mandated) as minimum requirement for membership.
1950	Nomineeship required plus examinations, written and oral, before advancement to Membership with some exceptions for candidates with "Extraordinary Qualifications." Up to 1951, written exam essay was typical.[26]
1951	Written objective examinations held in 50 cities for Nominee advancement to Membership. The writing of case reports instead of a thesis becomes typical for advancement to Fellowship.[27]
c. 1960	Special provision made for admission of program faculty.[28]
1965	Annual Revision of written exam starts.[29]
1966	Introduction of structured, oral interview with rigorous standards.[30]
1967	Baccalaureate degree now required for admission, plus 3 years' experience (Baccalaureate equivalency no longer allowed).[31]
1969	Nominee and Membership periods extended by one year each.[32]
1970	Admission of non-hospital health administrators allowed.[33]
1972	66% of College membership now has Master's degree or more.[34]
1974	In-depth review of oral examination for Membership.[35] The administrative residency eliminated as fulfilling a year of administrative experience.[36]
1975	August 18, Regulations Governing Admission and Advancement approved. These remained in effect with revisions into 1993.[37]
1977	Change in entry level, allowing admission of lower level administrators.[38]
1978	96.5% of new Nominees have at least a Master's degree.[39]
1978	April 29, Board of Governors endorses and authorizes proceeding with development of a continuing education lifelong learning program.[40]

TABLE 6.2
Continued

1981	Rapid growth in the number of student associates (3600).[41]
1981	August 31, Revision of Regulations for Advancement[42]
1982	New category of affiliation "Candidate for Nomineeship"[43]
1984	Adoption of Recertification program for Members and Fellows gained approval for two additional fellowship projects, mentorship and continuing education seminars. Development of a new membership exam with a generic core exam and five specialty tracks.[44]
1987	453 Fellows and 552 Members became recertified during the first year of the program.[45]
1988	August 8, Recertification added to Regulations Governing Admission and Advancement. New category of affiliation "Faculty Associate"[46]
1992	Credential Task Force established to recommend changes in Admission, Advancement, and Recertification Regulations.[47]
1993	New Regulations Governing Admission, Advancement, and Recertification.[48]

Admission and Advancement Procedures Upgraded: 1945–1965

In 1944, the College retained an educational psychologist to upgrade admission and advancement procedures.[51] She reported that it would be difficult to improve procedures without a defined criterion of competency in hospital administration. With the help of Ralph W. Tyler, Dean of Graduate Education, University of Chicago, proposals were developed leading to a Kellogg Foundation grant to improve educational courses and to develop more effective procedures for selection and advancement of personnel in the field of hospital administration. This project was undertaken by the ACHA-AHA Joint Commission on Education with Charles Prall serving as the Senior Staff Member.[52]

In 1947, the Educational Policies Committee, chaired by Dr. Robin Buerki, proposed a fund raising effort to develop short course institutes; improve master's degree and internship training; provide scholarships; and improve criteria for selection of hospital administrators. Although little funding was available for this later component, the College continued to work on improving its admission and advancement criteria.[53] In the early 1950s, the Professional Examination Service (PES) was contracted with to develop even more sophisticated examinations. This relationship with the College was to continue.

In 1947, the Junior Membership category was replaced by the Nominee category. Entry into the College required a baccalaureate degree or its equivalent. An R.N. was considered equivalent to two years of college training. In 1950, one college year was equivalent to

TABLE 6.3
American College of Hospital Administrators Examination for Membership, Sample Questions, 1952

Part I.

(Time: One Hour)

Note: Answer numbers 1 and 5 plus any other three questions.

 I. You are the administrator of a 150-bed hospital which operates its own essential facilities or departments, including pharmacy, laundry, bakery, cafeteria, etc. You desire to show the lines of authority and interrelationship of the various departments of your hospital in order that your department heads may fully understand the organization plan. Draw a schematic chart outlining the various relationships from the Governing Board to each of the departmental activities in the hospital.

 II. What is a Medical Audit? From an administrative standpoint, what are its chief advantages?

 III. Outline the essentials of an effective Public Relations Program for the hospital.

 IV. Enumerate briefly the steps which should be taken by the administrator in the preparation of the hospital budget.

 V. Name five evils or abuses in hospital practice against which the administrator must be constantly alert.

 VI. Distinguish between the responsibilities of the Hospital Administrator and the responsibilities of the Governing Body.

 VII. What are the basic causes for shortages of nurses. (etc.)

[A selection of true/false questions from a total of 25 on the exam.*]

TRUE OR FALSE

1. Education is THE principal function of a hospital.
2. The administrator is acknowledged to be the head of the hospital responsible for the physical plant and every act committed therein.
3. The legally constituted governing body has supreme authority for the administration of the hospital.
4. It is considered good policy for a member of the Active Medical Staff to be also a member of the Board of Trustees.
5. Under no circumstances may a patient leave the hospital without the consent of the attending physician.
6. All employees who handle hospital funds should be bonded.

Part III.

(Time: 30 Minutes)

Administrative Problems

(Answer both Problems)

The following problems are given to elicit administrative judgement and analysis in situations which come within the purview of a hospital administrator. There is no one classic solution to either problem. You will be graded solely on the practicability of your answer. ALLOW yourself 15 minutes for each question.

TABLE 6.3
Continued

1. You are the administrator of a hospital and have just been informed of the death of a patient from a serious over-dosage of a potent drug administered by a general duty nurse. It is alleged that the death occurred as a result of an error in the nurse's interpretation of a doctor's correctly written order for the drug. What steps would you take in the complete handling of this death case.
2. You are the administrator of a 150-bed voluntary non-profit general hospital in a midwestern city of 25,000 population.

    Your hospital maintains a favorably known and accepted school of nursing, also an internship and residency training program, although it has no direct university or medical school affiliation. At present the pathologist and the chief of staff in internal medicine are jointly engaged in a modest research study which has been subsidized in part by a grant from a national foundation.

    Your hospital is a major beneficiary of the community chest. In connection with the annual community fund drive, you have been asked "to portray your hospital's picture" to a large mass meeting. Your audience, being a fair cross-section of the community, is quite remote from considerations of medical and nursing education and medical research.

    Someone in the audience wants to know how you justify the teaching and research program at your hospital, the expense of which is not entirely related to patient care. What would you tell the audience?

The correct answers were: Question (1) False, (2) True, (3) True, (4) False, (5) False, (6) True.

a year-and-a-half of administrative experience; two years as an assistant administrator or business manager; and three years as an administrative assistant, supervisor, or department head. Administrative experience outside of healthcare could not count for more than two years. People with master's degrees in hospital administration (one year academic, one year residency) were required to have an additional year of experience. Kipnis stated:

> These comparatively stringent requirements for the rank of Nominee—rank which no longer even brought Membership in the College—indicate the remarkable advance in qualifications which the College had been able to insist upon in less than twenty years. Few professions have been able to make such rapid progress in so short a time. . . .[54]

By 1950, Nomineeship was the required first step, with some exceptions given for candidates with extraordinary qualifications. Prior to 1960, special provision was made for faculty members of approved courses in hospital administration who would otherwise have met the usual requirements of hospital experience required of all other candidates.[55]

In 1951, with the aid of Dr. Lillian Terris, Honorary Fellow, a written examination drawing on 300 true/false questions was developed. These examinations were given in 50 cities in 1951 for advancement from Nomineeship to Membership.[56] This examination remained in place until 1966, when Richard Stull initiated steps to completely overhaul the exam. Table 6.3 illustrates the 1950 examination for admission to Membership. Table 6.4 demonstrates the stages of College affiliation and requirements for advancement as of 1960.

1966–1992

In 1966, after "a year of intensive study," a structured oral interview was introduced and the written exam revised. Prior to this time, the failure rate was only 6 percent. With the new version, failures rose to 28 percent, and remained from 18 to 26 percent for several years after. In 1967, the last group of non-Baccalaureate degree candidates entered Nomineeship. From that time on, all affiliates were required to have an undergraduate degree; no more Baccalaureate equivalencies were accepted.[57]

In 1969, the Council of Regents approved an additional year of tenure as necessary for advancement. So, in 1971, there were no Nominees or Members eligible for advancement, unless they had already accumulated the required seniority.[58] In 1970, the admission criteria were changed to allow the acceptance of candidates holding administrative positions in health-related organizations:

> Health delivery was evolving as a system of many components with varied forms of leadership, but all with a significant impact on the operations of hospitals and health institutions. It was felt that this total leadership should be incorporated under the umbrella of professionalism as represented by the College in order to expedite and facilitate communications and relationships essential for our common goals. . . .[61]

In 1974, admissions requirements were amended:

> . . . calling for the elimination of the residency as fulfilling the requirement for the one year of administrative experience. The genesis of this amendment was a change in the educational practice of the graduate programs. Many of them began offering two years of academic study without a residency and a considerable number continued to offer one year of graduate study and one year of residency education. In a sense, the College's regulations, before they were

TABLE 6.4
Stages of College Affiliation and Requirements as of 1960[59]

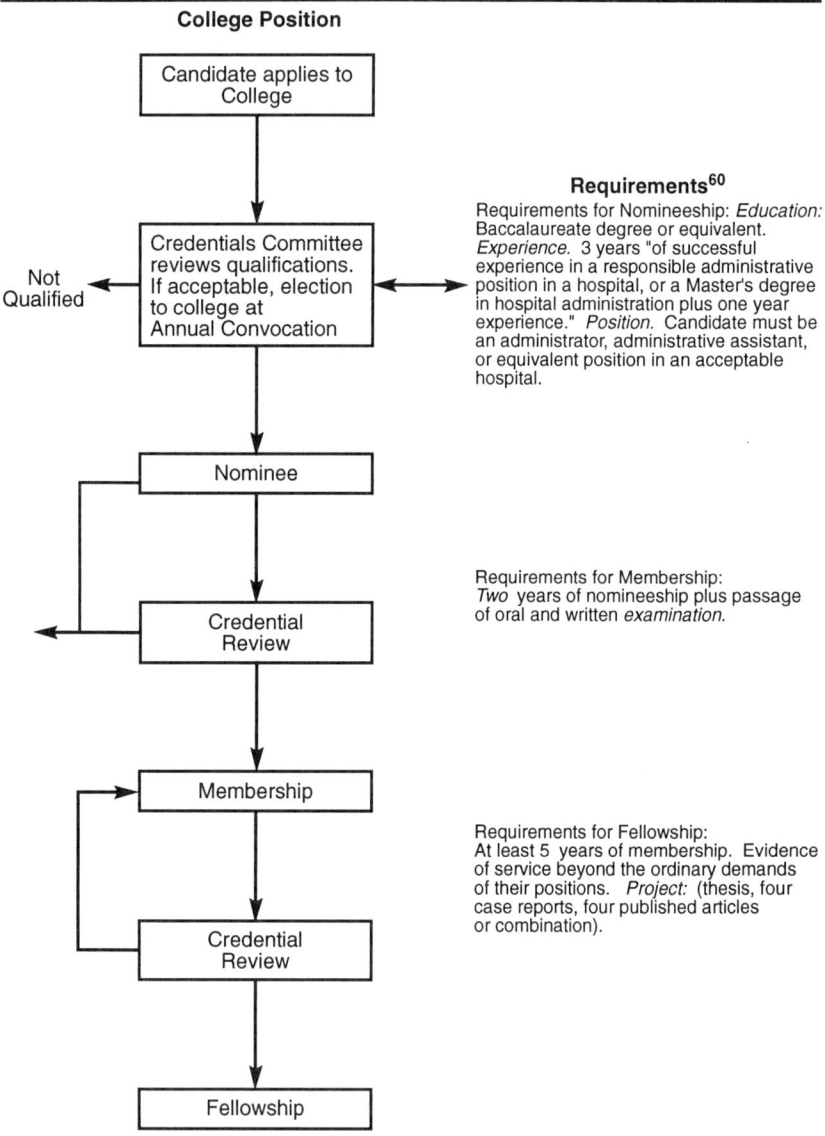

College Position

Candidate applies to College

Requirements[60]

Credentials Committee reviews qualifications. If acceptable, election to college at Annual Convocation

Not Qualified

Requirements for Nomineeship: *Education:* Baccalaureate degree or equivalent. *Experience.* 3 years "of successful experience in a responsible administrative position in a hospital, or a Master's degree in hospital administration plus one year experience." *Position.* Candidate must be an administrator, administrative assistant, or equivalent position in an acceptable hospital.

Nominee

Credential Review

Requirements for Membership: *Two* years of nomineeship plus passage of oral and written *examination.*

Membership

Credential Review

Requirements for Fellowship: At least 5 years of membership. Evidence of service beyond the ordinary demands of their positions. *Project:* (thesis, four case reports, four published articles or combination).

Fellowship

amended, discriminated against the two-year programs, since students of the other programs automatically fulfilled the experience requirement. Similarly, with the waning of interest in the residency on the part of the graduate programs, the experiences of the students, in some cases, were becoming less meaningful; it was doubtful, in fact, that it could validly be given consideration as a measure of expected performance, since it was so basically educational in nature.[62]

In 1977, the admissions requirements were modified to allow acceptance of candidates at lower administrative levels.

This amendment addressed the problems encountered by young men and women who were being graduated in substantial numbers and finding it increasingly difficult to obtain health service positions at a level which met the stipulated requirements of the College. Certainly when one considers the number of candidates competing for a limited number of managerial posts, the diverse factors impacting on the time schedule for ascension on the career ladder to responsible administrative positions, and the desire to involve young men and women early in the affairs of the College in order to inculcate them with the attitude and spirit of professionalism, this was a realistic move.

This amendment in the regulations also had another dimension: it effected a reconsideration of Nominee status in the College. What emerged was the belief that the Nominee period is a time of transition during which there is an opportunity to monitor their progress and adaptability as they proceed up the job ladder. In addition this period of Nomineeship also allows them time for broader exposure to the operations of institutions . . . In other words, Nominee status is to be viewed as a period of transition and development with the Membership examination becoming the real screening device to determine their eligibility for full status in the College and complete identification as a professional.[63]

Several changes were reflected in Richard Stull's words. The growing number of graduate programs made jobs more difficult to find; more junior level positions were taken. At the same time, hospitals grew in size and complexity. Some of the "lower level" jobs carried more responsibility than many senior positions did in the early years of the College. Finally, the number of years spent in middle management by health care administrators grew steadily. Proportionately fewer administrators could become a CEO.

The College reflected these concerns by encouraging the development of local Young Administrator Groups, starting in 1971. By 1978, there were between 58 and 60 of these groups.[64] The College also became more interested in providing job and career information, beginning with the "Career Mart" feature in the *ACHA News* in 1970.[65] By the 1990s *Career Mart* was a separate publication available by subscription.

By 1978, 96.5 percent of all new Nominees had master's degrees or a higher level of academic qualification. In 1947, Kipnis viewed with astonishment the requirement that all new members of the College would have a baccalaureate degree or equivalent. The years between 1947 and 1978 brought another equally remarkable change: by January 1, 1981, the number of student associates reached a record number of 3,600.

By 1992, the College had the following affiliation categories: Nominees, Members, Fellows, Life Members, Life Fellows, Honorary Fellows, as well as Candidates for Nomineeship, Student Associates, and Faculty Associates.[66]

Student Associates after graduation are encouraged to become either Candidates for Nomineeship or Nominees. Graduates who have not been Student Associates can also apply. After three years a nominee may advance to Membership. This requires references, current work in the field, demonstrated leadership, education and the completion of the Board of Governors Examination in Healthcare Management. This examination has 200 general multiple choice questions and 50 questions in a specialty area. There is also an oral interview.[67] The Mock Questions from the Board of Governors Examination of 1992 are shown in Table 6.5.

The Board of Governors Examination questions are grouped into ten categorical function areas. In addition to the generic core exam, there are seven specialty exams of 50 questions each. The importance of the functional areas to the specialties are shown in Table 6.6. There are three functional areas that relate only to the Consultant Specialty.

Membership recertification is now required. A formal application is used. Continuing education of 25 hours of ACHE credits and 25 added hours of College or non-College credits are required over five years. Evidence of participation in health care affairs and community affairs is required along with 6 years tenure as a Member.[69]

Application for Fellowship requires references, work in the field, leadership, education, continuing education and membership for at least six years.[70] A Fellowship project is also required and can take one of three forms: a thesis of about 50 pages, four case reports of 10 to 12 pages each, or two years of structured mentorship with quarterly reports. About 10 percent of applicants choose the thesis, 85 percent choose the case reports and 5 percent choose mentorship.[71] Fellowship recertification is required after ten years of Fellowship. Ninety hours of continuing education are required over the previous nine years in addition to participation in health and community affairs.[72]

TABLE 6.5
1992 Board of Governors (membership) Examination

Written Examination: Mock Questions

1. In a dispute between two staff physicians, the primary role of the chief executive officer is to:
   1. ask a representative of the governing authority to mediate the dispute.
   2. avoid any involvement in the dispute.
   3. meet with both parties as soon as the problem is identified.
   4. request the appropriate chief(s) of service to investigate and report back.
2. Environmental changes, including shifts in public attitudes, community health needs, provider practices and actions of competing institutions, may alter a healthcare institution's direction. Healthcare executives will be forced to:
   1. reduce levels of patient care to the level of payments received.
   2. scrutinize all new ventures from a variety of perspectives, including financial, environmental, ethical and quality of care.
   3. eliminate patient-care programs that do not pay for themselves.
   4. place ceilings on those financial categories of patients that pay less than full operating costs.
3. As a result of the Health Care Finance Administration's action to reimburse healthcare facilities on a prospective basis, action taken in healthcare facilities today is *best* described by the statement that:
   1. governing authorities and physicians are investigating new ways to develop sources of income through joint ventures.
   2. managers and physicians are collaborating in revising medical protocol and in restraining excessive use of tests and procedures.
   3. managers are increasing their marketing efforts to garner more support for new admissions from the medical community.
   4. physicians are reviewing new methods of caring for their patients that could result in lowered length of stay.
4. In selecting a new physician to join a healthcare facility, the chief executive officer should first:
   1. serve as liaison between the medical staff and the governing board.
   2. prepare a statement of duties and responsibilities for review by the governing board.
   3. be cognizant of current trends and practices related to the perquisites of institutional physicians.
   4. interpret to the governing board the significance and the appropriateness of the elements of the proposed contract.
5. Which one of the following classifications or groups of financial ratios would be most useful as a guide to long-range financial viability of an organization to undertake facility replacement?
   1. leverage ratios
   2. profitability ratios
   3. liquidity ratios
   4. composition ratios
6. The *primary* purpose of the quality assurance/risk management program is to:
   1. comply with licensure and accreditation standards as required by state and federal legislation.
   2. monitor medical staff practices in order to control the increases in malpractice rates.
   3. identify potential problems that will keep the hospital from being a party to litigation.
   4. monitor, control and direct the institution's efforts toward achieving delivery of the optimal level of care.

TABLE 6.5
Continued

7. The administrator's relationship with the board of directors should be one in which the administrator:
   1. minimizes board involvement in any operational issues.
   2. draws upon skills of board members to facilitate appropriate discussion and decision-making.
   3. identifies those topics with which the board should involve itself.
   4. serves as the functionary for implementing all board of director's decisions.
8. In consultation with the board, the administrator has decided that an effort must be made to increase the level of involvement among management personnel in quality assessment and assurance. Which one of the following options is most likely to achieve the desired results?
   1. Send all key management personnel to quality assessment workshops over the next year.
   2. Delegate quality assessment functions in question to the medical records committee.
   3. Delegate quality assessment education functions to the utilization review coordinator.
   4. Develop an in-house program using trained key personnel to present and discuss quality assurance and its implications to the organization.
9. A healthcare facility can best meet its social and economic goals by:
   1. developing a realistic and coordinated approach to long-range planning.
   2. devoting most of its efforts to the development of efficient operational practices.
   3. having a good public relations program, which will focus the facility in the community.
   4. providing all reimbursable services desired by the community.
10. The governing body of a healthcare institution meets its responsibility for the quality of patient care by:
   1. delegating accountability for patient care to the committee appointed by the governing body which provides formal administrative liaison between the governing body, the administration and the medical/professional staff.
   2. delegating to the chief executive officer the responsibility for developing criteria to make certain that effective medical/professional audit is carried out.
   3. establishing, maintaining and supporting through the medical/professional staff and management staff an ongoing program of review and evaluation of patient/client care and action on findings.
   4. establishing an effective system for utilization review, medical/professional audit activities and credentialing of the medical/professional staff.

In late 1993, major changes to the regulations were passed; these appear in Appendix A. Table 6.7 and Appendix B summarize the resulting stages of affiliation.

The highlights of the 1993 Credentialing Program changes are as follows:

- All Nominees in the College are now called Associates.
- All Members in the College are now called Diplomates.
- An individual can remain an Associate without ever advancing to Diplomate, provided reappointment requirements are met every six years.

TABLE 6.6
1992 College Membership Examination Categorical Functions and Specialty Exams Allocation of Questions[68]

Categorical Function Area	Generic Core Exam	Specialty Examinations						
		Executive Management Specialty	Consulting	Addiction Treatment	Mental Health	Canadian Healthcare	Marketing	Planning
Governance and Organization	10%	16%	—	—	—	20%	8%	10%
Planning and Marketing	15	24	—	—	12	14	72	54
Human Resources	10	14	—	20	20	10	—	—
Financial and Assets Mgmt.	15	18	—	—	2	16	14	30
Plant and Facility Mgmt.	5	—	—	—	—	—	—	—
Information Systems	5	—	—	—	—	—	—	—
Quality Assessment, Improvement	15	28	—	32	24	24	—	—
Government Regulation and Law	5	—	4	12	12	10	6	6
Organizational Arrangements and Relationships	10	—	—	14	16	—	—	—
Professional Culture, Education, Research, and Ethics	10	—	16	22	14	6	—	—
Business Devel.	—	—	20	—	—	—	—	—
Project Mgmt. and Control	—	—	20	—	—	—	—	—
Consulting Techniques	—	—	40	—	—	—	—	—
Total	100%	100%	100%	100%	100%	100%	100%	100%

TABLE 6.7
Paths to College Admission, Advancement, and Recertification 1993[73]

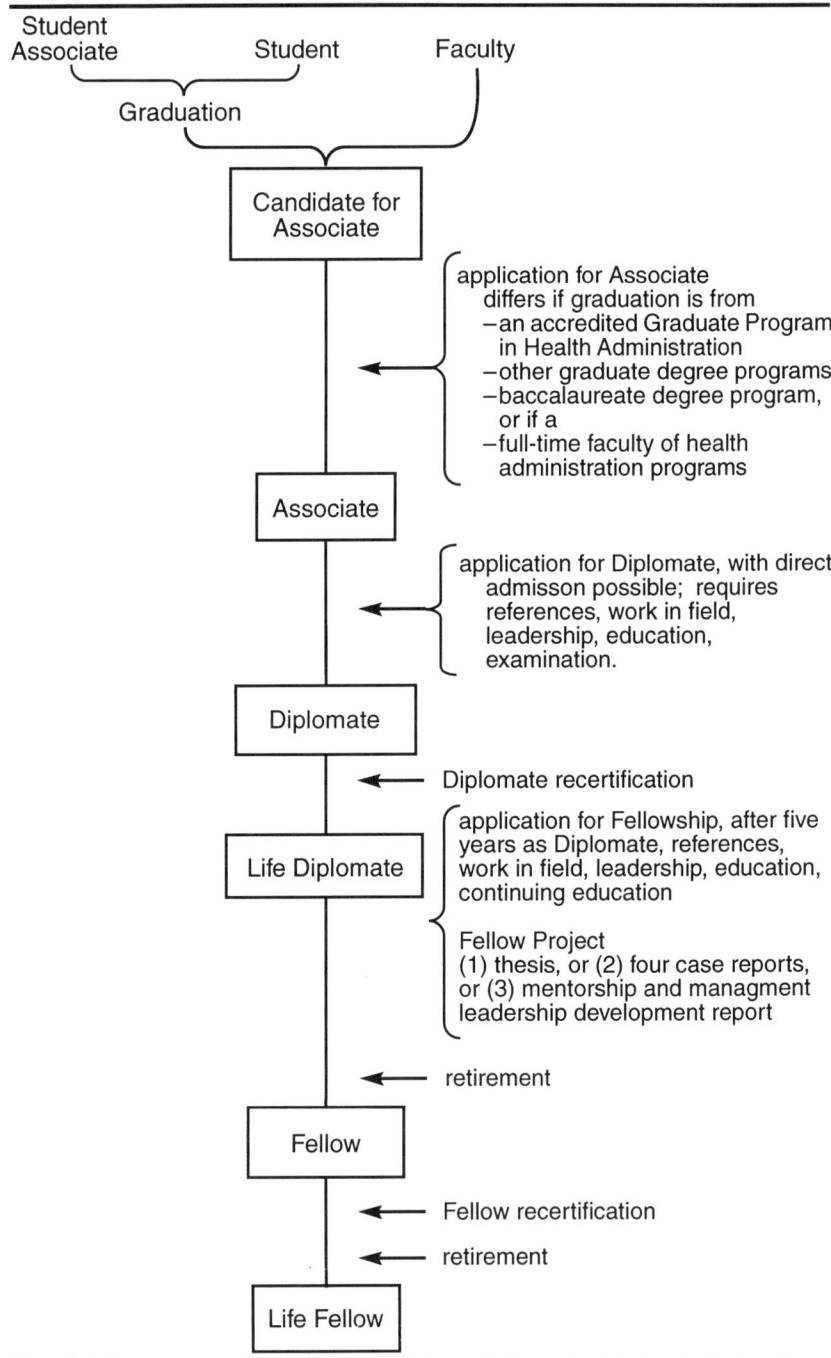

Student
Associate

Student

Faculty

Graduation

Candidate for Associate

application for Associate
differs if graduation is from
−an accredited Graduate Program
in Health Administration
−other graduate degree programs
−baccalaureate degree program,
or if a
−full-time faculty of health
administration programs

Associate

application for Diplomate, with direct
admisson possible; requires
references, work in field,
leadership, education,
examination.

Diplomate

Diplomate recertification

Life Diplomate

application for Fellowship, after five
years as Diplomate, references,
work in field, leadership, education,
continuing education

Fellow Project
(1) thesis, or (2) four case reports,
or (3) mentorship and managment
leadership development report

retirement

Fellow

Fellow recertification

retirement

Life Fellow

- Healthcare executives may join the College as Diplomates, provided the Diplomate eligibility requirements are met, including the successful completion of the Board of Governors Examination in Healthcare Management.
- Diplomates may use the "CHE" (Certified Healthcare Executive) credential after their names.
- An individual must be a Diplomate in good standing for at least five years to be eligible to advance to Fellow.
- ACHE and/or non-ACHE continuing education credits can be used to meet continuing education requirements for Diplomate status.

Self-Assessment

In 1967, the Committee on Membership discussed recertification. In 1969, the Council of Regents gave its first official recognition of the importance of this issue.[74] In the early 1970s, the Committee on Membership continued to pursue this issue, ultimately resulting in the "Proposed Program for Self Development and Recertification" of April 30, 1976. Table 6.8 summarizes the landmarks in the development of the College's self-assessment program. This proposal "embodied the accumulated wisdom of all the task forces, committee deliberations, planning sessions and staff resource information regarding the subject matter."[75]

> During its existence, the College has maintained a program of certification which directly affects at least the first nine years of an administrator's career. In more recent years intense interest and study has been given the concept of recertification.[76]

Recertification was seen as requiring "refined programs of on-the-job performance evaluation, coupled with self-evaluation and planned programs of career development." This proposal typically anticipated six five-year cycles of recertification over 30 years. Recertification would include on-site evaluation of the candidate, personalized counseling, and maintenance of all necessary data by the College.[77]

The program would consist of five parts: (1) self assessment; (2) professional development criteria; (3) continuing education; (4) career education development; and (5) follow-up. The proposed budget was $961,576.[78]

Although this proposal was endorsed by the Board of Governors on September 17, 1976, it underwent further modification and improvement and was resubmitted to the Governors on April 29, 1978.

TABLE 6.8
Self-Assessment Chronology of Events[82]

1965–1970	ACHA Committee on Admissions and Advancements (now the Membership Committee) discusses recertification.[83]
1969	The Council of Regents passes a motion stating that high level career-long education and credentialing are essential concerns of a professional society. The Regents directed the Membership Committee to study the recertification of Fellows.[85]
1970	The Committee on Membership requests a staff plan on recertification.
1971	Anton W. Kovacks' Master's thesis, using College data, provided basis for discussion by the Committee on Membership.[86]
1972	The Committee on Membership asks the Professional Examination Service to submit a proposal for development of a self-testing program.[87]
1973	The Committee on Membership asks the Board of Governors to provide funds for the development of a self-administered examination as an initial step toward career-long certification.
1974	Task Force Report on the Role of the ACHA in Ensuring Competence among Practicing Health Care Administrators.
1975	Task Force on Guidelines for Assessment of Administrative Performance.[88]
April, 1976	Proposed program for self-development and recertification.[89]
September, 1976	The Board of Governors endorses the proposed program of recertification. This leads to further refinement of this program.[90]
April, 1978	Board of Governors re-endorses the self-assessment component of the program.[91]
May, 1979	W. K. Kellogg Foundation funding obtained.[92]
May, 1981	Report on Enhancing Executive Competence.[93]
1981–1982	The development of trial self-assessment exercises jointly by ACHE and Professional Examination Service.[94]
1982	Seventeen self-assessment workshops held throughout the country. About 800 affiliates take the self-assessment.[95]
1983	W. K. Kellogg Grant to develop the Health Executive Self-Assessment workbook.[96]
1983	Development of Administrative Communication Techniques self-assessment (ACT).
March 1983	Congress on Administration organized around the four performance domains of the self-assessment program.[97]

168

TABLE 6.8
Continued

1986	Simulation Self-Assessment for Ambulatory Care and Medical Group Management developed jointly with the American College of Medical Practice Executives taken by about 150 affiliates and 100 ACHE/Practice Executives members yearly.[98]
1989	Revision of the General Management Assessment.[99]
1991	Administrative Communication Techniques (ACT) revised. Taken by about 200 affiliates yearly.[100]

It discussed self-assessment as an essential first step in lifelong learning and career development.[79]

All of these modifications related to the growth of College's educational programs. In 1966, the College provided eight educational sessions with 2,400 attendees; in 1976, the College produced 96 sessions with 5,350 attendees, plus six administrative forums with 3,000 attendees.[80]

There was also increased recognition of diversification in the profession: in organizations employing ACHE affiliates and in the number of functions—notably finance, law, engineering, planning, and marketing.[81]

This two-fold diversity meant that needed skills would vary situationally. Administrative competence would have to match both environment and function. Needs assessment would have to be individualized.

The proposed program of continuing self-assessment is a logical extension of College functions in professional credentialing and continuing education. The program will be designed to serve the following purposes:

- provide health services management personnel with a mechanism for assessing at various stages in their careers their knowledge and skill in practice-relevant areas, and for planning programs of continuing education oriented to career goals; and
- provide the College with a means for guiding and recognizing career-long learning in the profession, and for establishing priorities in the planning of continuing education.

Initially, participation in the self-assessment process was to be elective, open to affiliates of the College who had achieved certification as Members, and those who had advanced to Fellowship. Designing, constructing and testing the self-assessment mechanism was viewed as the next stage of a long-range strategy for extending and refining the certification function of the College, and for developing supporting programs of continuing education in the profession.[101] The proposed budget for the project was $400,000.[102] The Board of Governors approved this self-assessment program on April 29, 1978.

This project was funded by the W. K. Kellogg Foundation, starting in May, 1979, under the direction of a Steering Committee chaired by James D. Harvey.[103] The College project was "to establish a standard of competence and promote excellence in hospital and health administration."[104] It was to provide a confidential, noncompetitive assessment of knowledge and skill that could be used as the basis for developing a personal program for continuing education and lifelong learning.[105] The performance domains covered by the assessment included: Governance and Control; Resource Acquisition and Management; Service Delivery; and Environmental Relations. The Steering Committee convened Specialist Panels for each of these four areas. A random sample of College affiliates was surveyed as to the importance of the topics covered[106] in order to validate the relevance of the assessment content.

The self-assessment instrument consists of "scenario-based," multiple-choice questions. After completing the test, executives received a personalized report profiling their knowledge in 18 key management areas that compared their performance with others in the field.[107] These were reduced to 11 areas by 1990.[108] In addition, a separate track for ambulatory/medical group management was developed in 1986.

In addition, self assessment took several different forms, including an "in basket" exercise and executive writing skills.[109] Another assessment administered by the College during the 1980s as part of its student competition was a computer-based simulation game for six healthcare corporations in one town, with 10 interactions of play. This simulation was developed by faculty at Georgia State University. An important overall goal of these measurement tools was to create assessments that reflect the real work of the manager.[110]

Many linkages were developed through self-assessment. Executives matched their assessments to the skills needed to pursue their chosen career paths. The assessment indicated needed education to both maintain existing skills and develop new ones. For many, this was the basis for a planned educational strategy. Needs were defined, objectives set, and educational methods selected. If goals were met, then the plan was fulfilled.

Whether or not this personalized plan was fulfilled, the self-assessment process could be repeated at some future date. This implied that healthcare managers had shifting priorities for areas of competence that meet both their career objectives and personal needs. It also reflected the growing diversification in health care management. Finally, self-assessment could be the basis for a future move toward recertification for College affiliates.[111]

Self-assessment was also linked closely to career counseling, which became even more important as health care administrators spent more of their careers in middle management positions in multi-institutional systems.

The College's educational programs were keyed closely to self-assessment. The 50 seminars of the 1983 Congress on Administration were grouped according to the four major topic areas of the self-assessment program. Thus, the affiliate could match personally defined needs with seminar content.[112] These linkages continue today.

By 1993, recertification for continued affiliation has become an accepted part of College participation. In 1992, 2,293 affiliates had recertified. In sixty years, the College has worked to improve the way that excellence is assessed as prerequisites to Membership and Fellowship. Recertification and formalizing a commitment to lifelong learning are major steps in the College's future journey. Perhaps the concepts of quality in daily worklife, coming out of the continuous quality improvement movement, will be part of the coming decades.

APPENDIX A
Regulations Governing Admission, Advancement, and Recertification

Worth Noting

The *Regulations Governing Admission, Advancement, and Recertification,* formulated and approved by the Council of Regents, establish the specific procedures by which candidates are admitted, advanced, recertified and continued as affiliates of the American College of Healthcare Executives.

The Credentials Committee, one of the standing committees of the College, is assigned the responsibility to recommend to the Board of Governors the admission, advancement, and recertification of candidates, according to specific regulations and directives from the Council of Regents.

The Membership Committee serves as a resource committee for study and recommendations on special problems relating to the rules and regulations governing the eligibility, admission, advancement, and recertification of affiliates.

These *Regulations Governing Admission, Advancement, and Recertification* were adopted by the College's Council of Regents at its annual meeting on Monday, August 18, 1975, and amended with interpretations through August 10, 1993.

Objects of the College

The objects for which the College is organized are set in the Articles of Incorporation as follows:

To establish standards of competence, to promote excellence in healthcare management, and to formulate and maintain a code of ethics for the profession;

To elevate the standards of efficiency and effectiveness of healthcare management;

To develop and promote standards of education and training for healthcare executives;

To provide a method for conferring the status of Fellowship and to recognize individuals who have performed or have provided noteworthy service in the field of healthcare management;

To educate the public, healthcare professionals and members of governing bodies of healthcare organizations to understand the issues surrounding the practice of healthcare management, including the special role of education and experience;

To provide for healthcare executives the opportunity for gaining continuing education, peer recognition and expanded development in the profession;

To represent the professional interest of healthcare executives in the development and implementation of public policy in concert with appropriate organizations.

Responsibilities of Affiliates

In full recognition of the responsibilities and obligations imposed by position and affiliation with the College, the affiliate shall:

Abide by the Code of Ethics;

Pursue duties with diligence and faithfulness;

Perform executive functions without bias and in the best interest of the institution or agency served;

Avoid the commission of acts that would reflect on personal character or that in any manner would be detrimental to the College, to the community, to the healthcare field, or to the institution or agency;

Follow the recommendations of the College, so far as may be practical, in matters relating to the improvement of healthcare management;

Cooperate and assist in the conduct of studies and surveys undertaken or sponsored by the College by furnishing information, opinions, reports, or in such other manner as may be possible;

Prepare to qualify for advancement through a personal program of continuing education in healthcare management and executive skills;

Make contributions of articles for publication on some phase of healthcare management or on related subjects.

Regulations Governing Admission, Advancement, and Recertification

Affiliates of the American College of Healthcare Executives are categorized as:

Associates, Diplomates, Fellows, Life Diplomates Associate, Life Fellows, Honorary Fellows, Student Associates, Candidates for Nomineeship, Faculty Associates and International Associates. The following requirements govern admission, advancement, and recertification of Nominees, Members, Fellows, and Faculty Associates.

I. Associate
   A. General Requirements
      1. *Forms.* A candidate for admission to the College must submit a formal application on forms prescribed by the College.
      2. *Dates.* The application may be submitted at any time throughout the year. Recommendations for admission to the College are by the Credentials Committee on a continuing year-round basis. Formal admission ceremonies are conducted only at the annual Convocation.
      3. *Information.* The candidate must furnish complete information about the position held and about the organization in which currently employed.
      4. *References and Participation.* The candidate also must submit evidence of high moral character, ethical conduct, participation in health related association activities, and civic affairs. Each applicant must furnish two references from the following: a Fellow, or a Diplomate, or an employer, or a program director.
      5. *Education.* The applicant shall provide information about formal education and such other data as may be requested by the College.
   B. Applicants Holding Graduate Degrees from Accredited Graduate Programs in Healthcare Management
      An applicant who has earned a degree from an accredited graduate program in healthcare management may qualify if:

1. *Within Six Months Post Graduation.* At any time upon graduation from an accredited graduate program and within six months thereafter, the applicant meets the eligibility requirements prescribed by the College (see Interpretation 1).
2. *Six Months or More Post Graduation.*
   a. *Position.* The applicant is engaged in a responsible healthcare management position, or a healthcare management related position which would provide experience to qualify the applicant for a healthcare executive management position (see Interpretations 2, 3); and
   b. *Organization.* The applicant is employed by an acceptable healthcare parent or subsidiary organization or program, or acceptable organization or program influencing the operations, growth and development of organizations, services, and/or programs of the health delivery system (see Interpretation 4); and
   c. *Other.* The applicant in other respects meets the eligibility requirements prescribed by the College.
C. Applicants Holding Graduate Degrees from Other Than Accredited Graduate Programs in Healthcare Management

   An applicant who has not earned a master's degree in healthcare management from an accredited program, but has a graduate degree from a program, college, or university accredited by a regional or national accrediting body may qualify if:
   1. *Position.* The applicant is engaged in a responsible healthcare management position, or a healthcare management related position which would provide experience to qualify the applicant for a healthcare executive management position (see Interpretations 2, 3); and
   2. *Organization.* The applicant is employed by an acceptable healthcare parent or subsidiary organization or program, or acceptable organization or program influencing the operations, growth, and development of organizations, services, and/or programs of the health delivery system (see Interpretations 4); and

3. *Experience.* The applicant has had at least one year of acceptable experience in such a position; and

4. *Other.* The applicant meets all the other requirements prescribed by the College.

D. Applicants Holding Baccalaureate Degrees from a College or University Accredited by a Regional Accrediting Body

An applicant who has not earned a graduate degree from an accredited graduate program but has at least a baccalaureate degree from a college or university accredited by a regional accrediting body may qualify if:

1. *Position.* The applicant is engaged in a responsible healthcare management position, or a healthcare management related position which would provide experience to qualify the applicant for a healthcare executive management position (see Interpretations 2, 3); and

2. *Organization.* The applicant is employed by an acceptable healthcare parent or subsidiary organization or program, or acceptable organization or program influencing the operations, growth, and development of organizations, services, and/or programs of the health delivery system (see Interpretations 4); and

3. *Experience.* The applicant has had at least three years of acceptable experience in such a position; and

4. *Intention.* The applicant declares his or her intention to continue in the field of healthcare management; and

5. *Other.* The applicant in all other respects meets the eligibility requirements prescribed by the College.

E. Applicants Not Holding Formal Degrees

An applicant who has not earned at least a baccalaureate degree may qualify if:

1. *Position.* The applicant is engaged in a senior-level healthcare management leadership position and also meets the acceptable position definition as applied for advancement to Diplomate (see Interpretations 2b, 2c, 3); and

2. *Organization.* The applicant is employed by an acceptable healthcare parent or subsidiary organization or program, or acceptable organization program influencing the operations, growth, and

development of organizations, services, and/or programs of the health delivery system (see Interpretation 4); and

3. *Experience.* The applicant has had at least ten years of acceptable experience in such a position; and

4. *Participation, Leadership, Education.* The candidate must submit evidence of:
   a. Active participation in healthcare management, professional, and educational activities (see Interpretation 5);
   b. Service beyond the ordinary demands of position; and

5. *Other.* The applicant in all other respects meets the eligibility requirements prescribed by the College.

6. *Eligibility Period.* This option shall remain in effect only until August 9, 1994. Associates admitted under this option may advance to Diplomate at any time before or after August 9, 1994, if they have twelve years' healthcare management experience in a leadership position and have met all other requirements.

F. Faculty

Faculty, researchers, or directors of acceptable graduate and undergraduate programs in healthcare management, if holding full-time appointments within the programs, may be eligible for admission and advancement in the College.

G. Eligibility of Position for Advancement

Eligibility of a position for admission does not give prima facie indication that the same position may be eligible for advancement.

H. Essential Dates

1. *Application.* All technical requirements for admission must exist:
   a. At the time the application is filed; and
   b. At the time the Credentials Committee considers the application.

2. *Request for Advancement to Diplomate.* Upon completion of two years as an Associate, an Associate, at personal discretion, may request the Credentials Committee to determine the candidate's worthiness and eligibility for advancement, and to grant permission to complete the required Board of Gover-

nors Examination in Healthcare Management. Advancement to Diplomate is not mandatory for Associates to maintain affiliation in the College.

3. *Reappointment.* Reappointment to Associate status is required every six years. Applicants for reappointment must provide evidence of 25 hours of Category I (ACHE education) and 25 hours of Category I or Category II (non-ACHE education) credit over the previous five years, as well as evidence of participation in healthcare and community affairs (see Interpretations 5, 6). Two references are required. Fellows of the College, Diplomates of the College, employers and program directors from programs in healthcare management may serve as references.

II. Diplomate
   A. General Requirements
      1. *Forms.* A candidate must submit a formal application on forms prescribed by the College.
      2. *When to Submit.* It is not necessary for an individual to be an Associate before advancing to Diplomate, provided he or she meets all other requirements.
      3. *Deadline Date.* The application must be received by the dates announced by the College before the candidate will be allowed to take the Board of Governors Examination.
      4. *References, Participation, Leadership, Education.* The candidate must submit adequate evidence of:
         a. High moral character and ethical conduct; each candidate must furnish two references, one a Fellow and the second a Fellow or Diplomate of the College.
         b. Active participation in healthcare management, professional, and educational activities. A candidate is expected to participate in an average of 10 hours of continuing education annually. A total of 20 hours of Category I or II credit is required over the most recent two-year period. (see Interpretations 5 and 6);
         c. Service beyond the ordinary demands of position, and
         d. Fulfillment of Responsibilities of Affiliates as listed in the *Regulations Governing Admission, Advancement and Recertification* of the College.
            (Note: Refer to Section IV, Regulations Gov-

erning Advancement to Fellowship, for guidance in developing a program of professional maturity and growth.)

B. Eligibility Requirements

A candidate may submit application for Diplomate status following:

1. a master's degree plus two years' healthcare management experience; or

2. a bachelor's degree plus five years' healthcare management experience: or

3. twelve years' healthcare management experience in a senior-level leadership position, but no formal degree, effective only until August 9, 1994. Associates admitted under the no-degree option may advance to Diplomate at any time before or after August 9, 1994, if they have twelve years' healthcare management experience in a senior-level leadership position and have met all other requirements.

C. Specific Requirements

To complete advancement to Diplomate, a candidate must:

1. *Position.* Be engaged in a healthcare executive management position or a healthcare management related position of equal responsibility (see Interpretations 2 and 3); and

2. *Organization.* Be employed by an acceptable healthcare parent or subsidiary organization or program, or acceptable organization or program influencing the operations, growth, and development of organizations, services, and/or programs of the health delivery system (see Interpretations 4); and

3. *Information.* Furnish complete information about position and the organization in which presently employed, and such other data as may be requested by the Credentials Committee. The application and the evidence thereon must meet fully all requirements prescribed by the Council of Regents as evaluated by the Credentials Committee.

4. *Examinations.* Complete satisfactorily the Board of Governors Examination in Healthcare Management. The candidate must be authorized by the Credentials Committee to take the examinations to proceed with advancement to Diplomate.

5. *Other.* Meet all other requirements prescribed by the College.
D. Essential Dates
   All technical requirements for advancement to Diplomate must exist:
   1. At the time the Request for Advancement to Diplomate is filed;
   2. At the time the Credentials Committee considers the Request;
   3. At the time the Board of Governors Examination in Healthcare Management is taken by the candidate (see Interpretation 7).
III. Diplomate Recertification
   A. General Requirements
      1. *Forms.* A Diplomate must submit a formal application on forms prescribed by the College.
      2. *When to Submit.* The application must be submitted after five years of Diplomate status or recertification of Diplomate status.

         (Note: For purposes of initial implementation of the recertification regulations, the application must be submitted in accordance with the following schedule by Diplomates in active status at the time of recertification regulations approval. August 1986.

Months in active Diplomate status	Applications must be submitted by deadline date after Convocation
143 or more	1990
83–142	1991
35–82	1992
1–34	1993

Candidates advanced to Diplomate in 1986 and thereafter will begin a six year recertification cycle at the time of advancement.

All active Diplomates with at least 60 months in active status may submit an application. Diplomates who submit applications and complete the requirements at any time prior to their mandatory application submission date will be deemed to have met the requirements at the Convocation following their mandatory application submission date. Subsequent recertification of these Diplomates will proceed on a six year cycle.)

3. *Deadline Dates.* Applications must be received by the dates announced by the College prior to the sixth year following advancement to Diplomate or recertification of Diplomate status.

4. *Other.* The Diplomate must submit adequate evidence of fulfillment of applicable Responsibilities of Affiliates as listed in the *Regulations Governing Admission, Advancement, and Recertification* in the College.

B. Specific Requirements

To complete recertification at the Diplomate level, a Member must provide sufficient documentation and evidence of completing one of the following alternatives since the last advancement or recertification date.

1. *Advancement to Fellow.* Meet all requirements for advancement to Fellow.

2. *Continuing Education.* Earn five hours of Category I credit and five hours of Category II credit on average for each year of Diplomate status. Diplomates applying for recertification would be expected to have a total of 50 hours of continuing education over the previous five years, no less than half of which must be Category I credit.

Diplomates must also show evidence of participation in healthcare and community/civic affairs, although no specific number of hours is required. (see Interpretations 5, 6)

Because the College has communicated other options for recertification since 1986, the College will accept those options for recertification, if affiliates choose them by the end of 1997.

C. Essential Dates

All technical requirements for recertification at the Diplomate level must exist:

1. At the time the application for recertification is filed; and

2. At the time the Credentials Committee considers the application.

D. Waiver of Recertification Requirements for Candidates Age 60 Years or More.

Mandatory candidates age 60 or more may request a waiver of recertification. This waiver is offered on a one-

time, five-year basis upon request of the candidate. If
after that five-year period the mandatory recertification
candidate has not retired or met the recertification requirements, the candidate will be placed on inactive status.

IV. Fellow

(Note: A candidate, having met the criteria of admission,
may be eligible to proceed under the *Regulations Governing
Admission, Advancement, and Recertification* without regard to
academic background, provided the candidate meets other
requirements pertaining to advancement.)

A. General Requirements

1. *Forms.* A candidate must submit a formal application on forms prescribed by the College.

2. *Deadline Date.* Applications may be submitted any time
during the year. However, applications should be
received by the dates announced by the College prior
to the year at which advancement may be completed.

3. *References, Participation, Leadership, Education.* The
candidate must submit evidence of:

a. High moral character and ethical conduct. Each
candidate must furnish three references, all of
whom shall be Fellows of the College. The Credentials Committee may select at least three additional Fellows as references;

b. Active participation in healthcare management,
professional, and educational activities. A candidate is expected to participate in an average of
10 hours of continuing education annually (see
Interpretations 5, 6). A total of 50 hours of continuing education credit is required over the most
recent five-year period. At least 25 of these hours
must be Category I;

c. Service beyond the ordinary demands of position; and

d. Fulfillment of Responsibilities of Affiliates as listed
in the *Regulations Governing Admission, Advancement, and Recertification.*

4. *Other.* Meet all the other requirements prescribed by
the College.

B. Specific Requirements

To complete advancement to Fellow, a candidate must:

1. *Longevity.* Have been a Diplomate in good standing for at least six years (see Interpretations 8, 9); and
2. *Position.* The applicant is engaged in a healthcare executive management position or a healthcare management related position of equal responsibility (see Interpretations 2 and 3); and
3. *Organization.* The applicant is employed by an acceptable healthcare parent or subsidiary organization or program, or acceptable organization or program influencing the operations, growth and development of organizations, services, and/or programs of the health delivery system (see Interpretations 4); and
4. *Fellow Projects.* Complete a Fellow project. Active Diplomates may complete one of the following alternatives to satisfy the requirement for a Fellow project:
   a. *Write a Thesis.* A thesis is a presentation based on an investigation of a specific subject selected by the candidate. Simply abstracting or compiling data will not be acceptable. The subject may be directly in the field of healthcare management in other related fields. A thesis must follow the printed instructions outlined in the *Guide for the Preparation of Fellowship Projects,* which is available upon request. A thesis prepared for other than the American College of Healthcare Executives is not acceptable unless the other organization is a professional healthcare management society acceptable to the Board of Governors. In all respects, theses submitted under this regulation must meet the current project standards for approval to be granted.
   b. *Write Case Reports.* The candidate may prepare four Case Reports on some facet of healthcare management. A Case Report is a written account of an actual administrative problem encountered in the candidate's healthcare management experience. Case Reports must follow the instructions outlined in the printed *Guide for the Preparation of Fellowship Projects,* furnished upon request.
   c. *Conduct a Mentorship/Write a Management Leadership Development Report.* The candidate (a chief

executive, chief operating officer, or comparable position) may serve as a mentor to a junior level executive in the same organization for at least a two year period or may serve as a mentor to two one-year postgraduate fellows or one two-year postgraduate fellow. Selections of candidate to mentor must be subject to screening by the Credentials Committee. The Mentorship is a highly structured advanced management leadership development experience which documents involvement, judgment and leadership development capability of the candidate, while providing practical management development literature for the field. A Mentorship project must follow the printed instructions outlined in the *Guide for the Preparation of Fellowship Projects* which is available upon request.

d. *Project Approval.* Any time after advancement to status of Diplomate, approval of Thesis topics, Case Report topics or Mentorship proposal may be sought from the Credentials Committee. Topics or proposals must be submitted in accordance with the requirements outlined in the *Guide for the Preparation of Fellowship Projects,* furnished at the time of advancement to Diplomate or upon request.

e. *Submission of Projects.*

(1) *Thesis.* A completed Thesis may be submitted for evaluation by the Credentials Committee after the candidate becomes a Diplomate.

(2) *Case Reports.* Completed Case Reports may be submitted for evaluation by the Credentials Committee after the candidate becomes a Diplomate.

(3) *Mentorship/Management Leadership Development Report.* The plan and quarterly reports may be submitted after the candidate becomes a Diplomate and has received approval of the Mentorship proposal. A final management leadership development report must be submitted upon completion of the project. A Diplomate may formally withdraw from this project at any time, without prejudice.

f. *Deadline for Projects.* The Credentials Committee reviews completed Fellow projects between September 1 and May 1 each year. Projects must be submitted by May 1 of each year to participate in the Convocation ceremony that year.

g. *Acceptance of Projects.* Completed projects must meet the approval of the Credentials Committee before it may recommend completion of advancement.

h. *Publication and Presentation Rights.* A candidate who submits a Fellowship Project shall forfeit all publication and presentation rights to the College and shall grant permission to the College to publish and present this material. However, the College will cooperate with candidates who may have an opportunity to publish or present material based upon their project. Additionally, the College will respect proprietary rights of other professional healthcare management societies where these may previously exist and grant confidentiality of projects when required.

C. Essential Dates

All technical requirements for advancement to Fellow must exist:

1. At the time the Request for Advancement to Fellow is filed;

2. At the time that the Credentials Committee considers the Request; and

3. When the authorized Fellow projects are submitted for review by the Credentials Committee.

V. Fellow Recertification

A. General Requirements

1. *Forms.* A Fellow must submit a formal application on forms prescribed by the College.

2. *When to Submit.* The application must be submitted after nine years of eligible Fellowship or recertification of Fellow status.

(Note: For purposes of initial implementation of the recertification regulations, the application must be submitted in accordance with the following schedule for Fellows in active status at the time of recertification regulations approved, August 1986.

Months in active Fellow status	Applications must be submitted by deadline date after Convocation
227 or more	1990
155–226	1991
95–154	1992
59–94	1993
35–58	1994
1–34	1995

All active Fellows with at least 108 months in active status may submit an application. Fellows who submit applications and complete requirements at any time prior to their mandatory application submission date will be deemed to have met the requirements at the Convocation following their mandatory application submission date. Subsequent recertification of these Fellows will proceed on a ten year cycle.)

3. *Deadline Dates.* Applications must be received by the dates announced by the College prior to the tenth year following advancement to Fellow or recertification of Fellow status.

4. *Other.* The Fellow must submit adequate evidence of fulfillment of applicable Responsibilities of Affiliates as listed in the *Regulations Governing Admission, Advancement, and Recertification* in the College.

B. Specific Requirements

Earn five hours of Category I credit and five hours of Category II credit on average for each year as a Fellow. Fellows applying for recertification would be expected to have 90 hours of continuing education over the previous nine years, no less than half of which must be Category I credit.

Fellows must also show evidence of participation in healthcare and community/civic affairs, although no specific number of hours is required. (see Interpretations 5, 6)

Because the College has communicated other options for recertification since 1986, the College will accept those options for recertification, if affiliates choose them by the end of 2001.

C. Essential Dates

All technical requirements for recertification at the Fellow level must exist:

1. At the time the application for recertification is filed; and

2. At the time the Credentials Committee considers the application.

D. Waiver of Recertification Requirements for Candidates Age 60 Years or More.

Mandatory candidates age 60 or more may request a waiver of recertification. This waiver is offered on a one-time, five-year basis upon request of the candidate. If after that five-year period the mandatory recertification candidate has not retired or met the recertification requirements, the candidate will be placed on inactive status.

VI. Interpretations

1. *Accredited Program.* Accreditation by the Accrediting Commission on Education for Health Services Administration—for purposes of Admission only—is the criterion for a graduate degree from an accredited program in healthcare management.

2. *Position Eligibility.*

a. Entry level positions of department head, staff positions, and specialty are eligible for purposes of admission. All applicants and Associates must be informed that the positions found acceptable for purposes of admission may not be found acceptable for purposes of advancement to the status of Diplomate.

b. For purposes of advancement, the technically eligible positions may include chief executive officers, associate and assistant administrative officers, and administrative assistant positions as well as specialty management positions of comparable executive authority.

c. *Position Other than Chief Executive.* Eligibility of management positions other than the chief executive officer shall be determined on a functional basis. While the eligibility of the candidate shall be determined primarily by the duties performed and the responsibilities carried, the title of the position should indicate management responsibility.

d. *Postgraduate Fellowships.* Postgraduate fellowships or residencies in the practice world which relate to "assistant to" position descriptions and provide support to decision making may be eligible as acceptable positions. However, postgraduate fellowships as part of academic programs or curricula in pursuit of either an additional degree or development of a research paper are not acceptable for eligibility of position for admissions and advancements.

e. *Position—Permanent Part-Time.* Permanent part-time positions, based on job descriptions and at least a three day, full-day work week, may be eligible for purposes of admission and advancement.

3. *Related Healthcare Management Activity.* May include consultants, regulatory agencies, health associations, health centers, and emerging healthcare systems and organizations as well as academic appointments.

4. *Organization Acceptability.* Acceptability is determined on the basis of the organization's or program's function and mission related to the provision of healthcare services. Organizations whose primary mission includes direct patient or client care services are acceptable in keeping with the other provisions of these Regulations. Organizations or programs whose primary mission includes activities which influence the growth, development, or operations of healthcare organizations, such as healthcare associations, healthcare consulting firms, healthcare management or holding companies, among others, are acceptable. Non-healthcare organizations are acceptable if the candidate's program is a healthcare delivery component of the organization or a component which influences the growth, development, or operations of healthcare organizations. Examples include educational programs in healthcare management clinics, regulatory agencies, general management consulting companies with a discrete healthcare consulting practice, among others.

5. *Participation.* The candidate must present evidence of:

a. Participation in the affairs of the College or other community, state, regional, or nationally recognized activities in the health field—denoting interest and contribution in the specialized area of health services;

b. Service as a professional, leadership potential, and the capacity and devotion to further and improve management as a profession; and

c. Significant participation in local, state, regional, or national health affairs with any of a variety of recognized essential groups or agencies for the purpose of improving and advancing healthcare.

6. *Continuing Education.* It is mandatory that every candidate be concerned with, and give evidence of, continued personal growth and development through a program of continuing education designed to enhance management effectiveness and to broaden potential for contribution in a variety of professional endeavors related to the field of health. The candidate must present evidence of continuing education by registration as a participant or service as a faculty member in programs of continuing or postgraduate education offered by the College, universities or colleges, healthcare associations, or other professional organizations or educational groups which afford exposure to learning in areas of knowledge applicable to management in the health field.

a. *For Advancement and Recertification.* As of the date of admission, advancement, or recertification of current status, as applicable, a candidate is expected to participate in the required amount of contact hours of Category I and Category II continuing education.

A contact hour for face to face type programs is defined as 60 minutes of instructional time, and excludes time allotted to meals and breaks and other time not dedicated to instruction. A contact hour for self-directed programs is defined on the basis of equivalency of the particular program type to face to face type programs. Consideration is given to the level of participant effort required and effectiveness of the learning methodology.

Category I Programs:

i. any face to face continuing education programs, seminars, institutes, Congresses, or conferences conducted by the College.

ii. certain specifically designated College self-directed educational programs.

This classification is made because programs developed by the College have had content and instructional effectiveness for affiliates developed and thoroughly validated under direct supervision of the College's Division of Education.

Category II Programs:

All other face to face continuing education programs conducted or sponsored by any organization qualified to provide educational programming in management.

All Category II programs will be reviewed by the Credentials Committee at the time of advancement or recertification application review. The Committee will review program title, program provider and program length in contact hours for appropriateness.

b. *Other.*

(1) *General.* The requirement of continuing education for purposes of advancement and recertification including attendance at Category I education programs is applied uniformly and no waiver can be made based on formal academic education programs in lieu of the currently required attendance at Category I education programs, except as may be applicable for specific recertification purposes.

(2) *Acceptable Experience/Education Requirements.* The present criteria for an eligible position and for longevity of position will be maintained, as well as the criteria for continuing education; thus, pursuit of a doctoral program is not acceptable as management experience time, nor position, nor does it fulfill the requirement of a personal program of continuing education.

(3) *Company Sponsored Continuing Education.* Attendance at company-sponsored education programs would not fulfill the criteria for at-

tendance at Category I education programs except in the event a company contacted the College to provide an established Category I program for presentation to personnel; and company programs of in-service education be reflected as a part of the continuing education program of the individual candidate, but in-service education programs may not replace expected attendance at Category I or Category II continuing education programs.

7. *Admission or Advancement by Examination.* Under no circumstances will the Board of Governors examination requirement be waived, unless otherwise provided under these regulations or by a duly approved reciprocity agreement.

8. *Tenure as Diplomate.* To establish tenure as a Diplomate, the required years must be spent in a healthcare management position. The question of the acceptability of nonconsecutive years in an acceptable position will be left to the discretion of the Credentials Committee.

9. *Date of Advancement.* Candidates who meet all requirements for advancement to the status of Diplomate or Fellow will be granted Diplomate or Fellow status immediately. The certificate attesting to the status of Diplomate or Fellow will carry the date of the Convocation of that year.

10. *Eligible Longevity.* Periods of inactive status do not apply toward fulfillment of tenure requirements.

VII. Supplemental Information

1. *Identification—Key and FACHE Designation.* (Adopted policy)

   a. Fellows and Diplomates may wear the official key of the College.

   b. Fellows are encouraged to use the designation "FACHE" following their names on official stationary, articles for publication, and on other appropriate occasions. Diplomates are encouraged to use the designation "CHE" (Certified Healthcare Executive) following their names on official stationary, articles for publication, and other appropriate occasions. Associates are not privileged to use these or any similar designation.

   c. If a Fellow or Diplomate resigns, is expelled, or becomes inactive, the key shall be returned and the use of the designation FACHE or CHE shall be discontinued.

2. *Insurance Program.* Participation in the College's Association Group Insurance Program is available during active status in the College, or after transfer to inactive status and then, only when the affiliate is at least a Diplomate and 55 years of age or older. Otherwise, a conversion privilege may be invoked.

3. *College Year.* The College Year begins with adjournment of the Council of Regents annual meeting. Length of tenure is based on the date on which the applicant was admitted, advanced or recertified.

4. *Annual Dues.* Assessment of dues for new Associates will be on the basis of 1/12th of the annual dues per month, effective the first of the month following the month in which Associate status is conferred. Diplomate/Fellow dues become effective January 1 following the year in which Diplomate/Fellow is granted.

5. *Waiver of Associate Dues for Graduates of Accredited Graduate Programs in Healthcare Management Who Apply Within Six Months.* The pro-rata portion of annual dues will be waived for new Associates who are graduates of programs accredited by the Accrediting Commission on Education for Health Services Administration who have applied within six months post graduation.

6. *Waiver of Dues for Unemployed Affiliates.* An unemployed affiliate, who is actively seeking employment as a healthcare executive, and who is not working in any paid capacity with a healthcare organization, may, upon request, have dues waived while continuing to hold the same affiliate status for up to two years past the current year for which dues have been paid.

7. *Life Status.* A Diplomate or Fellow who meets the criteria for Life status may request this privilege at personal discretion. Conferral of Life status is not automatic nor retroactive.

   Bylaws of the College authorize conferral of Life status under the policies adopted by the Board of Governors and approved by the Council of Regents.

A Fellow or Diplomate may, of course, continue active status without regard to age. Life status (which is an active status) provides for continuation of all rights and privileges of the College (except that of being eligible for elective office), without payment of dues.

The purpose of Life status is to recognize the loyalty and support of affiliates who reach retirement and no longer are involved with earning income.

Criteria for Life Diplomate and Life Fellow are as follows:

Age	Full dues paying years as Diplomate and/or Fellow
60	25
61	24
62	23
63	22
64	21
65	20

Any Fellow or Diplomate who has suffered a permanent disability and is unable to work full-time is eligible for life status regardless of age or years of service.

8. *Inactive Status.*

   a. *Associate.* In the case of an Associate who does not complete reappointment by the end of six years as an Associate, the Board of Governors may designate inactive status. During inactive status the candidate may ask the Credentials Committee to determine technical eligibility to take the Board of Governors Examination for advancement to Diplomate. On successful completion of the examination, the candidate may be reinstated and proceed with advancement. The candidate may also ask the Credentials Committee to determine eligibility to be reappointed as an Associate, once reappointment requirements are met.

   b. *General.* In instances where the affiliate leaves the field of healthcare management, or for other valid reasons does not prefer to maintain active status, a request for transfer to inactive status may be made while dues are in a paid condition, to the

Board of Governors (see Interpretation 10). This may be done only while the affiliate is in good standing with paid dues.

c. *Inactive on Recertification.* In instances where a Diplomate or Fellow does not fulfill recertification requirements within the allotted time frame, the affiliate will be designated as inactive on recertification pending final action for this status by the Board of Governors. A Diplomate pursuing advancement to Fellow may request a one-year administrative extension (beyond the six year time frame) to complete advancement activities when the affiliate's Fellow project is deferred in the sixth year and avoid an automatic change to inactive on recertification status.

9. *Reinstatement*

a. *From Inactive Status—Associate and General.* Reinstatement to active status may be requested and may be granted when the inactive affiliate is in a position which would be determined to be technically eligible for advancement.

b. *From Inactive on Recertification Status.* Reinstatement to active status may be requested and may be temporarily granted when the inactive affiliate submits a recertification application prior to the final recertification application deadline date of the College year. The application must provide sufficient documentation and evidence that the affiliate has fulfilled the recertification requirements. Final action on reinstatement is subject to Board of Governors approval.

c. *From Suspended Status.* Reinstatement to active status may be requested and may be granted when the suspended affiliate is in a position which would be determined to be technically eligible for advancement.

d. *Dues.* From inactive or suspended status, reinstatement will be granted upon payment of pro-rated current year dues based on months in active status.

e. *Reinstatement—Severance by Ethics Action.* An affiliate dropped for ethical reasons may reapply for Associate, if the individual so wishes. The Credentials Committee may handle, on an individual basis without obligation to reinstate an individual at a former level, such reapplications for admission from persons dropped for ethical reasons.

f. *Ethics Committee Review.* Where the prior inactive, suspension or resignation action relating to the reinstatement request occurred "under a cloud" of potential action by the Ethics Committee, or where the applicant was previously dropped for ethical reasons, the Ethics Committee will first review the reinstatement request and make a recommendation to the Credentials Committee to support or deny reinstatement based on the applicant's ethical conduct up to the time of the Ethics Committee review of the request or application.

10. *Guidance for Advancement and Recertification.* You may refer to your personal copy of the *Log Book for Advancement/Recertification* for general guidance on advancement or recertification.

11. *Requests for Information.* Requests for information regarding any of the matters mentioned in this pamphlet may be directed to:
Division of Membership
American College of Healthcare Executives
840 North Lake Shore Drive
Chicago, IL 60611

APPENDIX B
Changes to the ACHE Credentialing Program

Following is information on the revised credentialing program adopted in August 1993, including requirements for each status. **The changes to the requirements are in bold type.**

I. **Associate** (Replaces Nominee Status)

The Associate title was adopted to more appropriately describe this entry-level, noncredentialed status. It is also consistent with the ACHE titles of Student Associate and Faculty Associate. In addition, it is hoped that the Associate title will be more attractive to experienced healthcare executives.

The most significant change related to this status allows an Associate to remain in this status without advancing as long as he or she meets reappointment requirements every six years. Requirements for **Associate** status are:

1. A. Master's degree plus one year healthcare management experience (experience requirement waived for graduates of programs accredited by the Accrediting Commission on Education for Health Services Administration), or

   B. Bachelor's degree plus three years' healthcare management experience, or

   C. No degree plus 10 years' healthcare management experience in a leadership position. This option shall remain in effect only until August 9, 1994.

   This change is intended to attract experienced executives who may be influential leaders in the field.

2. **Two references,** either from Fellows of the College, Diplomates of the College, employers, or directors of health services administration programs.

   One reference was required in the past. Because Associates may elect to remain in Associate status, the additional reference is required.

3. Position

   A responsible healthcare management position or a healthcare management related position that would provide experience to qualify the applicant for a healthcare executive management position. Entry-level positions of department head, staff positions, and specialty areas are eligible for purposes of admission.

4. **Reappointment**

   Reappointment to Associate status is required every six years. Associates applying for reappointment are expected to have a total of 50 hours of continuing education over the previous five years, no less than half of which is Category I (ACHE education) credit. The remainder may be Category I or Category II (non-ACHE education) credit. Evidence of participation in community and healthcare affairs is also required. Two references are required. Fellows of the College, Diplomates of the College, employers, and directors of health services administration programs may serve as references.

   (Reappointment will not be required until 1999.)

   This option eliminates mandatory advancement. Although encouraged to advance, Associates who do not advance will be allowed to retain all benefits of affiliation.

II. **Diplomate** (Replaces Member Status)

The Diplomate title was adopted to better recognize successful completion of the Board of Governors Examination in Healthcare Management. It also is consistent with the title bestowed on board-certified physicians and is well respected among the medical staff community.

Following successful completion of the Board of Governors exam, individuals are allowed to use "CHE" (Certified Healthcare Executive) after their names. The CHE designation is intended to be an incentive for advancement. It is also designed to increase the visibility of the credential among board members, the medical staff, and the public. Finally, it is consistent with the practice of the Canadian College of Health Service Executives.

Requirements for **Diplomate** status are:

1. A. Master's degree plus **two years'** healthcare management experience.

   (As an incentive for advancement, one less year of experience is required) or

   B. Bachelor's degree plus **five years'** healthcare management experience.

   (As an incentive for advancement, one less year of experience is required) or

   C. **No degree plus 12 years' healthcare management experience in a leadership position. This option shall remain in effect only until August 9, 1994.**

   This change is intended to attract experienced healthcare executives who may be leaders in the field.

2. Two references, one from a Fellow and the second from a Fellow or Diplomate of the College.

3. Position

   A healthcare executive management position or a healthcare management related position of equal responsibility.

4. Continuing education

   20 hours of Category I (ACHE education) credit or **Category II (non-ACHE education) credit over the previous two years.**

   This change gives experienced healthcare executives with Category II credit only the opportunity to enter directly into Diplomate status.

5. Evidence of participation in community/civic and healthcare affairs.

6. Successful completion of the Board of Governors Examination in Healthcare Management.
7. Diplomate recertification

     Recertification of Diplomate status is mandatory every six years. Diplomates applying for recertification are expected to have a total of 50 hours of continuing education over the previous five years, no less than half of which is Category I (ACHE education) credit. The remainder may be from Category I or Category II (non-ACHE education) credit. Evidence of participation in community and healthcare affairs is also required.
III. Fellow

Fellow status is reserved for healthcare executives who have made significant contributions to the field. Fellowship in the College is the highest level of distinction.

Requirements for **Fellow** status are:
1. Longevity

     Applicants must have been a Diplomate in good standing for at least **five** years.

     The longevity requirement has been reduced from six years to five years in response to affiliate requests to shorten the length of time an affiliate must wait to advance to Fellow.
2. Position

     A healthcare executive management position or a healthcare management related position of equal responsibility.
3. Three references, all from Fellows of the College.
4. Continuing education

     50 hours of continuing education, **25 of which must be Category I (ACHE education) credit** and the remainder of which may be Category I or Category II (non-ACHE education) credit.

     The previous requirement was 50 hours of continuing education, including a minimum of 20 hours of Category I credit. The remainder could be Category I or Category II credit. This change makes the continuing education requirement for advancement to Fellow consistent with the continuing education requirement for Diplomate recertification.
5. Evidence of participation in community and healthcare affairs.
6. Approved completion of Fellow project.

7. Fellow recertification

Fellow recertification is mandatory every 10 years. Fellows applying for recertification are expected to have a total of 90 hours of continuing education over the previous nine years, no less than half of which is Category I (ACHE education) credit. The remainder may be from Category I or Category II (non-ACHE education) credit. Evidence of participation in community and healthcare affairs is also required.

NOTES

[1] Agnew, 1939.

[2] Kipnis, 1955, p. 13.

[3] ACHA, *Minute Book*, Vol. 1, Oct. 7, 1932. Kipnis, p. 10.

[4] Kipnis, p. 12.

[5] *Ibid.*, p. 13.

[6] ACHA, *Minute Book*, Vol. 1, Feb. 14, 1933. Kipnis, pp. 14–15.

[7] The other members were Fred Carter, Robert Neff, John Smith, and Robin Buerki. Executive Committee Minutes, May 3, 1934. ACHA, *Minute Book*, Vol. 1. Also Kipnis, pp. 15, 31–32.

[8] John R. Mannix interview, 1982. Also W. Richard Kirk interview, 1983.

[9] Kipnis, p. 15. ACHA, *Minute Book*, Vol. 1, First Annual Report to the Board of Regents, 1937.

[10] Kipnis, p. 17.

[11] See Appendix at end of text for list of Charter Fellows.

[12] Kipnis, p. 20. Direct election to Fellowship for administrators of recognized standing would remain open to Jan. 1, 1940.

[13] ACHA, *Minute Book*, Vol. 1, p. 89. Board of Regents Meeting Sept. 23, 1934. Kipnis, pp. 19–20.

[14] This decision was re-reviewed with respect to changing the name of the College to Health rather than Hospital Administrators. *Modern Healthcare*, Oct. 1981, pp. 77–78. Wesbury, ACHA, April 1981.

[15] *Modern Healthcare*, op. cit., Oct. 1981, p. 77. Kipnis, pp. 65–66.

[16] Kipnis, pp. 65–66.

[17] ACHA, "Regulations Governing Admission and Advancement," 1982.

[18] 1934 Constitution and Bylaws. ACHA, *Minute Book*, Vol. 1. Kipnis, p. 13.

[19] Dewey Lutes did not graduate from the University of Chicago. It was the rare nurse then who attended a baccalaureate nursing program. There were still practicing in 1933 numerous pre-Flexner-reform physicians without college degrees.

[20] Dewey Lutes interview. This censure procedure was later to become formalized. See ACHA, *Code of Ethics*, 1973, pp. 8–10.

[21] *Bulletin of the ACHA*, Vol. 1, No. 1, circa 1934–1935. According to Kipnis, Lutes started the *Bulletin* in 1934. Kipnis, p. 58. It was to become the *ACHA News* in 1938.

[22] Kipnis, p. 120.

[23] Kipnis, pp. 13, 20, 66. ACHA, *Minute Book*, Vol. 1, Oct. 7, 1932, p. 3.

[24] The following dates are cited from Kipnis, 1933–34, pp. 10–13; 1934–35, pp. 18, 19–20, 127: Admission to Membership approved by the Credentials Committee in 1934, inducted in 1935; 1935, pp. 23–24; 1936, pp. 28–30, 64; 1940, p. 20; 1941, pp. 65–66; 1944, p. 88; 1947, pp. 118–119; 1950–53, p. 105; 1950, p. 119. Master's degree requirement suggested by Wilmar Allen, M.D., College president, 1949–50; 1951, p. 120.

[25] ACHA, Stull, "Historical Perspective of the American College of Hospital Administrators Certification Program," April 14, 1978, p. 1.

[26] Stull, op. cit., p. 2.

[27] *Ibid.* Stull says new objective exams were first given in 1952. See Table 6.3 for example of this exam.

[28] ACHA, *1960 Directory*, p. 13.

[29] Stull, op. cit., p. 2.

[30] ACHA, *1977–78 Annual Report*, p. 4.

[31] *Ibid.*

[32] ACHA, *An Interim Progress Report*, 1971, p. 7 (unpaginated).

[33] ACHA, 1977–78 Annual Report, pp. 4–5.

[34] ACHA, *Progress Report 1972–1973*, p. 10.

[35] ACHA, *The Year in Review 1974–75*, pp. 8–9.

[36] ACHA, *1977–78 Annual Report*, pp. 4–5.

[37] ACHE, *1991–1992 Annual Report and Reference Guide*, p. 38.

[38] *Ibid.*, p. 5.

[39] *Ibid.*, p. 6. This high percentage has fallen somewhat as an increased number of graduates of baccalaureate degree programs have, with experience, qualified for Nomineeship. Stuart Wesbury interview, 1983.

[40] ACHA, Stull, "A Summary Report on a Proposal for Developing the Self-Assessment Component of a College-Based Program . . .," April 29, 1978.

[41] ACHA, Wesbury, Jan. 28, 1981, p. 11.

[42] ACHA, *1983–1984 Annual Report*, p. 4.

[43] ACHA, *Annual Report* 1982–83, p. 4

[44] ACHA, *1985–86 Annual Report*, p. 21.

[45] ACHE, *1986–87 Annual Report*, p. 2.

[46] *Ibid.*, p. 50.

[47] ACHE, *1991–92 Annual Report and Reference Guide*, p. 4.

[48] ACHE, 1993.

[49] Today these positions can be vastly more complicated than they were in the 1930s.

[50] Kipnis, p. 64.

[51] Margaret R. Barnes, consulting psychologist, University Hospitals, Cleveland. Kipnis, p. 88.

[52] Kipnis, pp. 88–96.

[53] *Ibid.*, pp. 98–105.

[54] Kipnis, pp. 118–119.

[55] Approved courses later became accredited courses in hospital or health administration. Those faculty with neither 3 years of hospital administrative experience nor a master's degree and one year of administrative experience would not qualify. ACHA *1960 Directory*, p. 13.

[56] W. Richard Kirk interview. Kipnis, p. 120. "Dr. Lillian D. Terris Retires," *PES NEWS*, Vol. 4, No. 1, July 1979.

[57] ACHA, *1977–1978 Annual Report*, p. 4, "Milestones of Progress." This is a summary of important developments from 1965 to 1978 during the tenure of Richard Stull as executive vice president and president of the College.

[58] ACHA, *An Interim Progress Report*, 1971.

[59] ACHA, *1969 Directory*, pp. 12–13. Membership was open to administrators working outside of Canada and the United States; however, they had to be affiliated with an acceptable hospital—that is, one listed in the Directory Guide of the AHA. Once the candidate was acceptable as a Nominee, it was possible to continue advancement in the College if he or she was working in a health-related organization, such as a Blue Cross Association.

[60] The requirements here are not exhaustive. Ethical conduct, recommendations, payment of dues, and other conditions held too.

[61] ACHA, *1977–1978 Annual Report*, p. 4.

[62] *Ibid.*, pp. 4–5

[63] *Ibid.*, p. 5. In the original last-quoted sentence it reads "reviewed" rather than "viewed."

[64] *Ibid.*, p 7.

[65] ACHA, *An Interim Progress Report*, 1971.

[66] ACHE, *1991–1992 Annual Report and Reference Guide*, p. 38.

[67] *Ibid.*

[68] ACHE, "Examination Outline 1992," internal document, p. 8.

[69] ACHE, "Application for Membership Recertification," circa 1992.

[70] ACHE, "Application for Advancement to Fellowship," circa 1992.

[71] Interview, Cynthia Hahn, Nov. 1992.

[72] ACHE, "Application for Fellowship Recertification," circa 1992.

[73] ACHE, *1992–1993 Annual Report and Reference Guide*, pp. 53–61.

[74] W. Richard Kirk interview, March 14, 1983.

[75] ACHA, Stull, "Historical Perspective . . .," April 14, 1978, p. 3.

[76] ACHA, "Proposed Program of Self Development and Recertification," April 30, 1976, unpaginated internal document.

[77] *Ibid.*

[78] ACHA, "Suggested Program and Budget to Develop and Implement the Proposed Program of Certification and Self Development," April 30, 1976, unpaginated internal document. W. Richard Kirk as head of the Division of Membership was responsible for the preparation of the two documents of April 30, 1976. He said it was the first million-dollar proposal Stull had received. This request might have precipitated Stull's heart attack. W. Richard Kirk interview.

[79] ACHA, Stull, "Proposal . . .," April 17, 1978, p. 2.

[80] In 1966, the Annual Congress on Administration plus 7 regional meetings were held. In 1976, the Annual Congress on Administration, 4 regional conferences, and 91 seminars were held. ACHA "Educational Pathways to Career Development within the Profession of Health Services Administration as proposed by the ACHA's Director of Education," April 14, 1978. p. 4.

[81] *Ibid.*

[82] ACHA, Stull, "Historical Perspective on the American College of Hospital Administrators Certification Program," April 14, 1978, p. 4.

[83] *Ibid.*, p. 2.

[84] ACHA, Stull, "A Word of Explanation. . . .," May 5, 1978. W. Richard Kirk interview, March 14, 1983.

[85] ACHA, Stull, April 14, 1978, op. cit., p. 2.

[86] *Ibid.*, p. 2. Kovack, "Periodic Recertification: Striving for Excellence," Washington University, St. Louis, master's thesis, 1971. ACHA *1981 Directory*, p. 465.

[87] ACHA, Stull, April 14, 1978, op. cit., p. 3.

[88] *Ibid.*

[89] ACHA, "Proposed Program of Self Development and Recertification" and "Suggested Program and Budget to Develop and Implement the Proposed Program of Certification and Self Development," April 30, 1976, internal document.

[90] ACHA, Stull, "A Summary Report on a AR Proposal for Developing the Self-Assessment Component of a College-Based Program . . .," April 17, 1978, p. 2.

[91] ACHA, "Board of Governor's Action, April 29, 1978, Meeting," May 1978, one-page internal document.

[92] ACHA, *1979–1980 Annual Report*, p. 8 (unpaginated).

[93] ACHA, "Enhancing Executive Competence," May 1981.

[94] Smith, I. Leon. "PES Develops a Self-Assessment Testing System for Hospital and Health Service Executives," *PES NEWS*, Vol. 7, No. 3, Fall 1982, pp. 3–6. Professional Examination Service, New York, NY. This firm worked with the College on this project.

[95] ACHA, *1981–1982 Annual Report*. ACHA, *1982–83 Annual Report*, p. 2.

[96] ACHA, *Twenty-Sixth Congress on Administration, March 1–4, 1983*. Interview with Cynthia Hahn and Arthur Strobeck, Nov. 1992.

[97] ACHA *Twenty-Sixth Congress on Administration, March 1–4, 1983*. Hahn and Strobeck interview.

[98] Hahn and Strobeck interview.

[99] *Ibid.*

[100] *Ibid.*

[101] ACHA, "A Proposal to Develop a Program for Continual Evaluation and Career-Long Authentication of Performance Expertise in the Profession of Health Services Administration," May 2, 1978, internal document, p. 1.

[102] *Ibid.*, p. 4.

[103] ACHA, *1979–1980 Annual Report*.

[104] ACHA, *1980–1981 Annual Report*.

[105] *PES News*, Vol. 7, No. 3, Fall 1982, pp. 3–6.

[106] ACHA, "Enhancing Executive Competence-Educational and Practice Perspectives, May 1981, p. 82. Foreword by Richard Klein and Carol Mickey.

[107] ACHA, "Health Executive Self-Assessment: A System for Professional Development," In-Basket Exercise I, Management Simulations Books I and II, and facilitators manual, 1982.

[108] Richard Klein interview, January 1983.

[109] ACHA, *Annual Report 1981–1982.*

[110] Hahn and Strobeck interview, Nov. 1992.

[111] Richard Klein interview, Jan. 1983.

[112] ACHA, Twenty-Sixth Congress on Administration, March 1–4, 1983.

7

The Evolution of Management and Healthcare Management Thought

"I do not believe . . . that the work of the hospital superintendents is all in potatoes and floor polish."

1913[1]

A history of medicine could hardly be written without describing physicians' changing ideas about disease and its causes. Hospital management also has an evolving intellectual history. The College has been continually involved in the definition and transmittal of the body of knowledge involved in, first, hospital and then healthcare management, as well as its philosophy, theory, and techniques.

Several themes run through this chapter. General management thinking has changed, due in part to more global historical changes. In the first half of the twentieth century, literature on hospital management remained distinct from general management theory, although the ideas of scientific management had an effect on hospital accreditation. However, by the time the College began, these ideas were so well diffused as to be scarcely recognizable.

Hospital management theory changed as hospitals evolved and required new methods of management. The College reflected and encouraged the merger of these two seemingly separate paths of general management and hospital management theory. This merger was also mirrored in—and fostered by—the changing education of hospital managers. The evolution has been so profound that many of today's more commonplace ideas are found nowhere in the earlier literature.

203

GENERAL MANAGEMENT THEORY

The evolution of general management theory is summarized in Table 7.1. As noted, a gap exists between first publication of an important work and its widespread adoption and acceptance by the field. Frederick W. Taylor's ideas, although first formulated in the early 1900s, were carried on into the 1920s and 1930s and persisted into the 1980s as basic skills for the industrial engineer.

Although Henri Fayol's work appeared in his native language in 1916, it was not published in English until 1929. The Hawthorne studies began in 1927, but the major summary of these studies appeared in 1939. Ideas about the informal organization became widespread only after World War II.

University education in business administration has been a phenomenon of the last 100 years, starting with the Wharton School at the University of Pennsylvania. Up to the 1890s, managers took a paternalistic view of the workers.

The Pullman Company provided a company town for its workers 100 blocks south of the Chicago Loop. In 1894, the Pullman workers rebelled against this paternalism in a violent strike that received national attention. The army was called up and 800 railroad cars were burnt. This event probably helped create a climate for the acceptance of Taylor's new ideas of scientific management in the first decade of this century.

The passage in 1889 of the New Jersey General Incorporation Law[45] allowed corporations to hold stock in other corporations for the first time. This served as the legal foundation for the growth of big business through mergers from 1895 to 1910: the era of "the Trusts." Except for the railroads, the army, and cotton mills, few large organizations existed before that time.

Taylor took a mechanistic view of worker time and motion studies, and encouraged piece rate incentives to make workers more efficient and productive. Frank Gilbreth also developed a classification of hand movements as a basis for time and motion studies which he modestly called "Therbligs" (Gilbreth spelled backwards). Some of Gilbreth's early time and motion analysis was applied to surgery.[46]

The standard textbooks on the history of management theory ignored the concepts of standardization which had played such an important role in the healthcare field from 1915 to 1930. At the core of these concepts was the notion that a standard should be defined and used as a yardstick to measure actual with ideal performance. These ideas related to the Flexner reforms and the hospital standardization program of the American College of Surgeons. They remain with us today in the practices of the Joint Commission on the Accreditation of Healthcare Organizations and in every hospital's budgeting process and internal control systems.[47]

The 1930s also saw the development of a group of writers now known loosely as the classical management theorists. Like Henri Fayol, they were concerned with the formal organization: unity of command,[48] hierarchy, span of control, departmentalization, coordination, and policies and procedures. They ignored the view of the people as individual personalities with human motivations. The Russian Revolution legitimized the works of Karl Marx. For others, the study of V. I. Lenin (revolutionary organization) and Joseph Stalin (five year plans), created another literature on organizations.[49] However, the "red scare" of 1918 put this literature out of the reach of managerial writers in this country.

The Hawthorne studies of the 1930s generated remarkable changes. The Depression encouraged a new questioning of managerial ideas. The growth of labor unions after the Wagner bill of 1935 made it clear that workers often had different opinions than managers. The Hawthorne studies of worker group dynamics confirmed this fact, and they became the departure point for the human relations literature of the 1940s and beyond. Morale, motivation and the informal organization became central concepts which flourish even today as "organizational behavior."

Combined with human relations concepts, World War II led to research on the authoritarian personality and participatory management. Both became foundations for the social psychology of organizations and small group research which is the basis for much of the consulting done in organizational behavior.

The translation by Talcott Parsons and others of the German writings of Max Weber in 1947, was a fundamental basis for sociological research on organizations. Weber's ideal bureaucratic organization affected the writings of Talcott Parsons, and Peter Blau and W. Richard Scott. An increasingly educated labor force probably also encouraged sociological research on professionals in organizations, the management of research, and organizational innovation. During World War I, Weber was a hospital administrator in charge of a large military hospital in Heidelberg, Germany. Perhaps this experience aided him in his writing on organizations.[50]

Although Herbert Simon wrote a 1946 paper on decision-making in organizations, the organizational decision-making school of Simon, March, and Cyert flourished in the 1950s and after. This was an era when computers entered organizations. Simon also became interested in artificial intelligence and computers. In 1978, he won the Nobel

TABLE 7.1
Landmarks in General Management Thinking[2]

Date	Individual**	Major Ideas	Related Events
1881	Joseph Warton[3]	Gives $100,000 to start the first university-based business school at the University of Pennsylvania. By 1911 there were 30 such schools	1894: The Pullman Strike challenges the idea of managerial paternalism.[4]
1903, 1911	Frederick W. Taylor[5] Frank Gilbreth	Scientific Management, time and motion studies, Therbligs, managerial engineering, efficiency	1895–1910: The Growth of Big Business, The Trusts,[6] Corporate Mergers, The Progressive Era.
1915–1930		The Standardization Movement[7]	
1916, 1929*	Henri Fayol[8]	First complete theory of Management, Unity of Command	1919: "The Red Scare" helps turn U.S. away from organization theories of Marx and Lenin.
1930–1943	J. Mooney, Gulick, Urwick[9]	The classical theorists: The formal organization, departmentalization, span of control, hierarchy coordination	1930–1938: The Depression
1927–1932, 1939*	Elton Mayo[10] Roethlisberger and Dickson[11]	The Hawthorne Studies; the Human Relations School; informal organization, morale, motivation.	1935: The Wagner Act: the basis for labor union expansion in industry.
1940s on	Argyris,[12] Likert,[13] Katz & Kahn,[14] Leavitt,[15] Sayles[16]	Social Psychology of Organizations; the authoritarian personality, participatory management, leadership	1940–1944: The war against fascism and totalitarianism
1920s, 1947, 1956	Max Weber[17] Talcott Parsons[18] Blau and Scott[19]	The Sociology of Organizations Bureaucracy Professionals in Organizations	

Date	Authors	Topics	Context
1946–1965	*Simon*,[20] March and *Simon*,[21] Cyert and March,[22] *Johnson, Kast, and Rosenzweig*,[23] Walton[24]	Decision Making in Organizations Systems Theory applied to organization	1950s on Development and Application of Computers Professional Workers, the most rapidly growing sector of the labor force 1960s: The growth of Multinational Conglomerates
1960s	Georgopoulos and Mann[25]	Quantitative Research on Organizations	
1967	*Lawrence & Lorsch*,[26] Woodward,[27] Becker,[28] Chandler,[29] *Herzberg*,[30] Blake & Mouton[31] Crozier[32]	Contingency Theories of Management International Comparisons	1980s: Growth of interest in Japanese industrial management techniques as a result of their success in manufacturing[33]
1970s	Walton,[34] Drucker,[35] Anthony and Herzlinger,[36] *Steiner and Miner*,[37] Sayles[38]	Effectiveness, Choice Control, Policy, Strategy Performance, Decision making	
1980s	Peters and Waterman[39] *Levenson and Rosenthal*[40] Leavitt[41] Kouzes & Posner[42]	Change Leadership Turbulent Times Vision and Values	1980s Growth of Interest in Japanese Management Techniques Wall Street "Go-Go" Era (Junk Bond Era)
1990s	Senge[43] Deming[44]	System Thinking Continuous Quality Improvement Total Quality Management	U.S. Baldrige Award

* Italicized dates indicate wide dissemination in English of the writer's main work.

** Italicized authors received ACHE James A. Hamilton Book Award.

Prize in economics for his work on the decision-making process within economic organizations.

These diverse strands of thinking were partially synthesized by contingency theorists such as Paul Lawrence and Jay Lorsch in 1967. They believed that there was no one right way to organize. Rather, a mesh is needed between organization and environment. This idea, which seems rather obvious today, helped resolve major intellectual divisions in management thinking and also provided a new rationale for the uniqueness of hospital administration.

The 1980's were the era of organizational change, mergers, leveraged buy outs, and corporate restructuring. It was the era of Michael Milken, junk bonds, and the predators ball. Such turbulent times called attention to corporate strategy, change, and leadership.

In the late 1980's and early 1990's there was an explosion of interest in continuous quality improvement and total quality management. Ideas developed originally by W. Edwards Deming, Joseph Juran, and others in the United States were ignored here and adopted in Japan. With the success of Japanese industry, these ideas were adopted widely in American industry and then spread to the health field through the efforts of Paul Batalden and Donald Berwick[51]

HEALTHCARE MANAGEMENT THEORY

The separation of hospital literature from general management literature in the 1950s is hardly surprising considering the educational background of most administrators in nursing, medicine, and religion, rather than business administration. The early, one academic year graduate programs in hospital administration were practitioner-oriented and often did not stress general management theory.

The Era of Creation of New Hospitals: 1880–1915

Up until the 1920s, books on hospital management were largely concerned with hospital architecture, construction, and design.[52] The typical book of this era included floor plans for hospitals (see Table 7.2).

There were two reasons for this emphasis. From 1880 to 1915, thousands of hospitals were created; the need for books on equipment and architecture was widespread. Though the peak in the creation of new hospitals was prior to 1915, many small hospitals appeared and disappeared after that date. In the prosperous 1920s, hospitals that started in large private houses were rebuilt and reorganized.

TABLE 7.2
Early Books on Health Management (Prior to the ACHE List of 1939)

Aikens, Charlotte. *Hospital Management*. Philadelphia: W. B. Saunders Co., 1911.

Billings, John S. *Description of the Johns Hopkins Hospital*. Baltimore: Johns Hopkins Press, 1890.

Billings, John S. *Ventilation and Heating*. New York: The Engineering Record, 1893.

Billings, John S. and Hurd, Henry M. (editors). *Hospitals, Dispensaries and Nursing*. International Congress of Charities, Correction and Philanthropy. Section III. Baltimore: Johns Hopkins Press, 1894.

Billings, John S., Folsom, Norton, Jones, Joseph, Morris, Caspar and Smith, Stephen. *Five Essays Relating to the Construction, Organization and Management of Hospitals for the Use of Johns Hopkins Hospital of Baltimore*. New York: William Wood & Co., 1875.

Burdett, Henry C. *The Cottage Hospital*. London: J & A Churchill, 1877.

Burdett, Henry C. *Hospitals and Asylums of the World*. 4 volumes. London: J & A Churchill, 1891–1893.

Davis, Michael M. *Clinics, Hospitals and Health Centers*. New York: Harper & Brothers, 1927.

Davis, Michael M. and Warner, Andrew R. *Dispensaries: Their Management and Development*. New York: The Macmillan Co., 1918.

Galton, Douglas. *On the Construction of Hospitals:* London: Macmillan & Co., 1869.

Hornsby, J. A. and Schmidt, Richard E. *The Modern Hospital: Its Inspiration, Its Architecture, Its Equipment, Its Operation*. Philadelphia: W. B. Saunders Co., 1914.

MacEachern, Malcolm T. *Medical Records in the Hospital*. Chicago: Physicians Record Company, 1937.

Morrill, Warren P. *Hospital Manual of Operation*. New York: Lakeside Publishing Co., 1934.

Nightingale, Florence, *Introductory Notes on Lying-In Institutions*. London: Longmans, Green, Longmans, Roberts & Green, 1871.

Nightingale, Florence. *Notes on Hospitals*. Third edition. London: Longmans, Green, Longmans, Roberts & Green, 1863.

Ochsner, Albert J. and Sturm, Meyer J. *The Organization, Construction and Management of Hospitals*. Chicago: Cleveland Press, 1907.

Rankin, W. S., Hannaford, H. E., and Van Arsdall, H. P. *The Small General Hospital*. Charlotte, North Carolina: Trustees of the Duke Endowment, 1928 (revised March 1945).

Stevens, Edward F. *The American Hospital of the Twentieth Century*. New York: The Architectural Record Company, 1918, 1921, 1928.

Woolsey, Abby Howland. *Hand-book for Hospitals*. State Charities Aid Association. New York: G. P. Putnam's Sons, 1883.

Willie, W. Gill. *Hospitals, Their History, Organization, and Construction*. New York: D. Appleton & Co., 1877.

Peabody, Francis Weld. *Doctor and Patient*. Papers on the Relationship of the physician to men and institutions. New York: Macmillan, 1930.

Mackintosh, Donald J. *Construction, Equipment and Management of General Hospitals*. London: Hodge & Co., 1916.

Stone, Captain J. E. *Hospital Organization and Management*. London: Faber & Gwyer, 1927.

The second reason for this focus was the central problem of hospital infection called "hospitalism." There were two conflicting theories about this condition. The miasmatic theory stated that infection was caused by bad climate, bad location, or lack of fresh air. The contagion theory held that disease was spread by carriers. The great works of Robert Koch (tuberculosis in 1879 and cholera in 1883) and Louis Pasteur (anthrax in 1877) on the germ theory of disease eventually convinced physicians that the contagion theory of disease was correct. But the battle between these two ideas lasted well into the twentieth century.[53]

At the turn of the century, what is now the *New England Journal of Medicine* regularly reported the local weather conditions, thought to be related to disease. New hospitals in Boston were built on top of hills to get fresh air. The pavilion style of hospital architecture put long distances between patient wards in the hopes of reducing contagion. The Nightingale ward for inpatients had high ceilings and lots of window space. The treatment of tuberculosis was rest and fresh air, as represented by the early years of the then famous Trudeau Sanatorium (1884 to 1954).[54]

In short, the philosophy was that if the hospital was located and designed correctly, "hospitalism" would be reduced. Thus, architecture was the basic answer to the central problem of the hospital. Once built, it was believed that only rigorous discipline was needed to run an institution successfully.

The Era of the Superintendent: 1915–1945

The College Defines the Administrator's Library

As early as 1938, the American College of Hospital Administrators began to define the appropriate and relevant literature for the hospital administrator.[55] Of course, the College's institutes and its encouragement of graduate education also indirectly promoted the definition of relevant managerial ideas.

In his dual capacity as Executive of the College and Associate Director of the Hospital Administration course in the School of Business at the University of Chicago, Gerhard Hartman said:

> We feel privileged to bring before our members a project as farsighted and stimulating as a reference library in hospital administration at the University of Chicago. This library will be kept apart from the general library. Such a library will serve a twofold purpose:
> 1. It will make available to graduate students in the hospital administration course and to advanced students at institutes the literature of the hospital field. Arrangements will be made

> whereby the texts and other materials will be sent from the library at the University of Chicago to the universities at which institutes are being conducted, this material to be for the exclusive use of administrators attending the institutes. The library is thus of immediate and practical importance.
> 2. As additional accessions are made and the library grows, it will serve as a research base for hospital administration students who will contribute further progress in the hospital field, for it is only through continued probing of the achievements of the past that the keen insight necessary to the solution of present problems is obtained. The library is thus of lasting and enduring value.

Hartman then called on College members to contribute books to the library. "We feel that in doing so they will be personally adding to the strength and solidity of the educational program they endorse through their membership in the American College of Hospital Administrators," he said.

In the *ACHA News* of September, 1939, the administrator's library was defined:

> The great lack of books on hospital administration is gradually being overcome. Ten years ago there were only a handful of worthwhile hospital texts. Today there are a score or more good books available and nearly a dozen more in course of preparation.[56]

The books "that should be found on every administrator's library shelves" were listed (see Table 7.3). All of these books were specifically related to healthcare and not concerned with general management theory.

Not one of these essential books made any reference to the general management literature summarized in Table 7.1, and almost none had footnotes or references to other literature. The earliest book in Table 7.3 was Joseph Weber's text on how to organize a new hospital, an important topic in an era when many new hospitals were being created.

Then, as now, law was important, as reflected by the books of John Lapp and Dorothy Ketcham and Emanuel and Lillian Hayt, which were to be republished several times. Judging by these books, the administrator was expected to know legal details, rather than the general theory of legal reasoning.

The Committee on the Costs of Medical Care (1927–1932) was a landmark effort to define healthcare. About 20 reports were published, many with extensive statistical descriptions. More recently it has been known for its early advocacy of health insurance and medical

TABLE 7.3
The ACHA List of Essential Books for the Hospital Administrator in 1939[57]

Older Books[58]

Michael M. Davis	*Hospital Administration: A Career*. New York, NY: privately published, 1929.
Frank E. Chapman	*Hospital Organization and Operation*. New York, NY: Macmillan, 1924.
Joseph J. Weber	*First Steps in Organizing a Hospital*. New York, NY: Macmillan Co., 1924.
John A. Lapp and Dorothy Ketcham	*Hospital Law*. Milwaukee, WI; Bruce Pub. Co., 1926.
Emmet B. Bay	*Medical Administration of Teaching Hospitals*. Chicago, IL: University of Chicago Press, 1931.
C. Rufus Rorem	*The Public's Investment in Hospitals*. Chicago, IL: University of Chicago Press, 1930.
Sir Arthur Newsholme	*Medicine and the State*. Baltimore, MD: Williams and Wilkins, 1932.[59]
Committee on the Costs of Medical Care	"Medical Care for the American People." *Final Report of the Commission on Medical Education*. Chicago, IL: University of Chicago Press, 1932.

Recent Books[60]

Malcolm T. MacEachern, M.D.	*Hospital Organization and Management*. Chicago, IL: Physicians Record Co., 1935 (second edition 1946).
Emmanuel Hayt and Lillian Hayt	*Legal Aspects of Hospital Practices*. New York, NY: Hospital Textbook Co., 1938.
Haven Emerson, M.D., et al.	*Report of the Hospital Survey for New York*. Three volumes. New York, NY: United Hospital Fund, 1937, 1938.
Frances Weld Peabody, M.D.	*The Care of the Patient*. Cambridge, MA: Harvard University Press, 1927, p. 48
Thomas R. Ponton, M.D.	*The Medical Staff in the Hospital*. Chicago, IL: Physicians Record Company, 1939.
Committee on the Grading of Nursing Schools	*Nursing Schools Today and Tomorrow*. New York, NY: 1934, privately published.
American Foundation	*American Medicine—Expert Testimony Out of Court*. New York, NY: The Foundation, 1937.[61]
Alden B. Mills	*Hospital Public Relations*. Chicago, IL: Physicians Record Co., 1939.

group practice. Many of its researchers went on to notable academic, government, and administrative careers.

Haven Emerson's three volumes described the hospitals of New York City in great detail.

C. Rufus Rorem, a long-time faculty member at the University of Chicago, was one of the most prolific writers on hospital economics and was associated with the Committee on the Costs of Medical Care. Francis Peabody's short book provided wise advice to medical students on the humane treatment of patients. Public relations of the day was concerned with philanthropic fund raising for the hospital, and this was covered in Mills' book on this topic.

Just as the profession of medicine defines its contents through its textbooks, the College defined hospital administration through its own list of texts. This was particularly true with respect to Malcolm MacEachern's book which went through several editions and grew to enormous size.

It was, for many years, the definitive textbook on hospital administration and in active use into the 1960s. Appropriate forms for medical records and patient information were reproduced for the era of small hospitals when the administrator had to know details of nearly all hospital work.

Since 1939, from time to time the College and the AHA Resource Center (library) have published essential or core bibliographies for health care executives. These lists can be seen as defining the changing core intellectual content of healthcare management. From 13 books in 1939, these lists have become larger and larger. The 1989 Core Collection assembled by the AHA Resource Center staff and published in the College journal lists 147 books and 87 journals.[62] To own such a library would have cost about $10,000 then. Table 7.4 lists nine of these

TABLE 7.4
Essential and Core Bibliographies for the Healthcare Executive

1939	ACHA List of Essential Books (see Table 7.3)
1943	Bachmeyer and Hartman, *The Hospital in Modern Society*
1948	Bachmeyer and Hartman, *Hospital Trends and Developments*
1972–78	"Administrator's Collection" AHA
1979	"A Selected Bibliography for the Well Read Health Services Manager" ACHA
1985	"Current Management Resources" AHA
1986	"Current Management Resources for Health Care Professionals" AHA
1989	"Health Care Administration: A Core Collection" *H&HSA* 34:4
1989	"Resource Bibliography" in ACHE *General Management Assessment* workbook, Section 6.

bibliographies from 1939 to 1989 spanning half a century. The later lists are far too long to reproduce here.

Standardization, Scientific Management, and the Accreditation of Hospitals

By the 1939 College list, the ideas of scientific management were not explicit. No references to the general literature on management are made in these books. The influence of scientific management is there but it was hidden and "underground." The ideas of scientific management probably had an impact on MacEachern by way of hospital accreditation and E. A. Codman (see below).

Dr. Robert L. Dickinson, founding member of the American College of Surgeons,[63] presented a paper to a joint meeting of the New York Taylor Society and the Harvard Medical Society,[64] which was later published in the *Bulletin of the Taylor Society* as "Hospital Organization as Shown by Charts of Personnel and Powers Functions." This was probably the first published organization chart for a hospital.[65] There were comments by Frank Gilbreth, one of the leaders of scientific management, and Ernest Amory Codman.[66]

Frank Gilbreth presented another paper at the 16th Annual Convention of the American Hospital Association in 1914 on "Scientific Management in the Hospital."[67] His wife, Lillian, presented a paper entitled "Efficiency in the Care of the Patient" at the same St. Paul, Minnesota meeting.[68] Lillian Gilbreth was made an Honorary Fellow of the ACHE in 1961.

Codman was influenced by the ideas of scientific management. He wanted his private "End Result" Hospital to be a standard for hospital efficiency. Data on patient outcomes after discharge were classified and related back to possible errors while patients were still in the hospital.[69]

Codman's one-page autobiography in his medical textbook, *The Shoulder*,[70] symbolized his interest in scientific management. However, he was also interested in graphical presentations of data even as a student at Harvard Medical School. He and the later noted neurosurgeon, Harvey Cushing, created the idea of graphically displaying patient signs during an operation, thus, starting a practice that is now universal among anesthesiologists.[71]

Codman was interested in technology and worked with x-rays soon after Roentgen's publication came to Boston. His unpublished book of x-rays was quite possibly the first book of its kind in the country.[72]

Codman's background probably made him very sympathetic to the ideas of scientific management. On January 6, 1915, as Chairman of the Surgical Section of the Suffolk District Medical Society, Codman organized a meeting to discuss "Hospital Efficiency."[73] The speakers were: Frank Gilbreth, the efficiency expert, and Robert L. Dickinson, M.D., the surgeon-gynecologist, discussing hospital efficiency from a surgeon's point of view. Dr. Herbert Howard, of the Peter Bent Brigham Hospital, spoke on behalf of hospital superintendents. Two trustees spoke, along with none other than His Honor, Mayor James M. Curley, a legendary Boston politician who was the model for *The Last Hurrah*.[74] *Cheaper by the Dozen*,[75] the story of Frank and Lillian Gilbreth's twelve children, was also made into a movie.

Codman brought his ideas on hospital efficiency to the American College of Surgeons, where he was Chairman of the Hospital Standardization Committee from 1912–1917.[76] "The Standard of Efficiency for the First Hospital Survey of the College," published in the *Bulletin of the ACS*, March, 1918, contained many of Codman's ideas,[77] including standardization, efficiency, and case records on a standardized form. The article noted: "In conclusion, the College would emphasize the importance of adequate records. They are in effect a pledge to the public for the integrity of all work done in the hospital."[78]

The requirements of adequate medical records and a well-organized medical staff persisted as core concepts in hospital accreditation when Malcolm MacEachern took charge of this program for the American College of Surgeons. Thus, the ideas of scientific management were imbedded in the background of hospital standardization.[79]

However, by 1938,[80] many of Codman's core ideas had disappeared. Hospital accreditation did not carry on the idea of after-hospital discharge assessment and routine listing of errors. "Efficiency" as a concept also faded into the background. Time and motion studies, Therbligs, and functional foremanship ideas taken directly from scientific management had no place in the ACHE's library of 1939.[81] However, MacEachern kept flow diagrams and organization charts.[82] Chapman's book also contained several hospital organization charts.[83]

The Era of the Hospital Administrator: 1945–1965

With the growth of hospitals and the professionalization of many areas, the roles of administrators changed. Until the 1940s, they needed an extensive knowledge of detail. Later, they sought competent specialized experts and created a climate for positive performance. The trained dietician, medical record librarian, laboratory technician, business officer, and nurse supervisor, took on much of the work formerly performed by the administrator. The work of the administrator thus evolved into the management of professionalized workers in an increasingly large, complex, and decentralized institution.

The College did not update its 1939 list of essential books; World War II intervened. In 1943 and 1948, Arthur Bachmeyer and Gerhard Hartman edited two collections of reprinted articles about hospitals and their management, *The Hospital in Modern Society*[84] and *Hospital Trends and Developments*.[85]

Bachmeyer was President of the ACHE in 1940–41, as well as Director of the University of Chicago Clinics and Director of Chicago's hospital administration course. Hartman held the equivalent two positions at the State University of Iowa after having been Executive Secretary of the ACHE from 1937 to 1941.

Of the 149 Chapters in their 1948 book, at least 35 were written by people who held leadership or honorary positions within the College. They included Bachmeyer, Ray Brown, Howard Bishop, Fred Carter, James Hamilton, Basil MacLean, and Joseph Norby, all ACHA Presidents. G. H. Agnew, Guy Clark, S. S. Goldwater, V. M. Hoge, Emanuel Hayet, Thomas Parran and Lillian Gilbreth were all Honorary Fellows. E. M. Bluestone was a Charter Fellow; George Bugbee, a First Vice President; Ray Amberg a Regent; and both Otho Ball and Malcolm MacEachern were Honorary Charter Fellows. Many of these articles were written in the late 1930s. In his 1938 address to the College convocation, S. S. Goldwater said, "It is to the credit of the College that in the vast literary output on hospital topics, the contributions of its members hold a conspicuous place."[86]

Only a handful of articles were by management theorists: Lillian Gilbreth, relating back to scientific management; Margaret Mead, writing of cultural anthropology; and Herbert Simon,[87] introducing a new era of thinking about organizations.

This book included no sample forms which were the hallmark of the earlier era. Unlike the previous era, there were extensive bibliographical references and even the first regression analysis, heralding the more quantitative statistical analysis of the future.[88] However, there was no mention of the human relations school of the coming years. This book was developed, in part, for students in "a number of our leading universities throughout the country," preparing for careers in hospital administration.

In 1939, Gerhard Hartman published "Problems and References in Hospital Administration" at the University of Chicago. "It may well have been the first teaching document for graduate education" in hospital administration.[89] This book was used as the basis of the 1952 College book written by Ray Brown and Richard Johnson entitled *Hospitals Visualized*.[90] *Hospitals Visualized* was intended for the use of hospital administration students as they began their field experience. The revised version of 1957 contains roughly 2,000 questions that students might ask in 32 hospital departments. The answers to these questions, presumably from knowledgeable department heads, would hopefully result in an understanding of the hospital's functioning.

Some questions were simply descriptive: "To what extent are the following fuels used in cooking: gas, steam, electricity?"[91] or, "What uniform does the social service worker wear? Is it required?"[92] Many other questions focused on hierarchical relationships: Who controls? Who is in charge of? Who is responsible for . . .? Other questions related to work flow: Policies, procedures, budgeting, and personnel policies.

In part, this book related back to the concern of classical management theorists with the formal organization. There were no human relations questions that illuminated the informal organization. Instead, it harkened back to the superintendent's era of knowledge of details. But, unlike the nurse administrator of a 40-bed hospital in the 1930s who had to teach staff, there were now hospital department heads to impart knowledge to students. *Hospitals Visualized* went out-of-print in the mid-1960s.

The new ideas of human relations were reflected in the College's "Human Relations Conferences for Hospital Administrators." The first of 17 such two-day conferences was held in March, 1951; they continued until 1955, with an average attendance of 40 participants.[93]

The inaugural issue of the College's journal, *Hospital Administration*, was published in the Fall of 1956. A College journal was proposed in 1942, but was not initiated due to lack of funds.[94]

The journal illustrated the entry of new management ideas into the field. The first issue, for example, included articles on "Human Relations" by Oswald Hall, Samuel Stauffer, and Robert Tannenbaum.[95] Human relations concepts were evident on a frequent basis in subsequent years, including effective motivation,[96] motivating hospital employees,[97] the primary group,[98] human relations,[99] organization man,[100] informal organization, organization as a social system,[101] motivation and morale,[102] shared communications symbols,[103] personality and organization, and the social context of motivation.[104]

For 25 years, the journal was edited by Lynn Wimmer, who retired in 1982. Throughout this time, it continued to serve as the leading journal on the theory and practice of hospital and healthcare management.

The social sciences were represented, with references to the economics of patient care,[105] the contributions of social science to hospital administration,[106] and psychology for hospital administration.[107] That the social sciences could contribute to good hospital management was a revelation at that time. Operations research was also new in 1958,[108] and these ideas continued with operational gaming in 1963,[109] and operations research in 1965.[110]

The twenty-fifth anniversary of the College in 1958 also saw the start of the James A. Hamilton Hospital Administrator's Book Award.

The first recipient was Herbert Simon for *Administrative Behavior*.[111] The organizational decision-making concepts found in Simon's book were later represented in the College's journal.[112]

Later Hamilton book awards included now classic books derived from human relations and the social psychology of organizations: Chris Argyris (1959), Douglas McGregor (1962), Rensis Likert (1963), Daniel Katz and Robert Kahn (1968), and Harry Levenson (1970).[113] The first Hayhow Award in 1960 for the best article to appear in *Hospital and Health Services Administration* was given to Oswald Hall for "Motivation and Morale," which was of the genre.[114]

Along with a continued interest in the education of the hospital administrator, other new ideas included "power politics,"[115] "administration by objectives," (heralding management by objectives as a new idea),[116] ethics and moral philosophy,[117] and the management of research.[118]

Many of the articles cited above described general management theories and demonstrated their application to hospitals. The year 1962 saw articles on the differences between hospitals and other organizations,[119] especially in terms of management principles. Basil Georgopoulos and Floyd Mann built an organizational theory to explain the unique features of hospital organization.

Georgopoulos also won two Hamilton book awards in 1967[120] and 1974[121] for this work. Paul Gordon also won the ACHA article award in 1964 for his description of the management triangle of trustee, administrator, and physician that is unique to hospitals.[122]

A 1965 survey showed that the College journal, *Hospital Administration*, was well read, suggesting it to be an effective conduit for the delivery of new ideas to the practicing hospital manager.[123]

The Era of the Hospital Manager: 1966–1978

The emphasis on human relations from 1956 to 1966 within the journal matched the growing size and complexity of the hospital. It also complemented the growth of technically skilled professionals[124] who had been given the opportunity to develop many of the functionally differentiated departments of the average hospital. The era when the superintendent had to know all the details of hospital work was over.

The introduction of Medicare and Medicaid marked a new era. Rising hospital costs meant that there were more staff, procedures, and technology used on each patient admitted to a hospital.

New concerns appeared in the journal. The growing complexity of the external environment of the hospital was reflected in areawide planning,[125] collective bargaining,[126] regional medical programs,[127] the federal government in health,[128] and the crisis in American healthcare.[129] Nearly all of the Fall issue of 1969 was devoted to health planning.[130] New topics also included community participation,[131] public utility status,[132] regulation,[133] licensure,[134] regionalization,[135] and Certificate of Need and PSROs.[136]

The complexity of the external environment led quite a few hospitals to reorganize their top management into a corporate model of president (Mr. Outside), and executive vice president (Mr. Inside). The growing number of healthcare organizations was reflected in the journal's name change at the beginning of 1976 to *Hospital & Health Services Administration*.

An article in 1967 on the administrator's role in computer mechanization started a series of articles on the role of the computer in the hospital,[137] as well as the planning, scheduling, and modeling techniques requiring computers.

There were also a growing number of articles using an economic approach,[138] and occasionally, a political science perspective.[139]

With respect to articles about hospitals themselves, the focus was on their internal organizational configuration, matrix organization,[140] internal control, and budgeting.

This is not to say that the human relations ideas vanished. But they were combined with concepts concerning participation, efficiency, and performance, as reflected in the Hamilton Book awards of 1972, 1976, 1978, and 1980.

The Corporate Era of the CEO: 1979 to 1989

The managerial concern for internal hospital structure and environmental relations did not disappear, no more than did the concern for human relations. However, in recent years, a new series of ideas emerged: multi-institutional systems, marketing, corporate finance, antitrust, competition, and forecasting models. Is it still too early to tell where this new emphasis will lead—whether it is a momentary enthusiasm or the beginning of a long-term trend? The writer of the centennial history of the College in 2033 will surely have a more accurate answer.

Nevertheless, these words captured new developments in the field. Almost none were found in the indexes of the essential books of 1939, or in the Bachmeyer and Hartman texts in 1948. That is not to say that earlier topics disappeared completely. Instead, they were incorporated into the knowledge base of healthcare management. There were, however, two areas of continuing interest: the hospital governing board and education for health managers.

By 1980, the separation between management thinking and important concepts of hospital administration ceased to exist. Hospital administration evolved into general management applied to a unique field, called either healthcare management or health services management.

In 1979, the College produced "a selected bibliography for the well read health services manager." It listed 220 books, dealing with both general management and health services management. Of these 220 books, 15 were written by Fellows of the College. Of the 15, several were by full-time academics. The bibliography was published because "The outpouring of publications related to the profession of health services administration threatens to inundate the busy practitioner."[141]

Not only had content changed; the authors of the hospital administration literature changed, too. In 1979, Edward Eckenhoff and Stefan Harasymiw analyzed the authors of hospital literature in six journals from 1948 to 1973.[142] In 1948, over 35 percent of the articles were by administrators; by 1973 this was below 20 percent. Increasingly, professional writers were at work in magazines like *Modern Hospital* and *Hospitals*. Attorney authors increased; architects declined. Consultants increased from one percent to 15 percent, as did faculty members.

Writing for healthcare management has become a field for specialists. The same trend has occurred for general management. CEOs, for example, rarely write for *Forbes, The Wall Street Journal,* or the *Harvard Business Review.*

Reading the content of *Hospitals and Health Services Administration* brings out the major concerns of the 1980's. The dominant ideas are competition[143], case mix (DRGs),[144] financing,[145] multihospital systems[146] and marketing.[147] Three concurrent forces drove down hospital occupancy and fueled competition. These are the introduction of prospective payment by Medicare using diagnostic related groups (DRG's) which shortened length of stay, the growth of ambulatory care, ambulatory surgery, and hospice reduced admissions.[148] Managed care (HMO's and PPO's) also reduced admissions.[149] Fewer patient days and high fixed costs compelled a competitive stance. Marketing, physician–hospital partnerships,[150] strategic planning,[151] quality assurance,[152] productivity,[153] financing, corporate reorganization,[154] and the growth of multi-institutional systems were all part of the competitive response.

The hospitals' responses changed what its leadership paid attention to: transformational leadership,[155] decision making,[156] change,[157] product line management,[158] vertical integration,[159] human resource management,[160] and management stress.[161] The needs of the competitive environment of the 1980's did not sit easily with College members, as the growth of articles about ethics shows.[162]

The College's designation of distinguished articles and books has also defined the central ideas of healthcare management as judged by managers themselves. This was yet another way for the College to identify the intellectual content of the field.

The historian, with hindsight, might note some articles and books which the College did not mention: Nobel laureate, Kenneth Arrow's "Uncertainty and the Economics of Medical Care" in 1963,[163] and Martin Feldstein's 1967 book, *Economic Analysis for Health Services Efficiency*,[164] which marked the founding of econometric analysis of hospitals. These were the works of scholars aimed at their peers. Though difficult to read, they ultimately affected healthcare management; they were not works for the practicing CEO. The College's role was as a bridge, a vehicle through which working managers declared what was relevant and important. Many awards were given for works that appealed to both manager and scholar.

In 1988, the College started the yearly health management research award for research on healthcare management and career opportunities in the field.

The 1983 Congress on Administration listed 50 seminars. The titles, reflecting a competitive corporate world, included "Diversification and Preservation of Assets through Corporate Restructuring," "Competition in Health Care," "Physician Recruitment—A Marketing Approach," "Creative Alternatives for Hospital Capital Formation," "Health Care Computer Systems," "Incentive Compensation," "Financial Ratio Analysis," "Diversification Strategies," "Health Provider Advertising," "Preferred Provider Organizations," and "Image Management: Administration's Newest Responsibility." Eighteen percent of the presentations were by College Fellows.[165]

These topics demonstrated how the College successfully merged general management theory with the professional life of the hospital and health services manager by the time of its fiftieth anniversary.

The 1993 Congress reflected these and other concerns. Ninety-five management seminars were offered, including general management programs and a number of seminars designed specifically for CEOs and nurse, physician, long-term care, and managed care executives. Titles, reflecting the College's efforts to meet the needs of healthcare executives from diverse settings and disciplines, included "CEO Leadership in Medical Staff Succession and Transition Planning," Key Planning Criteria for Patient Care Units of the Future," "Developing Physician Support for Major Strategic Initiatives," "Long-

Term Care Facility Trends," and "Ongoing Management of Your Contract Relationships."

The 1990s: A New Era

By the 1990s, the intellectual content of the field had changed substantially. Total Quality Management, stemming from discussions of Japanese management methods[166] and quality circles[167] in the late 1980s, led to Continuing Quality Improvement[168] as a topic for publications and seminars. The 1992 Presidential campaign brought national health insurance back into the limelight and to vigorous political debate about healthcare system reform. Increasing diversity in the workforce stimulated thinking about hospital structures, and communities and networks became important.

NOTES

[1] Comment by Dr. Hurd on John Hornsby, "Standardization of Hospitals." *Transactions of the American Hospital Association*, Vol. 15, 1913, p. 184. The ellipses in this quotation replace the words "with Dr. Codman" referring to Dr. Ernest A. Codman, with whom he is agreeing.

[2] George, 1968. Mouzelis, 1968.

[3] "How Business Schools Began," *Business Week*, 1963. Rosett, 1982.

[4] Lindsey, 1964. Bendix, 1956.

[5] Haber, 1964. Kakar, 1970. Taylor, 1903. Taylor, 1911.

[6] Porter, 1973.

[7] See Chapter 4 for discussion and references.

[8] Fayol, 1967.

[9] Mooney and Reiley, 1931. Gulick and Urwick, 1937. Koontz and O'Donnell, 1955. Starkweather, 1967, p. 71.

[10] Mayo, 1933.

[11] Roethlisberger and Dixon, 1939.

[12] Argyris, 1953 and 1957 (1959 Hamilton Book Award).

[13] Likert, 1961 (1963 Hamilton Book Award).

[14] Katz and Kahn, 1966 (1966 Hamilton Book Award).

[15] Leavitt, 1958 (1960 Hamilton Book Award).

[16] Sayles, 1979 (1981 Hamilton Book Award).

[17] Weber, Max, 1947.

[18] Parsons, 1956.

[19] Blau and Scott, 1971.

[20] Simon, 1947, 1957. Simon won the first Hamilton Book Award in 1958 and the Nobel Prize in Economics in 1978. Some years before this, Simon was awarded an honorary doctoral degree in Sweden. In preparation of this he learned the Swedish language well enough in a few months to be able to give his hour-long speech entirely in Swedish. This made a great impression on that country (Edgar Borgenhammer, Ph.D., personal communication).

[21] March and Simon, 1958. This book along with Simon's *Administrative Behavior* were the two most frequently used books on organizational behavior in the graduate programs in 1971. Neuhauser, 1972.

[22] Cyert and March, 1963.

[23] Johnson, Kast, and Rosenzweig, 1963 (1965 Hamilton Book Award).

[24] Walton, Clarence C., 1969 (1971 Hamilton Book Award).

[25] Georgopoulos and Mann, 1962, and Georgopoulos, 1972 (Hamilton Book Award for 1964 and 1974, respectively).

[26] Lawrence and Lorsch, 1967 (1969 Hamilton Book Award).

[27] Woodward, 1965.

[28] Becker and Neuhauser, 1975.

[29] Chandler, 1962.

[30] Herzberg, reprinted in 1982 (1978 Hamilton Book Award).

[31] Blake and Mouton, 1964 (1980 Hamilton Book Award).

[32] Crozier, 1964.

[33] Yoshino, 1968. Dore, 1973. Ouchi, 1981. Shortell, 1982. Brown, Montague, 1982. Vogel, 1981.

[34] Walton, C., 1969.

[35] Drucker, 1974.

[36] Anthony and Herzlinger, 1975.

[37] Steiner and Miner, 1986.

[38] Sayles, 1979.

[39] Peters and Waterman, 1982.

[40] Levenson and Rosenthal, 1984.

[41] Leavitt, 1987.

[42] Kouzes and Posner, 1987.

[43] Senge, 1990.

[44] W. Edwards Deming. Although Deming has been at work on CQI for over 50 years, these ideas hit the health field only in the late 1980s. See Deming, 1986, and Walton, M. 1990.

[45] George, 1968.

[46] Gilbreth, 1916.

[47] See Chapter 3. For present uses of these ideas, see Anthony and Herzlinger, 1975 (1977 Hamilton Book Award) and Herzlinger, Moore, and Hall, 1973. Also Lawrence and Davis, Chapter 4, 1983.

[48] Unity of Command is advocated for hospitals by Ochsner and Sturm, 1907, pp. 44–45.

[49] Mouzelis, 1968, pp. 11–15.

[50] The author was unable to find the reference to the history of Max Weber's life.

[51] Paul Bataldan, M.D., was associated with the Hospital Corporation of America. The article by Donald Berwick, M.D. in the *New England Journal of Medicine*, 1989, was very widely read.

[52] Ochsner and Sturm, 1907, devote 147 pages to management principles and 472 pages to construction and architectural plans.

[53] Dowling, 1977.

[54] McNeill, 1976, pp. 265–291.

[55] Dowling, 1977, pp. 75, 170.

[56] *ACHA News*, 1938.

[57] *ACHA News*, 1939. Hartman, "The Administrator's Professional Library," 1940. These books are now very rare. Most can be found in the Rare Book Room of the Asa Bacon Library of the American Hospital Association or the National Library of Medicine in Bethesda, MD. These are probably the most complete libraries in the world with respect to the hospital management literature. However, the only copy of the Committee on the Grading of Nursing Schools I could find was in the personal library of John Mannix, now part of the AHA historical collections. Chapman's book had a press run of only 300 copies (Mannix interview, 1982).

[58] Michael Davis was the first Honorary Fellow of the College after the Charter Honorary Fellows. Frank Chapman was the administrator of Mt. Sinai Hospital in Cleveland. John Mannix was an assistant administrator here and helped with the book. Emmet B. Bay was a cardiologist at the University of Chicago Clinics and an early physician supporter of the hospital administration program there (M. Davis in Brown, Ray E., 1959). Davis wrote the introduction to this book. The Rorem book was part of the same series of the University of Chicago Press, as the Bay book, which Davis edited.

[59] See Arthur Newsholme's biography, *Fifty Years in Public Health: A Personal Narrative with Comments*. 1935, cited in Eyler, 1979, pp. 195–196.

[60] MacEachern, Emerson, and Emmanuel Hayt were Honorary College Fellows. Frances Peabody was a professor at Harvard Medical School. Thomas Ponton was a coworker and friend of MacEachern, working as his assistant at Vancouver General Hospital, 1918–23, and then for him in the American College of Surgeon's hospital survey program (Ponton, 1953).

[61] There are apparently two volumes of this work. See Burling, Lentz, and Wilson, 1956, p. 336.

[62] American Hospital Association Resource Center, "Health Care Administration: A Core Collection." *Hospital & Health Services Administration*, Vol. 34, No. 4, pp. 559–575.

[63] Davis, Loyal, 1960, p. 478. For more on Codman, see "Ernest Amory Codman, MD, and End Results of Medical Care," Neuhauser, D., International Journal of Technology Assessment in Health Care, Vol. 6, No. 2, 1990, pp. 307–325.

[64] Rosner, 1982, p. 61.

[65] Dickinson, 1917. A rival for the earliest organization chart can be found in Ochsner and Sturm, 1907, p. 43.

[66] Rosner, *op. cit.*, p. 206.

[67] Gilbreth, 1914. Also see his "Motion Study in Surgery," 1916, pp. 22–31.

[68] Gilbreth, 1914. Reverby, 1979.

[69] Codman, 1917.

[70] Codman, 1934, p. vi.

[71] Beecher, 1940, cited in Fulton, 1946, pp. 93–95.

[72] In Countway Library, Boston, MA.

[73] Announcement for the meeting. Boston, Jan. 6, 1915. Author's library.

[74] O'Conner, 1956.

[75] Gilbreth and Carey, *Cheaper by the Dozen*, 1948.

[76] Codman, 1934, p. vi. He also brought these ideas to the AHA in 1913; Codman, 1913.

[77] *Bulletin of the American College of Surgeons*, March 1918.

[78] *Ibid.*

[79] American College of Surgeons, *Manual of Hospital Standardization*, 1938.

[80] MacEachern, 1935.

[81] *ACHA News*, 1939, *op. cit.*

[82] American College of Surgeons, *op. cit.*, 1938.

[83] Chapman, 1924. Also see Ochsner and Sturm, 1907, p. 43.

[84] Bachmeyer and Hartman, 1943.

[85] Bachmeyer and Hartman, 1948.

[86] Kipnis, 1955, p. 51. The College General Education Session of 1940 in Boston included a talk by Alden Mills on "How to Write for Publication" (Mills, 1941).

[87] Simon. Chapter One of his *Administrative Behavior*, 1947, adapted from *Public Administration Review*, Vol. 4, Winter 1944, pp. 16–30.

[88] Bachmeyer and Hartman, 1948, p. 801, footnote 3.

[89] Hartman, *Problems and References in Hospital Administration*, 1938, p. 58 (with editing by Michael M. Davis and Arthur Bachmeyer). Lewis Weeks interview of Gerhard Hartman, 1982. Personal communication with Gerhard Hartman, March 29, 1983.

[90] ACHA, Brown and Johnson, 1952, 1957. Another precursor to this book is Foley, 1933.

[91] ACHA, Brown and Johnson, *op. cit.*, 1957, p. 38.

[92] *Ibid.*, p. 69.

[93] Kipnis, 1955, p. 141. These courses may have continued beyond 1955. The classic book of this era on the human organization of the hospital is Burling et al., *The Give and Take in Hospitals*, 1956.

[94] ACHA, *Minute Book*, Vol. 1, Oct. 12, 1942. Kipnis, p. 51.

[95] *Hospital Administration*, journal of the American College of Hospital Administrators, abbreviated below as *HA*, Vol. 1, No. 1, Fall, 1956. It changed its name in 1976 and is abbreviated below as *H&HSA*. Between 1981 and 1986, six issues a year were published with the help of the College's Mary W. and Foster G. McGaw Endowment Fund. ACHE *Foundations for Excellence*, 1982, Foreword.

[96] *HA*, Vol. 2, No. 2, Spring, 1957.

[97] *HA*, Vol. 2, No. 4, Fall, 1957.

[98] *HA*, Vol. 3, No. 3, Summer, 1958.

[99] *HA*, Vol. 3, No. 4, Fall, 1958.

[100] *HA*, Vol. 4, No. 1, Winter, 1959.

[101] *HA*, Vol. 4, No. 2, Spring, 1959.

[102] *HA*, Vol. 4, No. 3, Summer, 1959.

[103] *HA*, Vol. 4, No. 4, Fall, 1959.

[104] *HA*, Vol. 5, No. 1, Winter, 1960.

[105] *HA*, Vol. 3, No. 4, Fall, 1958.

[106] *HA*, Vol. 6, No. 1, Winter, 1961.

[107] *HA*, Vol. 6, No. 2, Spring, 1961.

[108] *HA*, Vol. 3, No. 2, Spring, 1958.

[109] *HA*, Vol. 8, No. 1, Winter, 1963.

[110] *HA*, Vol. 10, No. 4, Fall, 1965.

[111] Simon, 1957.

[112] *HA*, Vol. 3, No. 2, Spring, 1958; Vol. 4, No. 4, Fall, 1959; Vol. 10, No. 4, Fall, 1965.

[113] Argyris, 1957. McGregor, 1960. Likert, 1961. Katz and Kahn, 1966. Levenson, 1968.

[114] Hall, 1956.

[115] *HA*, Vol. 5, No. 4, Fall, 1960.

[116] *HA*, Vol. 6, No. 1, Winter, 1961.

[117] *HA*, Vol. 2, No. 4, Fall, 1957; Vol. 5, No. 2, Spring, 1960; Vol. 7, No. 3, Summer, 1962; Vol. 7, No. 4, Fall, 1962. Golembiewski, R. (1967 Hamilton Book Award).

[118] *HA*, Vol. 6, No. 4, Fall, 1961; Vol. 8, No. 2, Spring, 1963; Vol. 9, No. 4, Fall, 1964.

[119] *HA*, Vol. 7, No. 4, Fall, 1962. Georgopolous and Mann, "Hospital as a Organization." *HA*, Vol. 9, No. 3, Summer, 1964.

[120] Georgopoulos and Mann, 1962.

[121] Georgopoulos, 1972.

[122] *HA*, Vol. 9, No. 2, Spring, 1964. Gordon P., 1964 and in *Hospitals*, "The Top Management Triangle in the Voluntary Hospital."

[123] ACHA, *1965 Progress Report*, pp. 45–46. Seventy-three percent of the 2,153 affiliate respondents said they spent an hour or more reading each issue of *Hospital Administration*. They passed it on to other managers in their hospital, and the overwhelming majority of respondents found it helpful.

[124] *HA*, Vol. 10, No. 2, Spring, 1965. Cordes, 1965, which won the ACHA article award for 1965.

[125] *HA*, Vol. 10, No. 2, Spring, 1965; Vol. 23, No. 4, Fall, 1978.

[126] *HA*, Vol. 12, No. 3, Summer, 1967; Vol. 17, No. 2, Spring, 1972; Vol. 18, No. 1, Winter, 1973; Vol. 19, No. 2, Spring, 1974; Vol. 19, No. 3, Summer, 1974; Vol. 19, No. 4, Fall, 1974; Vol. 21, No. 2, Spring, 1976.

[127] *HA*, Vol. 13, No. 4, Fall, 1968.

[128] *HA*, Vol. 14, No. 2, Spring, 1969; Vol. 17, No. 1, Winter, 1972.

[129] *HA*, Vol. 14, No. 3, Summer, 1969.

[130] *HA*, Vol. 14, No. 4, Fall, 1969; Vol. 16, No. 1, Winter, 1971.

[131] *HA*, Vol. 16, No. 1, Winter, 1971; Vol. 16, No. 4, Fall, 1971.

[132] *HA*, Vol. 16, No. 4, Fall, 1971.

[133] *HA*, Vol. 19, No. 4, Fall, 1974.

[134] *HA*, Vol. 20, No. 2, Spring, 1975.

[135] *Ibid.*

[136] *HA*, Vol. 20, No. 3, Summer, 1975; Vol. 23, No. 4, Fall, 1978.

[137] *HA*, Vol. 12, No. 2, Spring, 1967; Vol. 13, No. 3, Summer, 1968; Vol. 17, No. 4, Fall, 1972; Vol. 18, No. 3, Summer, 1973; Vol. 20, No. 1, Winter, 1975; Vol. 24, No. 4, Fall, 1979.

[138] *HA*, Vol. 13, No. 1, Winter, 1968; Vol. 19, No. 1, Winter, 1974; Vol. 19, No. 4, Fall, 1974; Vol. 20, No. 1, Winter 1975; Vol. 20, No. 2, Spring, 1975.

[139] *HA*, Vol. 20, No. I, Winter, 1975; Vol. 21, No. 2, Spring, 1976. Special Issue #2, 1980.

[140] *HA*, Vol. 17, No. 4, Fall, 1972; Vol. 21, No. 1, Winter, 1976; Vol. 21, No. 4, Fall, 1976.

[141] ACHA, *A Selected Bibliography for the Well Read Health Services Manager*, Jan. 25, 1979, p. 50. Of the 15, this does not include Honorary Fellows. There is one ACHA publication on the list.

[142] Eckenhoff and Harasymirv, 1979.

[143] *H&HSA*, Vol. 28, No. 1, 28:3, 28:5, 29:4, 30.4 (2 articles), 33:4, 35.3, 36:2.

[144] *H&HSA*, Vol. 28, No. 2, 29:1, 29:4, 30:1, 30:3, 30:6, 31:1 (pp. 62, 75), 31:3, 31:4, 33:2, 36:4.

[145] *H&HSA*, Vol. 29, No. 1 (2 articles) 29:3, 30:1, 30:6, 31:1, 31:2 (2 articles), 32:2, 32:4, 35:1, 36:2.

[146] *H&HSA*, Vol. 28, No. 4, 29:2, 30:2, 30:6, 31:2, 32:2, 33:3, 35:1, 35:2.

[147] *H&HSA*, Vol. 28, No. 3 (whole issue); 29:1, 30:6, 31:2, 31:4, 31:6, 32:2 (2 articles), 33:1, 33:2.

[148] *H&HSA*, Vol. 28, No. 2, 28:5, 29:4, 35:2, 36:3.

[149] *H&HSA*, Vol. 30, No. 3 (p. 44), 32:3, 35:4.

[150] *H&HSA*, Vol. 28, No. 2, 28:3, 28:5, 29:3, 29:6, 30:3, 30:6, 31:2, 32:2, 33:1, 35:1.

[151] *H&HSA*, Vol. 28, No. 3, 28:6, 29:4 (pp. 21, 50, 79), 31:6, 32:2, 33:1, 33:2.

[152] *H&HSA*, Vol. 28, No. 2, 28:6, 31:6, 34:4, 35:1, 35:2 (2 articles).

[153] *H&HSA*, Vol. 30, No. 4 (10 articles), 32:3 (3 articles), 33:1, 35:4, 36:4.

[154] *H&HSA*, Vol. 28, No. 6, (p. 21) 29:3, 31:5, 31:6.

[155] *H&HSA*, Vol. 34, No. 2, 36:4.

[156] *H&HSA*, Vol. 28, No. 3 (p. 38), 32:2, 34:1, 35:4, 36:2, 36:4 (2 articles).

[157] *H&HSA*, Vol. 29, No. 6 (p. 7), 31:2.

[158] *H&HSA*, Vol. 33, No. 2, 35:3.

[159] *H&HSA*, Vol. 32, No. 3, 33:1, 33:3.

[160] *H&HSA*, Vol. 30, No. 1 (3 articles) 30:3.

[161] *H&HSA*, Vol. 3, No. 5 (3 articles).

[162] *H&HSA*, Vol. 28, No. 2 (pp. 15, 81), 29:2 (pp. 84, 102, 120), 30:3, 30:5 (4 articles), 31:2, 31:3, 31:6, 35:3.

[163] Arrow, 1963.

[164] Feldstein, Martin, 1967.

[165] ACHA, *Twenty-Sixth Congress on Administration, March 1–4*, 1983.

[166] *H&HSA*, Vol. 29:2, 32:2, 34:3.

[167] *H&HSA*, Vol. 29, No. 5 (four articles).

[168] *H&HSA*, Vol. 35:3, 37:2. Also, Kit Simpson and Curtis McLaughlin won the 1991 Health Management Research Award for "Diffusion and Adoption of Total Quality Managment"; and Robert Casalou won the 1991 first-place graduate division title in the Hill-Rom Management Essay Competition in Health Administration for "Total Quality Management in Health Care."

8

New Directions

The Mission of the American College of Healthcare Executives

The College's mission remains what it has always been: to enhance the practice of healthcare management and to ultimately build a more effective and compassionate healthcare system. No longer an organization comprised exclusively of hospital administrators, the College now works to represent and serve healthcare management professionals in all settings.

Setting Standards

The mission of the College is to increase the effectiveness of healthcare management by promoting high professional ethical standards.

Executing Excellence

The College advances management excellence by serving the professional and personal development needs of healthcare executives.

Inform and Advocate

The College is a key information resource and advocate for healthcare management. It represents the profession to diverse publics and brings management insight and a system-wide perspective to the dialogue on healthcare policy issues.

ACHE 1985

The mission of the American College of Healthcare Executives is to be the professional membership society for healthcare executives; to meet its affiliates' professional, educational, and leadership needs; to increase the effectiveness of healthcare management, and to advance healthcare management excellence.

ACHE, 1989[1]

In 1980–1981 the College developed its "programmatic thrusts" as a guide to planning and future development. These became the blueprint for College development in the 1980's. According to Stuart Wesbury, they were based on "Thoughts floating around."[2] These thrusts are summarized in Table 8.1. The largest activity according to Wesbury was the self-assessment project (professional development). It allows affiliates to assess their own skills and compare their performance to their peers. This became the basis for planned continuing education. The project was funded by the Kellogg Foundation and is described in chapter 5. This led to the creation of the Stull Learning Resource Center at the College which includes a library on health management. The initial idea of creating a resource directory became too much of an effort and was largely abandoned, with the remaining parts in the bibliographic references in the College's self-assessment manual.

Early Career development took several paths. One is the development of Student Affiliates to encourage early College membership.

The College developed a list of postgraduate clinical experiences. When most of the master's programs became two academic years, the administrative internship or residency largely disappeared. With the increase in program graduates, postgraduate fellowships returned to popularity. The *Directory of Postgraduate Fellowships and Management Development Programs in Health Services Administration* is published annually by the College.

Young administrator groups started independently from the College. They became the basis of the College's local healthcare executive groups. This was also true for the women's healthcare executive networks. The College developed policies for formal recognition of these groups and provides them support. The women's healthcare executive networks have been very valuable to some female affiliates, who value them highly; others, however, find that they imply separation. Although he worked hard at it, Stuart Wesbury says his one disappointment was his inability to link more closely with other specialized health management associations.

ORGANIZATIONAL CHANGE

The growth of the College diversity led to a change in the number of Regents to include At-Large Regents appointed by the Council of Regents to increase the number of regents who are women, minority members, or from nonhospital organizations.[4] As of 1993 there are 13 members of the Board of Governors (9 Governors), 92 Regents and about 99 Staff employed by the College.[5]

TABLE 8.1
Programmatic Thrusts 1980–1981[3]

Programmatic Thrusts—which were later incorporated into the Strategic Plans consisted of specific projects classified into seven special areas and designed to help affiliates in their continual challenge to enhance their administrative performance and improve their managerial competence.

A. Professional Development (Lifelong Learning)
   1. Self-Assessment (Diagnosis/Treatment)
      a. Methods
         Objective: To develop alternate assessment methodologies (e.g., in-basket exercises, structured work samplings) and to integrate the Georgia State University "Health Services Management Computer Simulation" into the College's Self-Assessment Program.
      b. Tracks
         Objective: To develop six "system" and "discipline" specific self-assessment tracks to permit the College to measure a professional's functional knowledge and skill in areas of management speciality. Examples include financial management, planning, etc. Objective profiles will be provided to participants as a basis for professional development.
      c. Resource Directory
         Objective: To develop, produce, and distribute a management-oriented directory of learning resources for hospital and health services executives including quality-validated references to the following:
         • current books
         • proceedings of meetings
         • audio and video cassettes
         • current management films (tentative)
         • current articles
         • continuing education seminars/workshops/programs
         • selected case studies
      d. Learning Resource Center
         Objective: To develop a learning resources capability where management executives can self-select resources and self-direct their energies toward enhancing their managerial strengths and correcting their weaknesses.

         To locate together, physical and functional resources, both as a non-duplicative extension to, and development of the Asa Bacon Library and, more important, to provide learning resource services on an outreach basis to professionals and centers of study in the field.

         To provide an organized professional development counseling aspect to learning resources available within the profession.

TABLE 8.1
Continued

2. Beginning and Early Career Development

   Objective: To create a Task Force to examine issues and make recommendations concerning ACHA and ACHA affiliate roles and responsibilities related to practitioner involvement in academic practicums and immediate post graduate experiences. Topical areas for study and recommendations include:
   - Practical Experiences in Academic Programs
   - Post-Graduate Clinical Experience
   - Entry-Level Employment
   - Position Referral Program
   - Mentoring

3. Governing Body Relationships (CEO Placement)

   Objective: To develop methodologies (e.g., publications, advertisements, conferences, etc.) to establish effective communication links with governing bodies.

4. ACHA Publications and Tapes

   Objective: To maintain effective communications with affiliates and others concerning ACHA services, project outputs, plans and educational programs using state-of-the-art communication techniques and approaches.

5. New Educational Approaches

   Objective: To effectively meet health administrators' constant need for new learning in the following areas:
   1. professional competency
   2. information resultant from scientific discoveries, new regulations, etc.
   3. personal growth issues, such as career enhancement, financial planning, etc.

B. Credentialing

   Objective: (1) To identify the needs for a credentialing process to interact with the changing health care delivery system; (2) to develop guidelines for credentialing based upon projections and predictions of future needs and expectations for health services administrators during the next ten years; (3) to develop specialty management examination tracks in the College certification program; and (4) to develop new approaches to publication of Fellowship cases and theses.

C. Recredentialing

   Objective: To develop guidelines and criteria for a system of recredentialing professionals to maintain an indication of contemporary relevance of a capacity for competence in management in the health delivery system, utilizing, among other processes, the self-assessment program.

D. Research

   Objective: To establish a continuing program of research on management roles in the health care delivery system. The research agenda would include:
   —collection and analysis of position descriptions and titles for management personnel in various types of organizations and at various levels in the management structure.
   —periodic surveys of compensation.
   —identification of career patterns in the profession.

TABLE 8.1
Continued

E. Public Policy

Objective: To establish a constructive and visible role for the College in bringing the expertise of the profession to bear on issues of public policy in health services delivery. The outcome would be a series of occasional position papers and support for testimony and statements related to public policy issues (see ACHA/AHA Accord—July, 1980).

F. Academia Relationships

Objective: To establish a permanent and specific programmatic activity to address our overall relationships with the academic community. Furthermore, the objective is to provide for staff and other financial support to allow the College to carry on an effective program of communication with faculty, graduate and undergraduate programs and the AUPHA in order to develop appropriate interfaces between practice and academia and to encourage the continued development of our Student Associate program.

G. Professional Organization Relationships

Objective: To establish a computerized, multi-organizational, health administration data base, compatible with the College's own "Health Administration Manpower Profile System," for purposes of conducting a broad and comprehensive program of research and special studies; and to maintain that multiorganizational data base by providing varied, supportive services to the organizational participants.

The diversity of membership led to the change in the name of the College. When it was first proposed, 65 percent of the Regents voted for it. One more vote would have resulted in the two-thirds votes needed for the change. Although this could have been done, such an important change would be better made with near unanimity. Four years later it was passed with near unanimity. Stuart Wesbury said, "we like to think that we made 'healthcare' one word." "Others followed our example."

The College was also reorganized. It was in 1980 a 501(c)3 non-profit organization. This does not allow for political involvement or public policy advocacy. The College was transformed into two corporations: the Foundation of the ACHE, classified 501(c)3, and the College itself, which is a 501(c)6 organization. The latter can include unrelated business income from the for-profit subsidiary, which in the case of the College is called Professional Society Services Incorporated (PSSI). It in turn held Career Decision, Inc. The Foundation includes Health Administration Press as well as the Division of Education.

Credentialing changes in the late 1980s and early 1990s include the development of management tracks. Membership exams now have a core component, plus specialty applications, tracks in ambulatory care, mental health, and planning. Recredentialing has become an accepted fact and is now mandatory. Affiliates must demonstrate: (1) current work in the field; (2) documented continuing education, (3) leadership, and (4) community involvement. By 1987, about a thousand affiliates had been recertified.[6]

Research has become a larger fixed activity resulting in an ongoing series of studies including the Delphi Studies and studies of CEO turnover. This has been aided by steady progress in computerizing the College affiliates data starting in 1973. The Directory became computerized in the 1970s. The result is that the College now has a unique database about healthcare executives.

Public policy issues fall into three broad categories:

1. Broad public issues which are "everyone's business," such as access to care. Many groups are involved here.
2. Issues related to healthcare executives as individuals, such as opposing employment discrimination. This is a distinctive area for the College.
3. Institutional issues, such as Medicare reimbursement and life safety codes, which are the domain of the AHA.

Public policy programs have included press releases that typically relate the results of research studies and an advocacy position. Surveys show that affiliates are in favor of greater public policy involvement by the College. New endeavors in the 1990s are described in Chapter 2.

Academic relationships were strengthened in the 1980s by development of student chapters at colleges and universities, Faculty Associates, and guidelines for faculty experience in healthcare settings. Academics are editors of *Hospital and Health Services Administration* and other journals published by the College through Health Administration Press. Further cooperation with AUPHA for joint publications and in reporting on beginning and early career development has also strengthened academic relationships.

Educational activities have changed. The yearly Congress is now the largest gathering of healthcare executives, with annual attendance exceeding 4,300. The 36th Congress was held March 1–5, 1993.[7] Long recognized as a place to see and be seen, career related activities, such as looking for a job and resume review, became an explicit part. The Congress offers many (95 in 1993) seminars, lectures, and other educational events.

Throughout each year, a variety of educational activities take place. The major activities are: conferences, which are usually two-day programs; institutes, which focus in-depth on a single topic; and seminars, which cover a number of topics, presented in a classroom setting.

The 1993 educational programs are described in Chapter 5, with more details on topics and participants.

Internship and Fellowship Programs at the College

In 1990, the College established an ACHE Minority Internship available to student associates of the College who have completed one year in an ACEHSA accredited graduate program. During three months the intern rotates through all major divisions of the College. The Stuart A. Wesbury Postgraduate Fellowship is a one-year program at the College open to student associates who have graduated from an accredited graduate program.

Health Administration Press

The College has been printing material from its first year and continues to do so. Richard Stull developed a working relationship with Aaron Cohodes, head of Teach'em and Pluribus Press. Cohodes' company records and distributes tapes of College Congress sessions. The College worked with Pluribus Press to publish the boxed, four-volume Fiftieth Anniversary Commemorative set in 1983.[8]

By 1984, Stuart Wesbury and Aaron Cohodes had started discussions about a joint publishing venture. An initial thought was to link the College, Pluribus Press, and Health Administration Press (HAP), but these had three distinctly different corporate cultures.[9]

By 1985, discussions with Pluribus Press had come to an end, but were continuing with John Griffith, Professor of Hospital Administration at the University of Michigan where Health Administration Press had been founded in cooperation with the AUPHA.[10]

The Health Administration Press had its origins in the early 1960's, when a notable group of faculty were drawn together at the University of Michigan hospital administration program under the directorship of Walter McNerney; included among them: John Griffith, Lawrence Hill, Beverly Payne, Donald Riedel, Thomas Fitzpatrick, Symond Gottlieb, Bernard Tresnowski, and others. (Their major research project culminated in the two volume report, *Hospital and Medical Economics: A Study of Population Service, Costs, Methods of Payment and Controls*, and published by the AHA's Hospital Research and Educational Trust in 1962.[11])

Other books followed from their research which the program arranged to have published. By 1972, this publishing effort had become formalized as the Health Administration Press with the support of a $50,000 grant from the Kellogg Foundation, obtained by Lewis Weeks, Gary Filerman of AUPHA, and John Griffith. The AUPHA withdrew from participation in 1984, after which time the Press was owned and operated by the University of Michigan. This University has its own Press, but also had about thirteen other publishing activities in various areas (for example, near eastern studies) one of which was HAP. All used the University Press warehouse, distribution and order processing system.

Planning for Cardiac Care[12] was the first book of the newly organized HAP and remained in print to 1984. The full-time directors were Lewis Weeks, Treville Leger, Robert DuBois and, since 1981, Daphne Grew. The governance arrangement until 1984 consisted of a three-person management committee of John Griffith, Gary Filerman and another person drawn from one of the other programs in health administration.

By 1984, the Press needed capital to expand. Foundations and the University were not interested, and thought was given to selling the Press.

In 1985, Stuart Wesbury and John Griffith developed a plan for the College to buy the Press, keeping the name, the staff, and the Ann Arbor editorial office, while incorporating its activities into those of the College. Although this arrangement was satisfactory, it took a long time to finalize the sale. The University had to agree, all author contracts had to be reviewed, and inventory evaluated. The Press is now a division of the College's Foundation (501(c)3 organization) and is managed like other College divisions except that it remains in a simple house in Ann Arbor rented from the University. According to Daphne Grew, this allows the Press to keep its experienced competent staff and its location in the "short-run printing capital of the country." A fax machine and day-long trips maintain communication between Ann Arbor and Chicago.

The Press has continued to grow, in part because the College has provided the working capital that has made expansion possible. The Press has a reputation for excellence in a field that has seen a number of publishers enter and leave. A conservative opinion would be that the Press is one of three leading publishers in this field. An enthusiastic opinion would be that it is the leader. The Winter 1993 Catalogue lists 122 books in print,[13] in addition to the four journals edited by the Press. The four journals include the College's *Hospital and Health Services Administration* (H&HSA). This journal, previously edited in the College offices by Lynn Wimmer and Joyce Flory, now has an external editor, starting with Professor Sam Levey, May 1987–1991,[14] and from 1991, Professor Richard Kurz. It has an external editorial board, as do all four journals and book series. The H&HSA board are all College members. The Press also publishes *Frontiers of Health Services Management*, edited in 1992–1993 by Douglas Conrad. The Press also publishes two scholarly journals, *Health Services Research*, Gordon DeFriese, editor, which is owned by the AHA's Health Research and Educational Trust and is the official journal of the Association for Health Services Research. The fourth journal is *Medical Care Review*, edited by Thomas Rundall, which celebrated its Fiftieth Anniversary in 1993. It was originally started by the Medical Care Department of the University of Michigan School of Public Health (see Table 8.2).

To fill orders for Health Administration Press books and other publications, the College established an Order Processing Center in Melrose Park, Illinois, a Chicago suburb. Six staff members work at this location, which includes a large warehouse for books as well as archives and other inventoried items. There is a computer system for processing orders and keeping subscription records. Other activities include printing and mailing of the newsletters and other documents sent to College affiliates, as well as packaging books and delivering supplies to the downtown office.

TABLE 8.2
Journals Published by Health Administration Press[16]

Hospital and Health Services Administration

Provides information on the latest trends, developments, and innovations in the industry. In concise articles, experts offer new approaches to the many areas of healthcare: management, policy and planning, quality issues, marketing, financing, and management information. The official journal of the American College of Healthcare Executives, it is free to College affiliates. (Quarterly)

Frontiers of Health Services Management

Each issue focuses on a single topic of immediate interest to forward-looking health services executives. One primary article leads the debate, followed by commentaries from outstanding scholars and practitioners in the field. Winner of the 1986, 1988, 1989, 1991, 1992, and 1993 Dean Conley Award. (Quarterly)

Medical Care Review

Features carefully peer-reviewed scholarly papers, along with commentaries, that analyze, critique, and synthesize the literature and research in areas such as: the financing of health services; organizational structure and behavior; physician-hospital relationships; patient behavior; and political issues. (Quarterly) [In late 1993, the College decided to cease its publication of this journal.]

Health Services Research

Published for the Hospital Research and Educational Trust. A multidisciplinary journal that provides those engaged in research, public policy formulation, health services administration, education, and practice, with advance information on new trends and the latest techniques of research and evaluation, enabling them to take advantage of current and significant research. Emphasizes not only scholarly research but the practical application of that research in the interest of improved healthcare delivery. (Bimonthly)

In 1992, the College concluded a new agreement for cooperative publishing with AUPHA. Thus, Press books are published with four different imprints. These are the ACHE Management Series for executives; the AUPHA Press/Health Administration Press for basic textbooks; the AHSR/Health Administration Press series for scholarly work, and Health Administration Press for books for the entire field. In addition the Press markets other College publications.

In February 1990, the College purchased the titles and name of Pluribus Press. This included 34 titles in inventory, added to the HAP list. Pluribus Press as a name no longer is in use. Some of the Press's best-selling textbooks include: Howard Berman, Lewis Weeks and Steven Kukla, *The Financial Management of Hospitals*, now in its eighth edition; *The Law of Hospital and Health Care Administration*, second edition by Arthur Southwick; *Information Systems for Health Services Administration*, fourth edition, Charles Austin; *Health Services Management*, fourth edition, compiled and edited by Anthony Kovner and Duncan Neuhauser, and *The Well-Managed Community Hospital*, second edition, by John R. Griffith.[16]

Long-term best-selling other books are: John Witt, *Building a Better Hospital Board* and John Eisenberg, *Doctor's Decisions and the Cost of Medical Care.*[17]

The Press has greatly increased the College role in the intellectual evolution of healthcare management. It is another bridge between the College, the scholarly community (AHSR) and academia (AUPHA). Its editorial boards are a way that academics play an active role in College affairs. Possibly every student in health administration is learning from publications of the Press and the College.

Career Decision, Inc.

In the early 1980s, Richard Dolan of the executive search firm of Witt and Dolan separated from this firm to create a new company that would provide outplacement services for healthcare executives.[18] He spoke about this at a College Congress, and Stuart Wesbury followed up with a visit to his office. Dolan saw a link with the College as an opportunity for better access to clients, while the College saw the acquisition of such services as consistent with the plan to be more helpful to affiliates. This lead to the College's acquisition of Career Decision, Inc. Dolan stayed with this firm for about three years; when he left, he was replaced by Michael Broscio, who continues to head the firm. Approximately 1,300 clients had been served by August 1993, since its founding in 1980.[19]

The College could not become involved in executive search activities because recommending one affiliate for an attractive position would

TABLE 8.3
ACHE Strategic Plan 1988[20]

Strategy

1. Address the critical management policy issues facing the health care delivery system, particularly as they affect the quality of leadership of executives.
2. Develop a broader spectrum of educational programming and of meeting the professional needs of affiliates and other health care managers in various settings with a variety of educational backgrounds and at various stages of their careers.
3. Explore alternatives including interest and/or specialty sections to respond to the increasing diversity of the College's membership.
4. Establish formal ties with Healthcare Executive Groups and Women's Networks so as to enhance affiliate involvement at the local level.
5. Enhance the recognition and value of becoming and remaining an affiliate of the College through increased recognition of the College and its affiliates as a professional society advancing the effectiveness of health care management through a national action plan.
6. Position the College to address the managerial ethics issues facing the health care executive.
7. Maintain and strengthen relationships with health administration education through additional and enhanced programs for faculty affiliates, student associates and student chapters.

Note: By 1991 item 4 was considered accomplished and this strategy was changed to "Enhance the College's efforts in the area of public policy." The wording of item 3 was changed in 1991 to "Explore alternatives to respond to the increasing diversity of membership."

probably distress others who were not chosen. Outplacement services and career counseling do not pose this problem.

The 1980–1981 programmatic thrusts were not revised, but instead, under the leadership of Alton Pickert, replaced by strategic plans in the mid-1980s. These plans were revised from time to time. Table 8.3 summarizes the College's 1988 strategic plan. These seven strategies continue the College focus on areas of importance such as public policy, educational needs, membership diversity, local networks, the value of membership, ethics, and educational relationships.

Chapter 10 will return to strategic plans for the 1990s.

NOTES

1. ACHE, *1985–1986 Annual Report*, p. 4; *1991–1992 Annual Report* (adopted 1989).
2. Stuart Wesbury interview, Dec. 29, 1992. Much of what follows in this chapter comes from this interview.
3. ACHE, *1985–1986 Annual Report*.
4. Wesbury interview, Dec. 1992.

[5] ACHE, Aug. 1993 "Fact Sheet."

[6] ACHE, *1986–1987 Annual Report.*

[7] ACHE, Nov. 1992 "Fact Sheet."

[8] This set includes *Coming of Age, Judgment in Administration* (Ray E. Brown), *Foundations for Excellence* (reprints of the Edgar C. Hayhow Award-winning articles from *Hospital Health Services Administration* from 1959—the year the first winner was chosen—through 1981), and *Challenging the Profession.* The Article of the Year Award started in 1958 and was renamed in honor of Conley in 1967. *Challenging the Profession* republished the first 25 award-winning articles, 1958 to 1983.

[9] Wesbury interview, Dec. 1992. Daphne Grew interview, Dec. 22, 1992.

[10] Daphne Grew interview, Dec. 22, 1992. Much of the section on the Press comes from this interview.

[11] Walter McNerney and Study staff, 1962.

[12] Clipson and Wehrer, *Planning for Cardiac Care*, 1973.

[13] Health Administration Press, *Winter 1993 Catalogue of Publications*, p. 20.

[14] Wesbury "Editorial," *Hospital & Health Services Administration*, May 1987.

[15] Health Administration Press, internal document, Feb. 3, 1988.

[16] Berman, Weeks, and Kukla, 1990. Southwick, 1988. Austin, 1992. Kovner and Neuhauser, 1990. Griffith, 1992.

[17] Witt, 1987. Eisenberg, 1986.

[18] Wesbury, inteview, Dec. 1992.

[19] ACHE, Aug. 1993, "Fact Sheet."

[20] ACHE, *1988–1989 Annual Report*, pp. 2–3.

9

The College: Its Leadership and Organization

For the man or woman who intends to make a career in hospital or health services administration, affiliation with the American College of Hospital Administrators is paramount. This is true for a number of reasons.

First of all, membership in the ACHA and participation in its programs readily provides professional identification in the field.

Secondly, hospital boards of trustees, governmental agencies and associations, more and more are restricting their key health care managerial positions to persons who hold affiliation in the College.

Finally, membership in the American College of Hospital Administrators is one obvious measure of a person's level of achievement in the health administration field and a reflection of one's interest in and commitment to self-development.

ACHA, 1979[1]

One means of viewing the evolution of the College and its organization is to consider the periods of its five previous chief executive officers. Dewey Lutes (1933–1937) and his friends created the organization. Gerhard Hartman, Ph.D. (1937–1941) brought more of the field's leaders into affiliation with the College and developed close links with university education for hospital administration. These two periods resulted in substantial growth in seminar education for hospital administration.

Dean Conley (1942–1965), the first full-time CEO of the College, provided stability and a formal structure for the College. His tenure saw a growth in the number of male administrators, in part promoted by World War II and the proliferation of graduate programs.

241

Richard J. Stull (1965–1979), brought financial solvency to the College and saw it through its corporate restructuring of 1965 and the growth of the hospital field in size, complexity, and costs.

Stuart A. Wesbury, Jr., Ph.D. (1979–1991) saw both growth and new directions in education, publications, and public policy.

Biographical data on these officers and those who were presidents or chairmen during their administrations appear in the College's biannual *Directory,* as noted in the References to this chapter.

The Years of J. Dewey Lutes 1933–1937[2]

Lutes, John Dewey[3]
Presidents (Chairmen) 1933–1937
1933–1934 Wordell, Charles[4]
1935–1936 Neff, Robert Emery[5]
1935–1936 Carter, Fred G., M.D.[6]
1936–1937 MacLean, Basil C., M.D.[7]

Lutes and his friends, Maurice Dubin, Ernest Erickson, L. C. Vonder Heidt and Charles A. Wordell, defined the College and saw to its creation.[8] As described in Chapter 1, the core components of the College were developed at the outset and remain in place to this day. The various levels of membership, periodic meetings, and the focus on continuing education remain at the heart of the College.

In the beginning, the organization of the College was conceived with a Board of Regents and an Executive Committee consisting of the President (later called Chairman), First Vice President, Second Vice President, and Director General (combining the functions of Secretary and treasurer) plus three other members.[9] In addition, there was a Committee on Constitution and Bylaws and a Nominating Committee,[10] plus a secret Credentials Committee which would soon have regional subcommittees.

Because expenses had to be limited, the Executive Committee handled problems of major consequence. Only later did the Board of Regents assume its full role in directing College affairs.[11]

On February 15, 1937, the Board of Regents approved the establishment of the first headquarters for the College at 18 East Division Street, Chicago. At that time, responsibilities of the Director General were so great that a full-time Executive Secretary was needed, a need that was not satisfied until 1942. Dewey Lutes spent a great deal of time travelling around the country, often at his own expense, in order to spread word about the College. At this February meeting, the Board agreed to pay him $100 a month.[12]

A typical example of continuity was the college key, originally designed by Dewey Lutes and made out of 10 karat gold. It was first sold for six dollars. Members were urged to buy one immediately because the manufacturer warned that the price might be raised due to the increased cost of gold. An ACHA *Bulletin* noted that the key "depicts education, learning and enlightenment by a rising sun in the background, with a lamp of knowledge resting upon books; service is depicted by a chevron; medicine by a caduceus and nursing by a cross. It has remained unchanged since the start of the College."[13]

The Years of Gerhard Hartman 1937–1941

Hartman, Gerhard[14]
Presidents (Chairmen)
1937–1938 Bishop, Howard Elmer[15]
1938–1939 Buerki, Robin Carl, M.D.[16]
1939–1940 Hamilton, James Alexander[17]
1940–1941 Bachmeyer, Arthur Charles, M.D.[18]

At the time Gerhard Hartman was appointed part-time Executive Secretary of the College, he was working on his doctorate degree in business administration at the University of Chicago, where he was a Teaching Assistant and Instructor with the Graduate Program in Hospital Administration.[19] From 1939 to 1942, he was Associate Director of this program under Arthur C. Bachmeyer, M.D. Hartman received his doctorate degree in 1942.

He described how he was given the job of Executive Secretary at the College.[20] Basil McLean, M.D., Chairman of the College, came to Chicago and asked to interview Hartman for the position. Hartman said:

> I very innocently appeared for the appointment and sat down on a settee. Basil was tall, elegant, and absolutely brilliant. He sat at one end of the settee, and I at the other. What I failed to notice, was that the door to the room was two inches ajar and the entire interview was conducted without the visible but with the actual presence of Dr. Fred Carter, Dr. Claude Munger, Miss Bernice Lawson, Bob Buerki, and I have forgotten, someone else.
>
> After the interview Basil said, 'What do you want for a salary?' I can't remember what I said. It was some modest sum, far less than what they were prepared to offer. I heard a roar of laughter. Then the door burst open and out came some of the others. That is the way my role in the College began.[21]

Hartman was appointed September 13, 1937, at a salary of $300 per month. According to Hartman, the founding fathers of the College were predominantly nonphysician executives concerned with the powerful position held by some of the leading physician administrators of the day.

It was not an anti-physician group, but they were concerned with achieving equality of pay.[22]

> My reason for getting the physicians into the College was that there was nothing to be gained by any symbolic or actual schism. Accordingly, when committees were formed we had one headed by Jim Hamilton (a non physician) and we had another one headed by Agnew (a physician).
>
> That kind of parity, if you look through the records, was one of the notable characteristics. To make real peace with the physicians, it wasn't difficult to get those that were in the American Hospital Association work, "but the real brilliant mind in the field was Dr. S. S. Goldwater. At that time, Dr. Goldwater was the Commissioner of Health for Mayor LaGuardia of New York. I might say that concurrently Goldwater was consultant to twenty eight large hospitals and medical centers. He had that kind of mind. Howard Bishop, administrator of Robert Packer Hospital in Sayre, Pennsylvania knew him. So Howard called Dr. Goldwater's secretary and said he would like to bring a fellow named Hartman in for an interview not to take more than twenty minutes. We stayed for an hour and a half. The exchange among us was truly entrancing. He not only accepted the opportunity to join ACHA, but within two months thereafter, he accepted an invitation to be the principal speaker at the 1938 Dallas convocation of the College. He gave one of his best addresses. The theme I will never forget. 'Hospitals Don't Practice Medicine, Doctors Practice Medicine in Hospitals.' It was just right. . . . He gave the College an aura that stood it in massively good stead. It was then that the journals like *Modern Hospital* and the rest accepted the publication of articles that we would digest from speeches that were given.[23]

One of the major purposes of the College was to build the professionalism of its members through its educational programs.[24] Hartman stated:

> Absolutely, that's why my Ph.D. studies and my University of Chicago appointment made me seem worthy. The College, born of controversy and conflict, also had a problem because I insisted that professionalism had to equate with educational identity.

Through Ray Amberg, Administrator of the University of Minnesota Hospital and Regent of the College, Hartman helped to organize the successful annual College-sponsored University of Minnesota Institute. The President of this university wrote on behalf of the ACHE to other university presidents, paving the way for other Institutes at Columbia, Duke, Berkeley, Tulane, Baylor and Harvard.[25]

At the College's Institute in Puerto Rico, Gerhard Hartman contracted malaria.[26] In 1942, he became the Administrator of Newton-Wellesley Hospital, outside Boston. Hartman said, "Fortunately, when Dean Conley succeeded me, he was of a far less aggressive sort than I. He was more of a coordinator . . ."[27] According to W. Richard Kirk, "Conley was the first true executive."[28]

The Years of Dean Conley, 1942–1965

Conley, Dean[29]
Presidents (Chairmen) 1942–1965
1941–1942 Wilson, Lucius Roy, M.D.[30]
1942–1943 Norby, Joseph[31]
1943–1944 Bishop, Robert H., Jr., M.D.[32]
1944–1946 Munger, Claude W., M.D.[33]
1946–1947 Bradley, Frank Richard, M.D.[34]
1947–1948 Hayhow, Edgar C., Ph.D.[35]
1948–1949 Turnbull, Jessie Junkin[36]
1949–1950 Allen, Wilmar Mason, M.D.[37]
1950–1951 Walter, Frank J.[38]
1951–1952 Erickson, Ernest I.[39]
1952–1953 Mooney, Fraser Dudley, M.D., C.M.[40]
1953–1954 Steele, Merrill Festus, M.D.[41]
1954–1955 Kerlikowske, Albert Carl, M.D.[42]
1956–1957 Swanson, Arthur John[43]
1957–1958 Groner, Frank Shelby[44]
1958–1959 Eckert, Anthony William[45]
1959–1960 Brown, Ray E.[46]
1960–1961 Sutley, Melvin L.[47]
1961–1962 Terrell, Burl Toliver[48]
1962–1963 Sutton, Frank Calvin, M.D.[49]
1963–1964 Bachmeyer, Robert Wesley[50]
1964–1965 Yaw, Ronald Donald[51]

Paul Fesler, Administrator of the University of Minnesota Hospital, brought both Ray Amberg and Dean Conley into hospital administration.[52] Fesler moved to Chicago; Ray Amberg replaced him; and Dean Conley became Administrator of the University of Minnesota student health service.

Conley contracted tuberculosis, although the diagnosis was not completely clear. By the time he was offered the ACHE position by Lucius Wilson, with the encouragement of Ray Amberg, Conley had a pneumothorax. Periodically, air was inserted into half the lung cavity to collapse that lung and, thereby, presumably stop the tuberculosis.

The committee of the College which interviewed Conley included Lucius Wilson, Joseph Norby, and Arthur Bachmeyer, M.D., formerly a chest physician who saw that Conley's disease was under control and would not hinder his work at the College.

Conley remembered Dewey Lutes as a dynamo who pushed himself hard. He remembered Hartman as precocious and personable, preaching and promoting educational activities. "Arthur Bachmeyer thought a great deal of him." Bachmeyer, according to Conley, was a serious, gracious, but somewhat inscrutable person.[53]

As of 1943, the committee structure of the College had expanded to reflect the larger range of College activities. In addition to the Executive Committee, there were Committees on Bylaws, Educational Policies, Code of Ethics, Defense, Poll of Current Issues, Nominating, Credentials, and Editorial Policies. See Table 9.1.

At the start, the annual dues were $25; the initiation fees were $25 for members and $50 for Fellows. As of September 1, 1933, the College had a cash balance of $1,510.29.[54]

By 1939, revenue from dues initiation and advancement fees was about $16,000. Expenditures were: $6,500 for salaries; committee expenses, $850; institutes, $15,000; convocation, $1,100; conventions, $1,500; printing, $700; office expenses, $800; and miscellaneous, $1,750, leaving a surplus of $1,500 for the year and a cash balance of $5,000.[55]

In June, 1943, the first contribution of record was received by the College to help support educational programs. Given by Dr. Otho F. Ball, Honorary Fellow and publisher of *Modern Hospital*, the contribution was for $1,000 and began a continuing flow of funds in the form of gifts or foundation grants.[56] The College had not sought government funding.[57] By 1945, the College's income was $39,034 and expenses were $30,013.[58]

The steadily expanding activities of the College were reflected in a growing committee structure. By 1957–58, (in addition to the Boards and Committees listed in the bylaws and described above, there were the following: Election Judges, Central Committee on Institutes, Code of Ethics Committee (jointly with the AHA), Budget Committee, Study Committee on Admissions and Advancements, Insurance, Administrative Relationship with Medical Staff (jointly with the AHA), and an AHA-ACHE Joint Committee.[60]

As of 1955, there were 15 regions of the College: 13 for the U.S. and two for Canada. As of 1957, there were 18 regions.

The active Members and Fellows of each region elected the Regent for their area for a term of three years; these 18 people comprised the Board of Regents.[61] The Regents, with the College officers serving ex-officio, held the powers of a Board of Directors. The President served as Chairman of the Board of Regents. The Regents approved policy,

TABLE 9.1
College Standing Committees and Dates as Known (Ad hoc Committees and Task Forces excluded)

American Hospital Association, ACHA-AHA Joint Committee; Committee on Hospital Associations [*1957–1965,* 1972,* 1983–]

ACHE-AUPHA Liaison Committee [1964–1965* ended before 1979]

Administrator Relationship with Medical Staff (with AHA) [1958,* not in 1963]

Board of Administrative Development [not in 1959, *1963–1964*]

Study of Admissions and Advancements [*1957–1965*]

Representation to ACEHSA [1987–]

Article of the Year [1959,* 1965,* *1979–]

Audit [not in 1965, *1972–1993; merged into Finance]

Awards and Testimonials, Board of Awards [not in 1959, *1963–]

Book of the Year, James A. Hamilton Hospital Administrators' Book Award [1959, 1964–]

Budget, Budget and Finance [not in 1943, *1953–1959,* not in 1962–1965, *1972–1993; merged into Finance]

Bylaws [*1943–]

Career Development [1993–]

Chief Executive Officers [1993–]

Representation to American Society of Clinical Pathologists [1985–1990]

Communications [1984–1988, 1992–]

Congress on Administration, Planning Committee [1959–1965*]

Representation to National Commission on Correctional Health Care [1991–]

Council of Regents Minutes Review Committee [1986–]

Credentials [*1943–1984*]

Defense [*1943*]

Directory [1959* ended by 1962]

Editorial Boards
  Frontiers of Health Services Management [1988–]
  Healthcare Executive [1987–]
  Hospital and Health Services Administration [1983–]
  ACHE Management Series [1989–]
  Medical Care Review [1986–]
  Association for Health Services Research/Health Administration Press [1986–]
  AUPHA Press/Health Administration Press [1992–]

Education, Education Policies, Board of Education Policy [*1943–]

Elections, Election Judges [*1943–]

Endowment [*1972–1974*], Special Fund Raising [1959*]

Environmental Assessment [1983–1985]

Ethics, Code of Ethics [*1943–]

Examining Committee [not in 1953, *1957]

Executive of the Year Committee [1964–1965*]

Finance [1993–]

Gold Medal Awards [*1979–1985*]

TABLE 9.1
Continued

Healthcare Executive Groups and Women's Healthcare Executive Networks [Ad Hoc 1990, 1991–]
Healthcare Executives in Investor-Owned Organizations [1993–]
Healthcare Executives in Not-for-Profit Healthcare Systems [1993–]
Higher Education Committee [1988–]
Hudgens Memorial Award, Young Hospital Administrator of the Year [*1979–]
Institutes, Central Committee on [not in 1953, *1957–1965,* ended before 1972]
Insurance [*1953–1986]
Joint Commission, JCAH, JCAHO Standards Review [1984–]
Long Term Care Executives [1993–]
Managed Care Executives [1993–]
Medical Staff Relations [*1957]
Membership, Membership Services [not in 1965, *1972–]
  Subcommittee membership examinations [1983–]
  Subcommittee membership recruitment [1987–]
Nominating [*1943–]
Nurse Executives [1993–]
Regents Committee on Organization Structure [not in 1959, *1963]
Personal Services [1985–]
Physician Executives [1993–]
Poll of Issues [*1943*]
Professional Assessment, (Ad Hoc Self Assessment 1981–1982), [1983–] subcommittee Ambulatory Care [1985–]
Board of Professional Reference [not in 1958, *1963–1964]
Public Policy [1983–]
Publications, Board of, Publications and Public Information [not in 1958, *1963–1984]
Publicity and Public Relations [not in 1965, *1972–1984]
Research, Research and Development [1965–1974,* not in 1979–1984, 1985–]
Scholarship [*1957, 1959,* not in 1963]
Silver Medal Award [1974–1991]

* Indicates that Committee may have existed before or after the given date.[59]

budget and financial statements, and admission and advancement policy; selected an executive director; elected Members and Fellows recommended by the Credentials Committee; and disciplined members for nonconformance with the Bylaws, but not without due process. The Regents appointed the Credentials Committee and the Regional Councils which represented the College in their various areas.

The officers of the College were: the President, President-Elect, Immediate Past President, First and Second Vice President, and Secretary-

Treasurer. Officers were elected by all present Members and Fellows at the annual meeting.[62]

The Executive Committee consisted of President, President-Elect, and Immediate Past President plus four Regents elected by the Board of Regents who would act between meetings of the Board of Regents.

Standing Boards or committees that were appointed by the Regents included: the Board of Credentials, consisting of Fellowship, Membership, and Nomineeship divisions, (consistent with the policy of 1933, the names of the members were not published).

The Board of Examiners, appointed by the Regents and having regional committees, supervised written examinations and conducted oral interviews for candidates for Membership.

The Board of Publications oversaw the quarterly journal, the monthly news bulletin, and *The Administrator's Digest*, which was only published in the early 1960s.

The Board of Professional References, oversaw the content of the *Directory* and *Roster*.

The Board of Awards formulated policy related to awards and testimonials.

The Board of Educational Policy oversaw all phases of hospital administration education.

The Board of Administrative Development promoted activities related to increasing the quality of hospital administration.

There was also a Committee on Bylaws and a Nominating Committee. Six members served three-year terms on the Nominating Committee. Each President appointed two new members. The Past President preceding the immediate past president was ex-officio chairman. This committee nominated candidates for President-Elect and First and Second Vice Presidents.[63]

By 1953, total income had grown to $139,000 with expenditures of $137,466. Of the expenditures, 48.8% went to salaries; 13.5% to travel; 7.4% to committees; 7.9% to special services; 2.6% to scholarship loans; 3.4% to meetings; and the rest to office costs and other.[64]

As of 1955, annual dues for Fellows, Members, and Nominees were $50; fees for admission or advancement were $50.[65]

Conley's era saw the heavy involvement of the College in Institutes, the post World War II influx of military administrators, the creation of the Annual Congress on Administration, overseas Fellows' seminars, and the initiation of the College's journal, edited by Lynn Wimmer. With the assistance of W. Richard Kirk, written Membership examinations were also begun.

Conley, with the help of Frank Bradley and Ada Belle McCleery, Administrator of Evanston Hospital, obtained the first of several W. K.

Kellogg Foundation grants. This grant was to support the study of education for hospital administration and would be directed by Charles Prall.[66]

According to W. Richard Kirk, a new generation of administrators gained prominence in the College by the mid-1960s. This group included Ron Yaw, Boone Powell, Robert Bachmeyer, and Richard and Everett Johnson. Boone Powell, in particular, led the restructuring of the College in 1965–1966.[67]

The Years of Richard J. Stull, 1965–1978

Stull, Richard J.[68]
President/Chairmen 1965–1978
1965–1966 Powell, Boone, Sr. [69]
1966–1967 Terenzio, Peter Bernard[70]
1967–1968 Cordes, Donald Wesley[71]
1968–1969 Thomas, Roy Zachariah, Jr.[72]
1969–1970 Swanson, Arnold Leonard, M.D.[73]
1970–1971 Booth, Orville Northrop[74]
1971–1972 Johnson, Everett Arthur[75]
1972–1973 Wallace, William Norrby[76]
1973–1974 Kidd, Gene[77]
1974–1975 Brines, William Stewart[78]
1975–1976 Harvey, James D.[79]
1976–1977 Jackson, Henry Xavier[80]
1977–1978 Burkett, Norman Dewitt, Sr.[81]
1978–1979 Woodham, Ray[82]

Gerhard Hartman did not see military service during World War II because of malaria; Conley did not because of tuberculosis; and Richard Stull did not because of football injuries sustained at Duke University where he was a member of the class of 1940. He completed the Duke program in hospital administration in 1942.

After serving as Administrator in Phoenix, Pennsylvania and Norfolk, Virginia, and as the Western Representative for James A. Hamilton Associates, Stull worked for the University of California from 1948 to 1960 as Director of University Hospitals and Founder, Director, and Professor of the Berkeley program in hospital administration. From 1961 to 1965, he was Vice President of the Brunswick Corporation and head of their Aloe Medical Division.[83] Stull said:

> Boone Powell was the first to contact me about the ACHA position. I talked with Ray Brown and told him I was thinking about getting out of Brunswick. The next thing I knew he had gotten hold of Boone

Powell and Ron Yaw and said, "Hey, you might be able to get Stull. He's in limbo, he can stay at Brunswick but I think he wants to get back into the health field."[84]

When Stull arrived, the finances of the College were in a serious state, in debt by half a year's income and steadily going deeper. It had a debt of $110,000 and a yearly income of $250,000. Within two years, Stull had wiped out the debt. By the time he stepped down in 1979, the College had over three million dollars in fund balances, clearly providing a firm financial foundation.[85] During his tenure, Stull raised about $2.5 million from outside funding sources. The largest gift of one million dollars was from Foster G. McGaw, founder of the American Hospital Supply Corporation.[86]

Richard Stull's arrival in July, 1965, coincided with the College's major reorganization. The former Board of Regents was divided into a Board of Governors and a new Council of Regents in order to improve communication at the grass roots. The relationship between these two groups was specified through the work of a 1965 joint study committee. Its recommendations were accepted by the Council in 1966, and resulted in the basic organizational structure of the College that continues today.[87]

The Council of Regents was composed of an elected representative from each state, Canadian province and territory, plus the District of Columbia. Every active Fellow in a state was invited to be a candidate for Regent. Members and Fellows voted for the Regent in their state or province by mail ballot. Unless one candidate received a majority of the votes, the top two candidates were voted on in a second, mailed ballot. If there was no Regent for a state or province, the members from that state were annexed to an adjacent state. There was also a Regent-at-Large elected from the U.S. uniformed services. Thus, the Council of Regents could have up to 64 members. Votes of Regents were weighted by the number of members in the state or province—one vote for every 50 members, but not exceeding five votes for any Regent. The Regents' terms were three years, and they met during the Annual Meeting of the College.[88]

The Council of Regents represented the membership and had the power to: approve dues and assessments; approve regulations related to admissions and advancements; make Bylaws changes; elect members of the Board of Governors (there could be only one governor from each of the seven districts); elect the Nominating Committee; approve or disapprove reports, actions, and resolutions; and designate the seven Districts. The Immediate Past Chairman of the College (formerly called the President), presided at meetings of the Council of Regents.

The Board of Governors, elected by the Regents, included one representative from each of the professional society's seven districts as well as its four officers: Chairman, Chairman-Elect, Immediate Past Chairman and President, who was a member without a vote. The Board of Governors had charge of the property of the College and had the authority to control and manage the affairs and funds of the College. It functioned as a Board of Directors, described in the General Not-For-Profit Corporation Act of Illinois, and was empowered to establish committees, grant Honorary Fellowships, bestow special awards, and accept grants and contributions.[89]

Governors were asked to communicate with and assist Regents; generate visibility for the College; identify potential affiliates for the College and help plan educational meetings; encourage the Young Administrators' Groups; and monitor College educational programs. They were also encouraged to contribute to the literature of hospital administration.[90]

According to the ACHE promotional piece: "Regents function as the principal on-line representative of the professional society in each state or province. In the last few years their duties and responsibilities have increased substantially as they have become the major link between the headquarters staff and their constituents."[91]

Regents made all legislative policy decisions; approved proposals related to dues assessments and fees; established and approved regulations governing admissions and advancement; approved changes in the Bylaws; elected officers, Board of Governors, and members of the Nominating and Bylaws Committees; approved and modified recommendations and reports; and made proposals and recommendations to the Board of Governors.[92]

Many regents call on affiliates in their jurisdiction to assist them as members of a Regent's Advisory Council. This increases affiliate participation, allows feedback from the diverse interests represented by affiliates and their participation in planning and goal setting. The creation and development of these Councils was spearheaded by D. Kirk Oglesby, Jr., and their existence is encouraged.

The officers of the College were the Chairman, Chairman-Elect, Immediate Past Chairman, President, Secretary, Treasurer, and if necessary, Assistant Secretaries and Treasurers. Thus, Dewey Lutes' original position was held by up to five people, all of whom were now appointed by the Board of Governors. The Council of Regents elected the Chairman-Elect, who also served as Chairman of the Budget and Finance Committee.

The Executive Committee of the Board included the Chairman-Elect, Chairman, Immediate Past Chairman and President (without vote), and could take action between Board of Governors' meetings. The Standing Committees were: Nominating, Bylaws, Credentials, and Audit. The Nominating Committee of 10 members (one from each District and three past Chairmen), proposed candidates to the Council of Regents for the office of Chairman-Elect, as well as the Board of Governors, and members of the Bylaws and Nominating Committees.

As of 1978, an additional committee included the Committee on Awards and Testimonials, which was the parent to committees on the Book of the Year, the Articles of the Year, and the Gold and Silver Medal Award for Excellence in Administration. The Committee on Budget and Finance oversaw the financial policies of the College. The Committee on Education oversaw the educational programs of the College. There were also the Committees on Elections, on Ethics, on Insurance, on Membership Programs and Services, on Publications and Public Information, and on the Hudgens Memorial Award for the Young Hospital Administrator of the Year.[93]

Stull revamped the educational effort of the College with support from the W. K. Kellogg Foundation by moving into a seminar series which continue to this day. The annual Congress grew even larger. The written examination was updated and the oral examination was restructured. With the support of Eli Lilly Co., funds were obtained by Conley and Stull to develop an oral interview manual and examination procedures.[94] Stull wrote:

> The results were a programmed manual of instructions for the interviewer and a base of questions with a rating system to be employed in the oral exam. The scoring was done by an outside independent agency. By 1976, the College had begun to embark on its program of self-assessment, self-development and life-long learning.[95]

With the growth of specialization in healthcare management, the College broadened its admission requirements while upgrading the educational requirements for membership.[96] According to Stull:

> There were some young guys who wouldn't go into government service (at the Department of Health Education and Welfare) because they couldn't get into the College. Planners, academics and all kinds of people were coming into the field in varying health institutions or non-institutional positions. They were accommodated by changing College regulations and requirements. The largest number in the membership were still in hospitals or in the emerging multiple hospital system structures.[97]

When Everett Johnson was Chairman (1971–1972), the College initiated a series of nine task forces to examine special topics of concern for the membership.[98] Task forces reports included: "The Regents Role in Medical Care Leadership," Donald W. Cordes, Chairman; "A Statement on the Productivity of Group Medical Practice," Sister Virginia Schwager, Chairman; "Principles of Appointment and Tenure of Executive Officers," "Specialized Management in Hospital Administration," Henry X. Jackson, Chairman; "Providing Primary Care in Community Hospitals," Charles T. Wood, Chairman; "The Chief Executives' Role and Responsibility for Administrative Development," Alton E. Pickert, Chairman; and "Recommendations on Standards to the Joint Commission on Accreditation of Hospitals," William S. Brines, Chairman.[99]

Stull was also responsible for computerizing the membership data known as the ACHE's "Administrative Profile" and the establishment of a Division of Project Development and Special Studies with Carroll M. Mickey, Ph.D., as its Director. With a grant from Mead Johnson and Co., the College helped launch Young Administrator Forums around the country.[100] He also initiated significant steps leading a broad approach to professional development, including the concept of self-assessment.

In Stull's words, "The College had progressed to a status of an accepted and respected professional society." In 1974, Stull had triple bypass surgery followed by a thoracotomy in 1976. His health slowed his pace and he stepped down from the College in 1979.[101]

The Years of Stuart Wesbury, 1979–1991

Wesbury, Stuart Arnold, Jr.[102]
Chairmen
1979–1980 Stocks, Chester Lee[103]
1980–1981 Newkirk, Donald Richard[104]
1981–1982 Wood, Charles Thomas[105]
1982–1983 Dresser, Earl George[106]
1983–1984 Pickert, Alton Eades[107]
1984–1985 Ross, Austin[108]
1985–1986 Johnson, William Elmer, Jr.[109]
1986–1987 Oglesby, D. Kirk, Jr.[110]
1987–1988 Cronin, Francis Joseph, Jr.[111]
1988–1989 Jeppson, David Hans[112]
1989–1990 Maysent, H.W.[113]
1990–1991 Hepner, James Orville[114]

Like Hartman, Conley and Stull, Stuart A. Wesbury, Jr., came to the College with strong university and academic connections. He received his Master's degree in hospital administration from the University of Michigan in 1960 and his doctorate from the University of Florida in 1972. He worked in several hospitals, including a period of service as the Director of the University of Florida's Shands Teaching Hospital and Clinics, before becoming the Director and Professor of the Graduate Program in Health Services Management at the University of Missouri–

Columbia from 1972 to 1978.[115] Thus, the close relationship between university education and the College continued.

The Wesbury era saw the development of the public policy agenda described in Chapter 8. Wesbury's interest in policy led him to resign from the College in 1991 to run for an Illinois seat in the U.S. House of Representatives. This era saw the development of self-assessment-based continuing education described in Chapter 5. It saw the development of closer links with academia through recognized affiliations with health management graduate programs, program faculty membership, and visiting faculty fellowships.

It saw the formal recognition of local healthcare executive groups and women's healthcare executive networks. The College's educational offerings continued to grow. In 1991, there were 5,836 paid attendees to about 180 seminars and programs, 1,150 to conferences and 3,681 to the Annual Congress; 789 self-directed learning modules sold.[116] This era saw the acquisition of Career Decision, Inc., and Health Administration Press as described in Chapter 8. It saw the interest in history (Table 1.2) continued.

The growth of the College can be measured by the number of Affiliates (Table 2.5) and by its financial reports. Table 9.2 summarizes the College finances for selective years from 1934 to 1991.

The organization of the College office employees has evolved over time. Table 9.3 summarizes the College's organization charts for 1978,

TABLE 9.2
The College Finances, 1934–1991, Selected Years[117]

Fiscal Year	Revenue	Expense	Assets/Liabilities	Fund Balance
1934	$ 2,215	$ 1,510	$	$
1937	9,116	7,334		
1941	19,033	18,868		
1945	39,034	30,013		
1950	135,925	76,548		24,623
1953	139,069	96,347		41,120
1957	134,109	103,804	78,868	77,552
1961	384,743	396,277	126,301	
1964	436,492	472,666	186,952	(5,193)
1971	1,193,439	1,178,389	1,096,788	714,429
1975	2,084,643	1,899,185	2,292,923	1,584,251
1979	2,786,623	2,575,833	4,319,498	3,248,882
1983	5,008,705	4,740,495	5,893,994	4,031,160
1985	5,606,643	5,844,127	6,597,717	4,476,056
1987	9,346,770	9,893,372	7,845,306	4,561,697
1991	12,313,424	12,234,576	9,936,944	4,802,644

TABLE 9.3
The Changing Staff Organization of the College 1978, 1983, 1993

1978[120]	President
	Directors of
	Publications and Public Information
	Membership Services
	Finance and Operations
	Education
	Project Development and Special Studies
	Eastern Regional Coordinator
	Western Regional Coordinator
1983[121]	President
	Vice President
	Directors of:
	Finance and Operations
	Publications and Public Information
	Education
	Development and Credentialling Programs
	Membership
	Project Development and Special Studies
	Research
	Self Assessment
	Policy Analysis
	Coordinators Regions A, B, C, D
1993[122]	President
	Executive Vice President, Senior Vice President
	Directors of:
	Career Decision, Inc. (Itasca, Illinois)
	Communications
	Education
	Finance and Administration
	Government Relations
	Health Administration Press (Ann Arbor, Michigan)
	Membership
	Regional Services
	Research and Development

1983, and 1992. In 1978, seven departments reported to Richard Stull (president). By August 1983, the College employed 52 staff persons. Of this group, 13 were healthcare management professionals by both education (master's degrees) and practical experience. Eleven other staff held professional degrees related to their College roles.[118] In 1981, a Vice President was needed. By 1993, there was a President, an Executive

Vice President, and a Senior Vice President. The College had seven internal departments, including Health Administration Press in Ann Arbor, Michigan. There was a Director for Government Relations. Career Decision, Inc. of Itasca, Illinois, was a corporate subsidiary.[119]

Stuart Wesbury developed the "programmatic thrusts" which became a feature of College planning and have been described in Chapter 8.

The Years of Thomas C. Dolan, Ph.D., 1991–

Dolan, Thomas Christopher[123]
Chairmen
1991–1992 Ellison, Paul Stribling[124]
1992–1993 Fanning, Robert Reece, Jr.[125]
1993–1994 Ronald G. Spaeth[126]

With Thomas Dolan's presidency, the links to academia continue. Dolan came to the College in 1986 from Saint Louis University in St. Louis, Missouri, where he had directed the Center for Health Services Education and Research. He had received his doctorate from the health administration program at the University of Iowa. Stuart Wesbury chaired the AUPHA in 1977–1978, while Tom Dolan chaired AUPHA in 1983–1984. The College initiatives for 1993 are described in Chapter 10; otherwise, an assessment of the Dolan years will await the next College history.

NOTES

[1] ACHA, "A Brief Description," 1979, p. 26.
[2] After the first edition of this book, John Mannix started work on brief biographies of all the College presidents (to 1972) and chairmen (1972 on). The material he collected can be found in the Mannix archives, AHA historical collection. The biographies and footnoted references build on his work.
[3] ACHA, *1972, 1984 Directory*. (In the notes that follow in this chapter, the ACHA and ACHE Directories are indicated by "D." followed by the appropriate date. Lutes, 1933, 1949, 1956. Mannix archives. Lutes' resume. Author's collection.
[4] D. 1944.
[5] D. 1968. Neff, 1951.
[6] D. 1948. Brown, Madison, 1984, p. 166. Carter, 1936, 1952, 1953. ACHA, Carter, 1938.
[7] D. 1962. Brown, Madison, 1984, p. 166. MacLean, 1950, 1957.
[8] Kipnis, 1955, p. 10.
[9] ACHA, *Minute Book*, Vol. 1, Feb. 13, 1933. President Charles A. Wordell, First V.P. Robert E. Neff, Second V.P. Joseph Norby, Director General J.

Dewey Lutes. The other members were Rev. Fritschel, John Smith, and Maurice Dubin.

10 ACHA, *Minute Book*, Vol. 1, Feb. 14, 1933. Constitution and Bylaws: Maurice Dubin, chairman; Robert E. Neff; John Smith; and Dr. F. G. Carter. Nominating Committee: Dr. Walter List, chairman; Howard Bishop; Dr. Herman Smith; and A. J. Swanson.

11 J. Dewey Lutes, "To the Members of the Board of Regents" (First annual report of the Director General). ACHA, *Minute Book*, Vol. 1, 1933.

12 ACHA, *Minute Book*, Vols. 1, 2, Feb. 15, 1937; Sept. 12, 1937; Sept. 13, 1937. Dewey Lutes interview, 1982.

13 *ACHA Bulletin*, Vol. 1, No. 1, 1934–35. Kipnis, p. 23.

14 D. 1972, 1984, 1992. Lewis Weeks oral history, 1984, Hartman, G. 1938, 1938, 1939, 1940, 1961, 1962, 1962, 1962, 1964, 1965. ACHA, Hartman, 1943.

15 D. 1966. Mannix archives.

16 D. 1972, 1981. Buerki, 1939, 1951, 1959.

17 D. 1972, 1984. Hamilton, 1938, 1939, 1957. ACHA, Hamilton, 1939. Lewis Weeks oral history, 1987.

18 D. 1948. Brown, Madison, 1984, p. 163. Bachmeyer, Arthur C., 1919, 1951. Bachmeyer and Hartman, 1943, 1948. ACHA, 1941 speech, "They Made Hospital History: Arthur C. Bachmeyer, MD" *The Modern Hospital*, Vol. 81, No. 5, Nov. 1953, pp. 65–66, 126–129. Mannix Archives.

19 Kipnis, pp. 35–36. Hartman was born in 1911; received his doctoral degree in 1942; was a teaching assistant, University of Chicago hospital administration program, 1936–37, and associate director, 1937–42; ACHA executive secretary to 1941 (reported dates vary). His last signed ACHA minutes are for June 6, 1941. He was absent due to illness Sept. 14 and on Sept. 15. The Board of Regents discussed a replacement for him. ACHA, *Minute Book*, Vol. 2. From 1942 to 1946 he was director of the Newton Wellesley Hospital, Newton Lower Falls, and became director of the University Hospitals (1947–71) and professor and director of the Graduate Program in Hospital Administration, State University of Iowa, 1947 through 1980. ACHA, *1960 Directory*, p. 178. *1981 Directory*, p. 353.

20 The following quotations come from the Lewis Weeks interview with Gerhard Hartman, Oct. 25, 1982, internal doc. Quoted with permission.

21 *Ibid.*, p. 11.

22 *Ibid*, pp. 13–14.

23 *Ibid.*, pp. 14–15.

24 These are the words of Lewis Weeks.

25 *Ibid.*, pp. 15–16.

26 *Ibid.*, p. 19. ACHA, "Institutes Inter-Americano Par Administradores de Hospitales," Dec. 1–14, 1940, San Juan, Puerto Rico.

27 Lewis Weeks interview of Hartman, p. 19.

28 W. Richard Kirk, interview, March 14, 1983.

29 D. 1972, 1984. Conley 1949, 1953, 1955, 1966. ACHA, 1942 speech.

30 D. 1972, 1979. Wilson, Lucius, 1952.

31 D. 1964. Norby, 1954, 1955.

[32] D. 1948. Brown, Madison, 1984, p. 166. Gottlieb, 1991. ACHA, 1943–1947 speeches.

[33] D. 1948. Brown, Madison, 1984, p. 166. Munger, C. 1939, 1950. ACHA, 1941–46 speeches. Brown reports Munger's death in 1949. *Modern Hospital* reports Feb. 3, 1950.

[34] D. 1972. Brown, Madison, 1984, p. 167. Bradley, 1953, 1958. ACHA, 1947 speech.

[35] D. 1948. Hayhow, 1952, 1956. ACHA, Hayhow circa 1938. Mannix archives.

[36] D. 1948. Turnbull was the only woman in 60 years to chair the College. Mannix archives.

[37] D. 1948. Brown, Madison, 1984, p. 167.

[38] D. 1964. Walter, 1953. Mannix archives.

[39] D. 1972. Erickson, 1952.

[40] D. 1972, 1984. Mooney, Fraser, 1951. ACHA, 1953 speech.

[41] D. 1972, 1979. Brown, Madison, 1984, p. 170. Hosick and Steele, 1951. Steele, 1957. ACHA, 1954 speech.

[42] D. 1972, 1984. Kerlikowske, 1953.

[43] D. 1960. Swanson, 1951, 1956.

[44] D. 1984, 1992. Groner, 1951.

[45] D. 1972, 1979. Eckert, 1951. Mannix archives.

[46] D. 1972. Brown, Ray E., 1955, 1959, 1983 (p. xv). *Ray E. Brown Lectures, Messages and Memoirs,* 1991 (listing his 206 publications). ACHA, Brown and Johnson, 1952, 1957, 1961.

[47] D. 1972, 1977. ACHA, 1961 speech by Sutley.

[48] D. 1972, 1981. Terrell, T., 1952, 1957. Mannix archives.

[49] D. 1972, 1981, 1984, 1992. Sutton, 1952.

[50] D. 1972, 1981, 1984, 1992. Bachmeyer, R. W., 1951. Robert Bachmeyer is the son of Arthur Bachmeyer.

[51] D. 1972, 1981, 1984, 1992. Yaw, 1950.

[52] Dean Conley interview, April 21, 1983. Hartman described Ray Amberg as follows: "Bob Buerki said that when you meet Ray Amberg don't be fooled. He said that Ray is half Irish and half Swede, that his speech may be as slow as a Swede's but his mind is as fast as an Irishman's." (Lewis Weeks interview, p. 16).

[53] Dean Conley interview, 1983.

[54] Kipnis, p. 14. ACHA, *Minute Book*, Vol. 1, 1933. "To the Members of the Board of Regents," p. 3.

[55] Kipnis, p. 63.

[56] *Ibid.,* p. 79.

[57] Stuart Wesbury interview, 1983. Wesbury said at the time that there was no College policy to avoid government grants or contracts.

[58] Kipnis, p. 131. Committees changed names and these are listed.

[59] Sources: Kipnis for 1943. College yearly annual reports, 1957 on. ACHA, *Minute Book*, Vol. 5, 1957.

[60] ACHA, *Minute Book*, Vol. 5, 1957.

[61] Kipnis, p. 128. ACHA, "Articles of Incorporation" and "Bylaws," Aug. 1960, pp. 11–12.

[62] ACHA, 1960, *op. cit.*, pp. 14–16.

[63] *Ibid.*, pp. 17–22.

[64] Kipnis, pp. 130–131.

[65] ACHA, "Articles of Incorporation" and "Bylaws," Aug., 1960, p. 9.

[66] Dean Conley interview, 1983.

[67] W. Richard Kirk interview, March 14, 1983. Dean Conley took early retirement at age 60 in 1965.

[68] D. 1972, 1981. ACHA, Stull, 1978. Lewis Weeks oral history, 1984.

[69] D. 1972, 1992. Powell, 1955.

[70] D. 1972, 1981, 1989, 1992. Terenzio, 1951.

[71] D. 1972, 1981, 1984, 1992. Cordes, 1957.

[72] D. 1972, 1981, 1989, 1992. Thomas, R. Z., 1957.

[73] D. 1972, 1981, 1984, 1992. Swanson, A. 1951, 1956.

[74] D. 1972, 1979.

[75] D. 1972, 1981, 1984, 1992. Johnson, Everett A., 1982.

[76] D. 1972, 1979. Mannix archives.

[77] D 1972, 1981, 1984, 1992. Kidd, 1955.

[78] D. 1972, 1981, 1984, 1992. Brines, 1958, 1959. Mannix archives.

[79] D. 1972, 1981, 1984, 1992.

[80] D. 1972, 1981, 1984. Jackson, 1980. Mannix archives.

[81] D. 1972, 1981, 1984, 1992. Burkett, 1959. Mannix archives.

[82] D. 1972, 1981, 1984, 1992. "Ray Woodham, A Tribute," 1983. Mannix archives.

[83] W. Richard Kirk interview. Stull brought in John O'Conner as the financial officer for the College. Stull recalls the College's assets at the end of his tenure as over $4 million, with $3.6 million invested. Lewis Weeks interview, p. 45.

[84] Lewis Weeks interview with Stull, 1983, p. 45.

[85] W. Richard Kirk interview.

[86] Lewis Weeks interview with Stull, 1983, p. 45.

[87] ACHA, *1977–1978 Annual Report*, p. 3. The distinctions between Governor and Regent were spelled out in detail in the ACHA publications *The Role of the Regent* (revised edition) 1978, and *The Role of the Governor*, 1977.

[88] ACHA, "Bylaws" of Aug. 7, 1972, amended in 1974, 1975, and 1979, published in 1980, pp. 7–11.

[89] ACHA, "A Brief Description," 1982, pp. 11–12.

[90] ACHA, *The Role of the Governor*, 1977, pp. 6–7.

[91] ACHA, "A Brief Description," 1982, loc. cit.

[92] ACHA, *The Role of the Regent*, 1978, pp. 5–6.

[93] ACHA, "Bylaws," 1980, pp. 11–25. "A Brief Description," 1982, *The Role of the Regent*, 1978, pp. 10–14.

[94] Lewis Weeks interview with Stull, p. 39. ACHA, "Manual for Interviewers," 1977.

[95] ACHA, "Proposed Program of Self Development and Recertification," April 30, 1976.

[96] Lewis Weeks interview with Stull, p. 40.

[97] *Ibid.*, p. 41.

[98] *Ibid.*, p. 43. W. Richard Kirk interview, 1983. Kirk said there were 9 Task Forces then, but there may have been 10.

[99] These reports appeared in 1972 and 1974. Some were published and some distributed internally. See Bibliography, American College of Healthcare Executives (non-periodic publications).

[100] Lewis Weeks interview with Stull, p. 44.

[101] *Ibid.*, pp. 45–46.

[102] D. 1972, 1981, 1984, 1992. Lewis Weeks oral history, 1986. Stuart Wesbury dissertation, 1972, 1992. ACHA, Wesbury, Jan. 1981; April 1981. Bast, Richard, and Wesbury, 1992.

[103] D. 1972, 1981, 1984. Mannix archives.

[104] D. 1972, 1981, 1984, 1992. Newkirk, 1959. Mannix archives.

[105] D. 1972, 1981, 1984, 1992. Mannix archives.

[106] D. 1992.

[107] D. 1972, 1981, 1984. Mannix archives.

[108] D. 1972, 1981, 1984, 1992. Mannix archives.

[109] D. 1992.

[110] D. 1992.

[111] D. 1992.

[112] D. 1992.

[113] D. 1992. Maysent, 1956.

[114] D. 1992. ACHA, Hepner, 1978, 1980.

[115] D. 1981, p. 903.

[116] ACHE, *1991–1992 Annual Report and Reference Guide*, pp. 18, 59.

[117] Years 1934–1953, Kipnis, p. 131. ACHA, *1958, 1962, 1965 Annual Report*. 1971: ACHA, *Progress Report 1972–73*, pp. 18, 19. 1975: ACHA, *The Year in Review 1974–1975*, pp. 18, 19. 1979: ACHA, *1979–1980 Annual Report*. 1983: ACHA, *1982–1983 Annual Report*, p. 29. 1985: ACHA, *Transactions; 1984–1985 Annual Report*, pp. 35–36. 1987: *1987–1988 Annual Report*, pp. 26–27. 1991: ACHA, *1991–1992 Annual Report and Reference Guide*, pp. 15–16.

[118] ACHA, *1982–1983 Annual Report. Coming of Age*, 1983, pp. 198–199.

[119] ACHE, *1991–1992 Annual Report and Reference Guide*, pp. 58–62. ACHE, "Organization Chart," April 1, 1993.

[120] ACHA, *The Role of the Regent* (revised edition), 1978, p. 113.

[121] ACHA, *1982–1983 Annual Report*.

[122] ACHE, *1991–1992 Annual Report and Reference Guide*, pp. 58–62.

[123] D. 1992, p. 272.

[124] D. 1992.

[125] D. 1992.

[126] D. 1992.

10

Past, Present, and Future

The professional must join and participate in those societies and associations which give him (or her) new ways to view his established practice. He must remove himself from practice from time to time for intensive periods of study, thereby not merely acquiring new knowledge but also gaining a broader perspective so that when he goes back into service again he views matters in a new light. He must in short use every means of continuing education available so that his work retains the lucidity and freshness of its early years.

ACHA, 1967[1]

"The College's mission remains what it has always been: to enhance the practice of healthcare management and ultimately to build a more effective and compassionate healthcare system."

—1992[2]

It is a challenge to describe the past, a struggle to keep pace with the present, and almost impossible to predict the future.

The Changing Environment

The development of the germ theory of disease, the emergence of clear supporting evidence for these ideas in the 1880s, and the resulting control of infectious diseases took decades to transpire. The acceptance of the vertical hospital, organized on principles of efficiency in the 1920s and 1930s, launched a new era for hospital management as represented by the birth of the College in 1933.

Will the discovery of the molecular structure of DNA in 1953[3] create an impact as great as the germ theory of disease? Will recombinant DNA technology transform medical care? Will there be a cure for cancer that will affect hospitals in the same way that drugs affected

263

tuberculosis and mental hospitals? The use of quantitative methods in physician decisionmaking—from careful reading of medical litera-ture, to medical technology assessment, to computerized diagnosis—have begun to change the way doctors look at the world.[4] As physician behavior continues to affect costs, how will hospital organization change?

The College was created by nurse, physician, religious, and lay administrators who believed that good management created the cli-mate for compassionate and humane patient care. Noted George Bug-bee, "Care of the sick has requirements which transcend the resources available and overshadow the importance of a balanced budget, or worse, a drive for mere profit."[5] The College recognized that a major ethical issue of the 1980s would be the delivery of high quality care amidst shrinking resources. A 1982 backgrounder issued by the Col-lege stated:

> Ethical issues affecting the delivery of health care in America have moved far beyond minor philosophical disagreements. Hospital ex-ecutives today face a broad list of ethical concerns that will impact directly on the way the system treats—or fails to treat—some pa-tients.[6]

America's population continues to age. Around 1975, the number of patients in nursing homes exceeded the number of patients in hos-pitals for the first time.[7] By 1986 community hospitals for the first time had more outpatient visits than inpatient days. By 1990, for the first time there were more outpatient surgical operations than inpa-tient operations in community hospitals.[8]

The July 1991, College strategic plan is explicit about expected changes in the healthcare environment.[9] These include the aging of the population due to increased longevity. Technologic advances will continue such as diagnostics, pharmaceuticals and genetic engineer-ing. These trends will challenge available resources. At the same time, there are pressures to control health care expenditures and questions about the best way to do this. Public health issues such as AIDS and infant mortality are significant. Corporate America is expected to be more involved in cost control efforts.

From Hospital to Health Care System

Hospitals have steadily increased in size, number of employees, assets per bed, costs per patient day, division of labor, complexity, and range of technology. As of 1983, the typical hospital shared services, while a third of community hospital beds were part of multi-institutional systems. Both vertical and horizontal integration of health services continued. Hospitals were both evolving into community health centers (vertical integration), and joining together in new and creative relationships (horizontal integration).

Is it possible that the hospital field continues to experience a transition similar to the automobile industry from the 1910s to the 1930s—starting with dozens of companies and evolving into a few very large ones? As of 1983, some CEOs of multihospital systems were bankers concerned with the stock market, Euro dollars, and the purchase of hospitals in other countries, but knew little about how hospitals work. Was this an anomaly or a sign of the future? Would there be the equivalent of a General Motors, Ford, Chrysler, or United Automobile Workers union in the future for healthcare? Or would a National Health Service once again become an issue?

By 1991, the College expected the following changes. Providers would be configured in new ways. Physicians would increasingly organize into groups.[10] Providers and payers would work together in more integrated systems to manage care. Future emphasis would be on outcome measures of quality of care. Delivery of care will continue to shift away from inpatient care. "It is estimated that 70 percent of health care expenditures will be for outpatient and home-based services." "Hospitals will become more involved in community-wide efforts and will take or reaffirm the leadership role in this regard." This will call forth the need for enhanced governance leadership. Competition between providers will be defined as achieving the best possible clinical outcome with the most efficient use of resources." This will change the management orientation. Measured quality will be the key to differentiation and competitive success.

From Administrator to Executive

In the 1910s and 1920s, hospitals were typically a cottage industry. Larger hospitals could choose a physician administrator right out of an internship like Dr. MacEachern in 1911,[11] or a department manager of a refrigerating company like Dewey Lutes in 1921.[12]

Even in the mid-1960s, one-third of community hospitals of 100+ beds in Chicago had no budget.[13] Medicare regulations compelled them to start budgeting. In the 1950s hospitals were large enough to have specialized department heads. The administrator learned the necessary human relations skills to work with these specialists. The growth of specialist health management societies in the '50s and '60s reflected this division of labor in management.

By 1991, the College strategic plan made the following assumptions about the profession. There would be a need for leadership in rationalizing the healthcare delivery system. Ethics issues would be important. Managers would be held responsible for the outcome of services rendered. The profession of healthcare administration would grow more diverse as more women and more minorities work in a growing variety of health settings. There would be more generalist MBA's entering the field. Executive turnover was expected to continue to be a problem.[14]

Changing Education

Will the future education of managers be in public health, business, or in medical and nursing schools? Probably all of these. As of 1983, graduate programs in health administration were increasingly oriented toward business management.[15]

In the 1910s and '20s, physicians often owned their own hospitals. In the Depression years of the '20s and '30s, some physicians could make no living in practice and found a "safe haven"[16] administering a hospital. Other physicians and administrators helped organize the College, which has had only two physician Chairmen since 1955.

The 1940s through the 1970s were years of prosperity for medicine. Private practice grew; research funds were abundant. With the anticipated physician abundance in the 1990s, more physicians may become interested in management, playing a potentially greater role in the activities of the College.

As of 1983, an increasing number of hospitals had full-time medical directors with responsibility for managing the affairs of the medical staff. These management specialists joined the vice president of finance, nursing, planning, and others as part of the senior management team. All might be eligible candidates for the top CEO spot. Physicians would likely rejoin the ranks of healthcare management rather than overwhelming it, as demonstrated by the background of senior managers in the largest multi-institutional systems.

Education in health management has gone through several transformations during the life of the College. Learning on the job was typical in the 1930's. The College Institutes provided short courses for working managers. The College participated in the growth of graduate programs in the 1950's and 1960's. By 1970, 85 percent of all new Nominees had masters degrees in health administration. By 1992, this had become only 52 percent, as more Nominees came with backgrounds of general MBA's, nursing, medicine or law.[17] Wide availability of graduate management education and rapid environmental change have called forth the demand and need for lifelong learning and recertification.

The 1991 strategic plan for the College assumed that healthcare managers would need greater continuing education and professional development assistance in more specialized areas, balanced with less time and money available for obtaining such education. The traditional career path would be challenged and executives would seek new abilities to remain competitive, particularly in the areas of technology, ethics, interorganizational management and outcome management.

Evaluating Excellence

It is hard to imagine a time when a single man, Malcolm MacEachern, M.D., not only knew every hospital manager, but also how well individual hospitals were run. He could therefore judge a person's worthiness for Membership or Fellowship in the College.

As early as the 1940s, the College sought expert advice on test construction for the membership examination. During 1981–1983, the College took a major step forward in focusing not just on a single entry exam, but on a program of lifelong learning tailored to diagnose and correct weaknesses in management knowledge and skill. By 1983, the College was involved in a wide range of approaches to evaluate excellence: an annual nationwide student computer game,[18] examinations for advancement to Membership, Fellowship case studies or theses, lifelong learning, and honorary awards for publications. The computer game is no longer being played. Now there is the Hill-Rom Essay Competition in Healthcare Administration which was established in 1989. Two $3,000 prizes are awarded each year, one to an undergraduate and one to a graduate student in health administration programs. These essays are published in the College Journal.

As of 1993, the College is rethinking criteria and categories of affiliation to accommodate the diversity of backgrounds, work environments and lifelong learning.[19]

Theory and Philosophy of Management

The College drew together the divergent views of hospital and general management. Only by reading between the lines of the "essential" literature on hospital management of the 1930s is the impact of general management theory, or of Taylor and the classical management theorists, evident. By the 1950s, human relations appeared in College seminars. The journal showed the steady, clear merging of general management with hospital administration theory. With each passing decade, more general management ideas were applied to hospital administration. Conversely, as medical care grew to 10 percent of the GNP and as healthcare corporations grew in size, professors of general business management were often drawn into the healthcare field as lecturers, consultants, or researchers. Through its book awards, the College recognized the work of these experts.

At the same time, a large active group of consultants and teachers in management had formed, devoting their entire careers to studying health services administration. The contingency and environmental theories of management provided an intellectual rationale for understanding the unique features of healthcare. The unique tasks of the profession, combined with the regulatory environment, reimbursement systems, and legal constraints, all pointed to healthcare management as a specialized area of competence.

This tension between managerial universalism and healthcare particularism will likely continue, to the benefit of all. One such example is the new interest in measured quality outcomes and their improvement. The health care field is developing distinctive ways to measure quality. Continuous quality improvement (CQI) coming from industry is being applied to health care. The College itself is responding to these ideas with systematic membership opinion surveys and using the results to shape and direct College programs. Mission statements, environmental assessments, clearly defined goals, and strategic planning became systematic in the 1980s.

New Directions

These changes are expected to have an impact on the College in the following ways. The traditional affiliates of the College, hospital CEO's, COO's and assistant administrators are expected to decline in number, to be replaced by a wide diversity of managers who will want a wider spectrum of education and have a diversity of needs. This diversification will result in greater competition for affiliates from other professional societies serving specialized needs. There will be more competition for educational programs, which is the College's specialty. Affiliates are expected to increasingly turn to the College to meet their career needs.[20]

With the growth of the College, there has been a declining probability of being involved in College governance. Even with expanded committees, according to Tom Dolan, there are only 375 committee appointments to allocate to 19,000 active affiliates, so that only about two percent of the affiliates are involved in College governance.[21]

Organization and Leadership

Organizational structure emerges from corporate objectives and environment. A definition of the future of the College will dictate its internal structure.

That the College of 1993 has more members than ever before suggests that it occupies a valued place in the professional lives of present and future executives. Judging by its membership, it is a young and growing organization.

According to Tom Dolan, the state of the College in 1993 was as follows.[22] There are now 92 Regents, 47 representing individual states and provinces. Larger states can have more than one Regent. Four regents represent over 1,600 military affiliates, and there are 7 at-large regents. They are limited to one 4 year term. The Board of Governors now consists of 13 members including a Governor for the uniformed services and an At-Large Governor. At the 1993 Convocation, the College added 2,745 new nominees, 552 new members, 193 new Fellows and recertified 717 Fellows and Members.

In 1991, the affiliates grew by 5.5 percent and by 6.1 percent in 1992, one of the highest growth rates in College history due in part to active recruiting. The membership exam is annually updated and has specialty tracks in executive management, planning, marketing, consulting, mental health, addiction treatment, and Canadian health-care. There are new tracks on ambulatory care, managed care, and long-term care.

Professional (self) assessment consists of three programs, now known as Executive Skill Builders: General Management Assessment, Medical Group Management–Ambulatory Care Assessment, and Administrative Communication Techniques. Recertification is now mandatory for all Members and Fellows. To assist unemployed affiliates the College will now waive their dues for 2 years. The College currently gives approximately 140 offerings of 26 different seminars around the country. In 1993, twelve cluster programs were offered. The Clusters consist of seven or more seminars offered over a five-day period at one location. For example, the January 25–29, 1993, Scottsdale, Arizona, Cluster program included twelve seminars on high performance internal operations, design and construction, executive skills, personal financial planning, communication, ambulatory care assessment, law and legislation updates, managing clinical resources, rebuilding the healthcare work force, total quality management, participative management, and return on investment.[23]

The College offers annual conferences: the Canada–United States Healthcare Executive Conference, which is mostly attended by Canadians; the Management Ethics Conference; the Fellows Conference; and the Eastern and Western Conferences, which are the largest. It also offers the Partnership Institute for Trustees, Executives, and Physician Teams, co-sponsored with the AHA and the American Medical Association. The 36th Annual Congress on Administration was held in March 1993, as always in Chicago.

The College has several self-directed learning programs which are based on books published by the Health Administration Press. These enable affiliates to earn continuing education credits without having to travel to conferences or seminars.

The Division of Research is as active as it has ever been, studying CEO turnover, gender and careers, a Delphi study of physician and hospital relationships, race and careers (in association with the National Association of Health Services Executives), and "Evaluating the performance of the Hospital CEO in a Total Quality Management Environment" (with the AHA).[24] The research department also conducts the annual affiliates' needs survey which is one basis for guiding the College's activities and planning.

The Health Administration Press continues to publish its journals and new books. Career Decision Inc. provides four services: executive outplacement, group outplacement, career planning and counseling, and management assessment.

Plans for 1993 included development of special interest groups, such as managed care and long-term care executives, and discipline groups (physicians, nurses, etc.). Public policy activities have been enhanced with the appointment of a Director of Government Relations who reports directly to the College President and the adoption of a plan of action for meeting affiliates' public policy needs.

College President Tom Dolan defined five goals for the College at the start of 1993.[25]

- The College must significantly advance its affiliates' careers.
- The College must serve the needs of its affiliates throughout their careers.
- The College must better represent its affiliates to trustees, physicians, government officials, and the public.
- The College must embrace diversity of gender, race, occupational setting, and educational background.
- The College must be on the cutting edge of new knowledge through education, publications, and research.

"If it aint' broke, don't fix it" has been replaced by continuous quality improvement.

The Future

We return to the quotation that began this volume. A corporate history should be general enough to define the key decisions of the past, show historic continuity, and, at best, serve as a guide to an evolving future. The College has always been a leader. It has drawn into its colleagueship and fellowship those administrators who have exemplified and directed the healthcare field. The College has been, is, and will be its affiliate body: who they are, how they learn, and how they function in a dynamic and challenging profession.

NOTES

[1] ACHA, Richard J. Stull ("Forward") quoting Cyril O'Houle, "The Lengthened Line of Education," June 1969.

[2] Dolan, July 1992, "College Update Speech," internal document.

[3] Watson, *The Double Helix*, New York: Signet Books, 1968.

[4] Neuhauser, 1980.

[5] George Bugbee, personal communication, Feb. 17, 1983.

[6] ACHA press releases "Healthcare Executives Must Prepare for Serious Ethical Conflicts" and "Ethics: A Critical Factor in Healthcare," Nov. 23, 1982. UPI, McCormack, "Life and Death Decisions: Ethical Dilemma for Hospitals," Nov. 30, 1982.

[7] U.S. Department of Health and Human Services, *Health United States 1981*, p. 172. In 1973–74, nursing home residents were at 1.075 million, rising to 1.303 million in 1977. During this time the census at all hospitals fell from 1.189 million in 1973 to 1.066 million in 1977: AHA, *Hospital Statistics 1982 Edition*, p. 4.

[8] AHA, *Hospital Statistics 1992–1993 Edition*, pp. XLVI; XLVII.

[9] ACHE, Strategic Plan, July 1991, internal document.

[10] *Ibid.*

[11] Davis, Loyal, 1960.

[12] Dewey Lutes resume, 1982.

[13] Neuhauser, 1971.

[14] ACHE, Strategic Plan, July 1991, internal document.

[15] Stephen Shortell, personal communication, 1983.

[16] Davis, Michael, 1929.

[17] Thomas Dolan interview, Dec. 30, 1992.

[18] Starkweather, David. He developed an elaborate computer-based simulation game for hospital managers. This game was played by students in many graduate programs.

[19] Oct. 26, 1992, "Credentials Task Force Recommendations for changes to the Regulations Governing Admission, Advancement and Recertification."

[20] ACHE, Strategic Plan, July 1991, internal document.

[21] Thomas Dolan interview, Dec. 30, 1992.

[22] Dolan, July 1992, "College Update Speech;" Dec. 30, 1992, interview.

[23] ACHE, 1993 Arizona Cluster, brochure.

[24] ACHE, *Evaluating the Performance of the Hospital CEO in a Total Quality Management Environment*, 1993.

[25] Dolan, op. cit.

Appendix

Contents:

CHAIRMEN OF THE COLLEGE 1933–1994*

1933–1934	†Charles A. Wordell	1962–1963	Frank C. Sutton, M.D.
1934–1935	†Robert E. Neff		
1935–1936	†Fred G. Carter, M.D.	1963–1964	Robert W. Bachmeyer
1936–1937	†Basil C. MacLean, M.D.		
		1964–1965	Ronald D. Yaw
1937–1938	†Howard E. Bishop	1965–1966	Boone Powell
1938–1939	†Robin C. Buerki, M.D.	1966–1967	Peter B. Terenzio
		1967–1968	Donald W. Cordes
1939–1940	†James A. Hamilton	1968–1969	R. Zach Thomas, Jr.
1940–1941	†Arthur C. Bachmeyer, M.D.	1969–1970	Arnold L. Swanson, M.D.
1941–1942	†Lucius R. Wilson, M.D.	1970–1971	†Orville N. Booth
		1971–1972	Everett A. Johnson, Ph.D.
1942–1943	†Joseph G. Norby		
1943–1944	†Robert H. Bishop, Jr., M.D.	1972–1973	†William N. Wallace
		1973–1974	Gene Kidd
1944–1946	†Claude W. Munger, M.D.	1974–1975	William S. Brines
		1975–1976	James D. Harvey
1946–1947	†Frank R. Bradley, M.D.	1976–1977	†Henry X. Jackson
		1977–1978	Norman D. Burkett
1947–1948	†Edgar C. Hayhow, Ph.D.	1978–1979	Ray Woodham
		1979–1980	†Chester L. Stocks
1948–1949	†Jessie J. Turnbull	1980–1981	Donald R. Newkirk
1949–1950	†Wilmar M. Allen, M.D.	1981–1982	Charles T. Wood
		1982–1983	Earl G. Dresser
1950–1951	†Frank J. Walter	1983–1984	†Alton E. Pickert
1951–1952	†Ernest I. Erickson	1984–1985	Austin Ross
1952–1953	†Fraser D. Mooney, M.D.	1985–1986	William E. Johnson, Jr.
1953–1954	†Merrill F. Steele, M.D.	1986–1987	D. Kirk Oglesby, Jr.
		1987–1988	Francis J. Cronin
1954–1955	†Albert C. Kerlikowske, M.D.	1988–1989	David H. Jeppson
		1989–1990	H. W. Maysent
1955–1956	†J. Dewey Lutes	1990–1991	James O. Hepner, Ph.D.
1956–1957	†Arthur J. Swanson		
1957–1958	Frank S. Groner	1991–1992	Paul S. Ellison
1958–1959	†Anthony W. Eckert	1992–1993	Robert R. Fanning, Jr.
1959–1960	†Ray E. Brown		
1960–1961	†Melvin L. Sutley	1993–1994	Ronald G. Spaeth
1961–1962	†Tol Terrell		

---

*Prior to 1972 identified as President
†Deceased

CHIEF EXECUTIVE OFFICERS OF THE COLLEGE 1933–1994

1933–1937	†J. Dewey Lutes, *Director General*
1937–1941	†Gerhard Hartman, Ph.D., *Executive Secretary*
1942–1965	†Dean Conley, *Executive Director*
1965–1971	†Richard J. Stull, *Executive Vice President*
1972–1978	†Richard J. Stull, *President*
1979–1991	Stuart A. Wesbury, Jr., Ph.D., *President*
1991–	Thomas C. Dolan, Ph.D., *President*

HONORARY CHARTER FELLOWS†

G. Harvey Agnew, M.D.
Otho F. Ball, M.D.
Richard P. Borden
Bert W. Caldwell, M.D.
Miss Margaret M. Cummings
Matthew O. Foley
Maurice F. Griffin
Thomas Howell
E. H. Lewinski-Corwin, M.D.

Emma Lucas Louie
Malcolm T. MacEachern, M.D.
Christopher G. Parnell, M.D.
John M. Peters, M.D.
C. S. Pitcher
Rev. Alphonse M. Schwitalla
Daniel T. Test
W. H. Walsh, M.D.

---

†Deceased

CHARTER FELLOWS†

Anderson, Victor
Anscombe, E. Muriel
Austin, Lawrence C.
Bachmeyer, Arthur C., M.D.
Bacon, Asa S.
Barker, W. D.
Barr, Mabel
Bartine, Oliver H.
Bates, F. Oliver
Benson, John G.
Binner, Mabel
Bishop, Howard E.
Black, B. W., M.D.
Bluestone, E. M., M.D.
Breitinger, W. M.
Brown, Burton A., M.D.
Buerki, Robin C., M.D.
Burlingham, L. H., M.D.
Calvin, Arthur M.
Candlish, Jessie M.
Cariss, Muriel McKee
Carter, Fred G., M.D.
Collier, E. M.
Copeland, John G.
Craig, Allan, M.D.
Cummings, Clarence C.
Davis, Carolyn E.
Decker, C. J.
Dinsmore, John C.
Doane, Joseph C., M.D.
Driver, Anna Lauman
Dubin, Maurice
Eickenlaub, Mark
Erickson, E. I.
Fesler, Paul
Fingerhood, Boris
Franklin, J. B.
Fritschel, Herman, Rev.

Hahn, Albert G.
Hahn, Mrs. Albert
Hanner, Guy M.
Haynes, Harley A., M.D.
Haywood, A. K., M.D.
Hedden, Henry, M.D.
Hewitt, S. R. D., M.D.
Hodge, Howard E.
Johnson, Clarence T.
Johnson, Lake
Jolly, Robert
Keller, Paul, M.D.
King, E. E.
Klopp, Henry I., M.D.
Lewis, Mary R., M.D.
List, Walter E., M.D.
Louis, Marie
Lutes, J. Dewey
MacLean, Basil C., M.D.
MacMaster, A. J.
Mannix, John R.
Matthews, Elmer E.
McGregor, Elizabeth
McNee, James
Mohler, Henry K., M.D.
Morrill, Donald, M.D.
Munger, Claude W., M.D.
Murray, Thomas T.
Neff, Robert E.
Nettleton, Robert A.
Norby, Joseph G.
Norris, James U.
O'Hanlon, George, M.D.
Oppenheimer, Russell H., M.D.
Remy, Charles E., M.D.
Rowan, Georgia
Rowland, Henry
Sexton, Lewis, M.D.

---

†All Deceased

Sheats, George D.
Shoneke, Austin J.
Slack, E. L.
Smelzer, Donald C., M.D.
Smith, Clinton F.
Smith, Herman, M.D.
Smith, John M.
Spry, Cecil T.
Stasel, Alfred G.
Steele, Merrill F., M.D.
Stephens, George F., M.D.
Stephenson, Mary V.
Sutley, Melvin L.
Swanson, A. J., M.D.

Turnbull, Jessie J.
Twitty, Bryce L.
Vollmer, Philip, Rev.
Vonder, Heidt, L. G.
Walker, Fred M.
Walter, Frank J.
Ward, Peter D., M.D.
Wilson, George W.
Wilson, Lucius R., M.D.
Witham, Robert B.
Woods, C. S., M.D.
Wordell, Charles A.
Wright, Carl P., Sr.

HONORARY FELLOWS 1933–1993

The Hon. J. Chaiker Abbis
('85)
Robinson E. Adkins ('61)
G. Harvey Agnew, M.D. ('33)
Mother V. Allaire ('47)
Guillermo Almenara, M.D. ('44)
Odin W. Anderson, Ph.D. ('67)
Major Gen. George E.
Armstrong ('53)
Major Gen. Harry G.
Armstrong ('53)
Arthur C. Bachmeyer, M.D.
('52)
Asa S. Bacon ('41)
Otho F. Ball, M.D. ('33)
Rt. Rev. Msgr. John W. Barrett
('49)
Karl D. Bays ('86)
Mme. L. De G. Beaubien ('39)
Stanley S. Bergen, Jr., M.D.
('92)
Rev. Hector L. Bertrand ('70)
Ella Best ('58)
Jack C. Bills ('91)
Rev. John J. Bingham ('44)
Jan E. G. Blanpain, M.D. ('77)
F. J. L. Blasingame, M.D. ('60)
Frances P. Bolton ('44)
Vice Admiral Joel T. Boone
('55)
Richard P. Borden ('34)
Nelles V. Buchanan ('62)
LeRoy E. Burney, M.D. ('59)
Bert W. Caldwell, M.D. ('33)
G. D. W. Cameron, M.D. ('64)
Charles A. Cannon ('67)
Guy J. Clark ('54)
L. T. Coggeshall, M.D. ('65)
John A. D. Cooper, M.D., Ph.D.
('82)
Lawrence T. Cooper ('77)

Paul B. Cornely, M.D. ('73)
Nelson H. Cruickshank ('58)
Margaret M. Cummings ('34)
Robert M. Cunningham, Jr.
('58)
Robert Cutler ('55)
Ward Darley, M.D. ('60)
Mrs. Maxwell Davidson ('79)
Graham L. Davis ('47)
Michael M. Davis ('35)
Michael DeBakey, M.D. ('90)
Mother Anna Dengel, M.D.
('62)
Marshall E. Dimock ('60)
Leland I. Doan ('55)
Avedis Donabedian, M.D. ('82)
William J. Driver ('68)
Leonard A. Duce, Ph.D. ('72)
Merlin K. DuVal, M.D. ('80)
Bernard J. Echlin ('88)
C. Wesley Eisele, M.D. ('66)
William J. Ellis ('35)
Paul M. Ellwood Jr., M.D. ('87)
Haven Emerson, M.D. ('50)
Lester J. Evans, M.D. ('59)
Robert S. Ewing ('83)
James R. Felts, Jr. ('78)
Edmund Fitzgerald ('58)
Rev. John J. Flanagan ('58)
Matthew O. Foley ('33)
Marion B. Folsom ('66)
Mrs. W. W. Fondren, Sr. ('63)
Thomas F. Frist, Sr., M.D. ('89)
Rt. Rev. Msgr. John G.
Fullerton ('57)
Mrs. S. Palmer Gaillard, Jr.
('73)
John W. Gates ('81)
Lillian M. Gilbreth ('61)
Maurice Goldblatt ('58)
S. S. Goldwater, M.D. ('38)

Ignatio Gonzalez, M.D. ('46)
Annie Goodich ('48)
The Hon. Willis D. Gradison, Jr. ('90)
Harald M. Graning, M.D. ('71)
Rev. Msgr. Maurice F. Griffin ('33)
Gunnar Gundersen, M.D. ('59)
Mrs. Albert G. Hahn ('48)
Jack C. Haldeman, M.D. ('65)
The Hon. Justice Emmett Hall ('80)
Paul R. Hawley, M.D. ('58)
Harley A. Haynes, M.D. ('48)
Emanuel Hayt ('58)
Lt. General Leonard D. Heaton ('60)
A. A. Heckman ('73)
Mrs. Clifford S. Heinz ('70)
Frederick T. Hill, M.D. ('62)
George W. Hill ('63)
Lister Hill ('54)
Vane M. Hoge, M.D. ('50)
Mrs. Chester A. Hoover ('59)
John F. Horty ('65)
Thomas Howell, M.D. ('33)
Sister John Gabriel (Ryan) ('35)
Lucius W. Johnson, M.D. ('57)
Robert W. Johnson ('62)
Richard M. Jones ('58)
Sidney R. Lamb ('36)
Eleanor C. Lambertsen, Ed.D. ('71)
Peter B. Laubach, D.B.A. ('84)
Lucille P. Leone ('57)
Edward H. Lewinski-Corwin ('34)
Lucile Emma Lucas Louie ('34)
James E. Ludlam ('66)
Malcolm T. MacEachern, M.D. ('33)
Arthur Mag ('58)
Charles W. Mayo, M.D. ('54)
William G. (Billy) McCall ('88)

Ada Belle McCleery ('47)
John F. McCreary, M.D. ('69)
Foster G. McGaw ('62)
Msgr. Andrew J. McGowan ('93)
Rev. Donald A. McGowan ('51)
John Alexander McMahon ('74)
Fred A. McNamara ('52)
William S. McNary ('64)
Richard L. Meiling, M.D. ('80)
Karl P. Meister ('56)
William S. Middleton, M.D. ('57)
J. Roscoe Miller, M.D. ('51)
Emory W. Morris ('55)
Richard Moses ('79)
Major General Oliver K. Niess ('61)
Maurice J. Norby ('58)
William A. O'Brien, M.D. ('43)
Rev. Joseph S. O'Connell ('39)
Basil O'Connor ('55)
Edward M. O'Herron, Jr. ('76)
Dennis S. O'Leary, M.D. ('92)
Sister M. Olivia (Gowan) ('36)
Herluf V. Olsen, Ph.D. ('58)
Christopher G. Parnall, M.D. ('34)
Thomas Parran, M.D. ('46)
Andrew Pattulo ('58)
Edmund D. Pellegrino, M.D. ('80)
Thomas L. Perkins ('66)
Earl Perloff ('70)
John M. Peters, M.D. ('34)
Marshall I. Pickens ('55)
W. Douglas Piercey, M.D. ('58)
Mrs. Viola Pinanski ('64)
Charles S. Pitcher ('34)
Charles E. Prall, Ph.D. ('59)
Rear Admiral Lemont Pugh ('53)
Richard L. Rand ('84)
W. S. Rankin, M.D. ('38)

Willard C. Rappleye, M.D. ('40)
Mary M. Roberts ('49)
Major Gen. Paul I. Robinson ('58)
David E. Rogers, M.D. ('87)
The Hon. Joseph D. Ross, M.D. ('67)
Charles G. Roswell ('65)
F. Burns Roth ('58)
Howard A. R. Rusk, M.D. ('63)
John T. Ryan ('58)
James H. Sammons, M.D. ('86)
Leonard A. Scheele, M.D. ('53)
Rev. Alphonse M. Schwitalla ('34)
James Shannon, M.D. ('65)
Vergil N. Slee, M.D. ('69)
Raymond P. Sloan ('53)
Winford H. Smith, M.D. ('42)
Anne Ramsay Somers ('74)
Herman Miles Somers, Ph.D. ('74)
Richard W. Soper ('37)
Henry J. Southmayd ('43)
Eric W. Springer, LL.B. ('78)
Nathan J. Stark, J.D. ('81)
Msgr. John C. Stauton ('72)
Sir Arthur G. Stephenson ('58)
Captain Joseph E. Stone ('47)

Jack I. Straus ('68)
Most Rev. Joseph Sullivan ('89)
William I. Taylor, M.D. ('66)
Lillian D. Terris, Ph.D. ('78)
Luther L. Terry, M.D. ('64)
Daniel D. Test ('34)
Paul H. T. Thorlakson, M.D. ('72)
Thomas M. Tierney ('67)
Rt. Rev. Msgr. Charles A. Towell ('54)
Col. Florence Turkington ('58)
Edward L. Turner, M.D. ('58)
Joseph F. Volker, D.D.S., Ph.D. ('79)
William H. Walsh, M.D. ('34)
Clarence A. Warden, Jr. ('64)
Frederic A. Washburn, M.D. ('40)
Malcolm Stuart McNeal Watts, M.D. ('75)
Lawrence L. Weed, M.D. ('75)
Lewis Weeks, Ph.D. ('85)
Lloyd B. Wescott ('67)
Homer Wickenden ('58)
Kenneth Williamson ('58)
Richard E. YaDeau, M.D. ('76)
Morley A. R. Young, M.D. ('63)

GOLD MEDAL AWARD*

1964
†Robin C. Buerki, M.D., CFACHE
Executive Director
Henry Ford Hospital
Detroit, Michigan

Pearl R. Fisher, FACHE
Administrator
Thayer Hospital
Waterbury, Maine

David Littauer, M.D., FACHE
Executive Director
Cedars-Sinai Medical Center
Los Angeles, California

†Tol Terrell, FACHE
Administrator
Shannon West Texas Memorial
   Hospital
San Angelo, Texas

1965
Frank C. Sutton, M.D., FACHE
Director
Miami Valley Hospital
Dayton, Ohio

1966
†Albert W. Snoke, M.D., FACHE
Executive Director
Yale-New Haven Hospital
New Haven, Connecticut

1967
†Charles P. Cardwell, Jr., FACHE
Vice President-Director
Hospital Division Medical
   College of Virginia
Richmond, Virginia

1968
Frank S. Groner, FACHE
Administrator
Baptist Memorial Hospital
Memphis, Tennessee

1969
†Ray E. Brown, FACHE
Executive Vice President
Northwestern McGaw Medical
   Center
Chicago, Illinois

---

*The Gold Medal Award was established in 1964 to recognize exceptional individuals who exemplify the highest standards and values of the profession. It is awarded to Fellows of the College who have demonstrated outstanding leadership and fostered excellence in healthcare management. In 1991, the Board of Governors approved the merger of the Silver Medal Award with the Gold Medal Award, authorizing up to two Gold Medal recipients annually. The award is presented during the College's annual meeting banquet. On the special occasion of the inauguration of the award in 1964, four awards were granted. All positions shown were those held by recipients at the time the award was bestowed.

†Deceased

1970
Boone Powell, FACHE
Executive Director
Baylor University Medical
  Center
Dallas, Texas

1971
T. Stewart Hamilton, M.D.,
  FACHE
President
The Hartford Hospital
Hartford, Connecticut

1972
James D. Harvey, FACHE
Administrator
Hillcrest Medical Center
Tulsa, Oklahoma

1973
Ronald D. Yaw, FACHE
President
Blodgett Memorial Hospital
Grand Rapids, Michigan

1974
George E. Cartmill, Jr.,
  FACHE
President
United Hospitals of Detroit
Detroit, Michigan

1975
Donald W. Cordes, FACHE
Executive Vice President
Iowa Methodist Medical Center
Des Moines, Iowa

1976
Peter E. Swerhone, FACHE
President
Health Sciences Center
Winnipeg, Manitoba
Canada

1977
Donald C. Carner, FACHE
Executive Vice President
Memorial Hospital Medical
  Center
Long Beach, California

1978
R. Zach Thomas, Jr., FACHE
Executive Director
Charlotte Mecklenburg Hospital
  Authority
Charlotte, North Carolina

1979
†William N. Wallace, FACHE
President
United Hospitals, Inc.
St. Paul, Minnesota

1980
Roy Rambeck, FACHE
Executive Director of Hospitals
University of Washington
Seattle, Washington

1981
Pat N. Groner, FACHE
President
Baptist Regional Hospital
  Systems
Pensacola, Florida

---

†Deceased

1982
Ray Woodham, FACHE
President-Emeritus
Southwest Community Health
  Services
Albuquerque, New Mexico

1983
Stanley R. Nelson, FACHE
Executive Vice President
Henry Ford Hospital
Detroit, Michigan

1984
Bernard J. Lachner, FACHE
President
Evanston Hospital
Evanston, Illinois

1985
Wade Mountz, FACHE
Vice Chairman & CEO
NKC, Inc.
Louisville, Kentucky

1986
H. Robert Cathcart, FACHE
President
Pennsylvania Hospital
Philadelphia, Pennsylvania

1987
†Samuel J. Tibbitts, FACHE
President
LHS Corporation
Los Angeles, California

1988
E. E. Gilbertson, FACHE
President
St. Luke's Hospital
Boise, Idaho

1989
Austin Ross, FACHE
Executive Administrator
Virginia Mason Medical Center
Seattle, Washington

1990
David H. Hitt, FACHE
President/CEO
Methodist Hospitals of Dallas
Dallas, Texas

1991
Sr. Irene Kraus, FACHE
President/CEO
Daughters of Charity National
  Health System
St. Louis, Missouri

1992
Horace M. Cardwell, FACHE
Senior Consultant
Methodist Hospital System
Houston Texas

John R. Griffith
*Andrew Pattullo Collegiate
  Professor in Hospital
  Administration*
University of Michigan
Ann Arbor, Michigan

1993
**James W. Holsinger, Jr., M.D.,
  FACHE**
Undersecretary for Health
Department of Veterans Affairs
Washington, D.C.

D. Kirk Oglesby, Jr., FACHE
President/CEO
Anderson Area Medical Center
Anderson, South Carolina

---

†Deceased

SILVER MEDAL AWARD*

1974
Stanley W. Martin, FACHE
Deputy Minister of Health
Ministry of Health
Ontario, Canada

1975
†Gerhard Hartman, Ph.D.,
  FACHE
Chairman
Graduate Program in Hospital
  and Health Administration
University of Iowa
Iowa City, Iowa

1976
Matthew F. McNulty, Jr., Sc.D.,
  FACHE
Chancellor
The Medical Center
Georgetown University
Washington, DC

1977
†Richard J. Stull, FACHE
President
American College of Hospital
  Administrators
Chicago, Illinois

1978
Walter J. McNerney, FACHE
President
Blue Cross and Blue Shield
  Associations
Chicago, Illinois

1979
O. Ray Hurst
President
Texas Hospital Association
Austin, Texas

1980
James O. Hepner, Ph.D.,
  FACHE
Director
Health Administration and
  Planning Program
Washington University
St. Louis, Missouri

1981
Donald L. Custis, M.D.
Chief Medical Director
Veterans Administration
Washington, DC

1982
George Bugbee, FACHE
Director
Veterans Administration Health
  Care Administrators' Forums
Chicago, Illinois

---

*The Silver Medal Award was established in 1974 to recognize outstanding executives who are not in hospital or hospital system positions. The award served as the counterpart to the professional society's Gold Medal Award until 1991. At that time, the Board of Governors approved the merger of the Silver Medal Award with the Gold Medal Award, authorizing up to two Gold Medal recipients annually. The 1991 Silver Medal Award was the last given. All positions shown were those held at the time the award was bestowed.
    †Deceased

1983
†**Robert M. Cunningham Jr., HFACHE**
Contributing Editor, *Hospitals Magazine*
Editorial Consultant, Blue Cross/Blue Shield Associations
Chicago, Illinois

1984
Richard L. Johnson, FACHE
President
Tribrook Group, Inc.
Oak Brook, Illinois

1985
†**David M. Kinzer**
President
Massachusetts Hospital Association
Burlington, Massachusetts

1986
J. Alexander McMahon, HFACHE
President
American Hospital Association
Chicago, Illinois

1987
RADM Lewis E. Angelo, MSC, USN
Chief, Medical Service Corps
Naval Medical Command
Washington, DC

1988
Donald R. Newkirk, FACHE
President
Ohio Hospital Association
Columbus, Ohio

1989
Everett A. Johnson, Ph.D., FACHE
Director, Program in Healthcare Administration
Georgia State University
Atlanta, Georgia

1990
Bernard R. Tresnowski
President
Blue Cross and Blue Shield Association
Chicago, Illinois

1991
Stuart A. Wesbury, Jr., Ph.D., FACHE
President/CEO
American College of Healthcare Executives
Chicago, Illinois

---

†Deceased

EXECUTIVE OF THE YEAR AWARD*

1961
Clarence B. Randall
Retired Chairman of the Board
Inland Steel Company
Chicago, Illinois

1962
George Romney
President
American Motors Corporation
Detroit, Michigan

1963
Clark Kerr, Ph.D.
President
University of California
Berkeley, California

1964
John A. Barr
Chairman of the Board
Montgomery Ward & Company
Chicago, Illinois

1965
General Robert W. Johnson
Member, Board of Directors
Johnson & Johnson
New Brunswick, New Jersey

1966
John W. Macy
Chairman
U.S. Civil Service Commission
Washington, DC

1967
Joseph L. Block
Chief Executive Officer
Inland Steel Company
Chicago, Illinois

1968
Ray R. Eppert
Chief Executive Officer
Burroughs Corporation
Detroit, Michigan

1969
George Champion
Chairman of the Board
The Chase Manhattan Bank
New York, New York

1970
Robert G. Dunlop
Chairman of the Board
Sun Oil Company
Philadelphia, Pennsylvania

---

*The Executive of the Year Award was introduced in 1961 and was presented annually at the College-sponsored Congress on Administration to an outstanding administrator outside the hospital field. In 1975 the award was discontinued at the recommendation of the Committee on the Executive of the Year, action endorsed by the parent Committee on Awards and Testimonials and the Board of Governors. All positions shown were those held at the time the award was bestowed.

1971
Edwin J. Faulkner
President
Woodman Accident and Life
  Company
Lincoln, Nebraska

1972
Walter K. Koch
Attorney-at-Law
Holme Roberts & Owen
Denver, Colorado

1973
**Reverend Theodore M.
  Hesburgh**
President
University of Notre Dame
South Bend, Indiana

1974
Archie K. Davis
Chairman of the Board
Wachovia Bank and Trust
  Company
Winston-Salem, North Carolina

ROBERT S. HUDGENS
MEMORIAL AWARD*

"Young Healthcare Executive of the Year"

1969
Donald C. Wegmiller
Administrator
Fairview-Southdale Hospital
Edina, Minnesota

1970
Monroe Mitchell
Administrator
A. Holly Patterson Home
Uniondale, New York

1971
Nelson Lewis St. Clair, Jr.,
  FACHE
Administrator
Riverside Hospital
Newport News, Virginia

1972
Robert L. Montgomery
Administrator
Alta Bates Community Hospital
Berkeley, California

1973
Gail L. Warden
Executive Vice President
Rush-Presbyterian-St. Luke's
  Medical Center
Chicago, Illinois

1974
G. Edwin Howe, FACHE
Director
Ohio State University Hospitals
Columbus, Ohio

1975
F. Kenneth Ackerman, Jr.
Administrative Director
Geisinger Medical Center
Danville, Pennsylvania

1976
Paul B. Hofmann, FACHE
Director
Stanford University Hospital
  and Clinics
Stanford, California

---

*The Robert S. Hudgens Memorial Award for "Young Healthcare Executive of the Year" was established in 1969 as a tribute to Mr. Hudgens—the College's First Vice President (an elected office)—by the Alumni Association of the Graduate Program in Health Services Administration of the Medical College of Virginia, Virginia Commonwealth University. It is awarded to an exceptional healthcare executive who is under 40 years of age and serving as a chief executive officer or chief operating officer of a healthcare organization.

Note: The Certified Healthcare Executive designation (CHE) was first authorized for use in August, 1993.

1977
James L. Farley
Executive Director
Pleasant Valley Hospital
Point Pleasant, West Virginia

1978
Jos. Michael Galvin, Jr.
Executive Director
Salem County Memorial
  Hospital
Salem, New Jersey

1979
Lloyd L. Cannedy, Ph.D.
Executive Director
Amarillo Hospital District
Amarillo, Texas

1980
Glen T. Randolph
Service Unit Director
Keams Canyon Indian Hospital
Keams Canyon, Arizona

1981
John T. Casey
President
Presbyterian/Saint Luke's
  Medical Center
Denver, Colorado

1982
Myles P. Lash
Executive Director
Medical College of Virginia
  Hospitals
Richmond, Virginia

1983
Jan R. Jennings
Executive Director
St. Luke's Memorial Hospital
  Center
Utica, New York

1984
David L. Bernd
President
Medical Center Hospitals
Norfolk, Virginia

1985
David J. Fine, FACHE
President
West Virginia University
  Hospitals, Inc.
Morgantown, West Virginia

1986
Mark E. Celmer
Director and CEO
De Graff Memorial Hospital
North Tonawanda, New York

1987
R. Timothy Stack
President
The South Side Hospital
Pittsburgh, Pennsylvania

1988
Mark Neaman, FACHE
President
Evanston Hospital
Evanston, Illinois

1989
John B. Grotting
Executive Vice President
Legacy Health System
Portland, Oregon

1990
Denise Williams
President
Roseland Community Hospital
Chicago, Illinois

1991
Michael J. Connelly, FACHE
Regional Executive/CEO
Daughters of Charity National
  Health System-West
Los Altos Hills, California

1992
Mark K. Wallace, FACHE
Executive Director/CEO
Texas Children's Hospital
Houston, Texas

1993
Kevin E. Lofton
Executive Director/CEO
Howard University Hospital
Washington, D.C.

DEAN CONLEY AWARD*

1958
"Principles of Administration"
By Wallace S. Sayre, Ph.D.
Hospitals

1960
"The Intellectual Development of the Operationalist"
By Rev. Robert J. Henle, S.J.
Hospital Progress

1961
"The Nature of Administration"
By Ray E. Brown, FACHE
The Modern Hospital

1962
"The Administrator Must Be Adept at Adapting"
By Ray E. Brown, FACHE
The Modern Hospital

1963
"Administrative Leadership in Hospital Research"
By Arnold L. Swanson, M.D., FACHE
Canadian Hospital

1964
"The Top Management Triangle in the Voluntary Hospital"
By Paul J. Gordon, Ph.D.
Hospitals

1965
"Proliferation of Hospital Professions Is New Challenge to Management"
By Donald W. Cordes, FACHE
The Modern Hospital

1966
"Administration Is Not a Numbers Game"
By Ray E. Brown, FACHE
The Modern Hospital

1967
"The Effective Hospital Administrator Leads Board and Community Thinking"
By Robert B. Ferguson, FACHE
Hospital Administration in Canada

1968
"New Consensus Health Care for Everybody"
By Harry Becker
The Modern Hospital

---

*The Dean Conley Award was established in 1958 to recognize outstanding articles on an administrative theme published in one of the major magazines or journals serving the healthcare management field. The award was named in tribute to Dean Conley, executive director of the College, serving from 1942 to 1965.

Note: The Certified Healthcare Executive designation (CHE) was first authorized for use in August, 1993.

1969
"Promoting Quality Care Through Evaluating the Process of Patient Care"
By Avedis Donabedian, M.D., HFACHE
Medical Care

1970
"The Notion of Hospital Incentives"
By Robert M. Sigmond
Hospital Progress

1971
"Hospital Costs and Payment: Suggestions for Stabilizing the Uneasy Balance"
By Anne Ramsay Somers, HFACHE
Medical Care

1972
"Reaching the Unreachable"
By H. Robert Cathcart, FACHE
Hospitals

1973
"Beyond Responsibility: Toward Accountability"
By Kenneth J. Williams, M.D., FACHE
Hospital Progress

1974
"Hospital Organization in the Post-Industrial Society"
By Gordon L. Lippitt, Ph.D.
Hospital Progress

1975
"Excessive Hospitalization Can Be Cut Back"
By Peter Rogatz, M.D., FACHE
Hospitals

1976
"The Promise of Multihospital Management
By Montague Brown, Dr. P.H., and William H. Money
Hospital Progress

1977
"Holding the CEO Accountable"
By Harold Koontz, Ph.D.
Hospital Progress

1978
"Reimbursement System Must Recognize Real Costs"
By David H. Hitt, FACHE
Hospitals

1979
"The Last Resort: Regulation by Law"
By Thomas M. Tierney, HFACHE
Hospital Progress

1980
"The 1980's: Rise of HMO's and the Marketplace Competition"
By Richard L. Johnson, FACHE
Hospital Progress

1981
"Rethinking Health Policy for the Elderly: A Six-Point Program"
By Anne Ramsey Somers, HFACHE
Inquiry

1982
"Predictions Too Rosy, Solutions Too Pat"
By David M. Kinzer
Hospitals

1983
"Hospital Strategic Planning Must be Rooted in Values and Ethics"
By Joseph P. Peters, FACHE, and Ronald C. Wacker
Hospitals

1984
"How To Create An Outstanding Hospital Culture"
By Terrence E. Deal, Ph.D., Allan A. Kennedy, and Arthur H. Spiegel III
Hospital Forum

1985
"Death of a Paradigm: The Challenge of Competition"
By Jeff C. Goldsmith, Ph.D.
Health Affairs

1986
"Medical Staff of the Future: Replanting the Garden"
By Stephen M. Shortell, Ph.D.
Frontiers of Health Services Management

1987
"How Companies Tackle Health Care Costs"
By Regina E. Herzlinger and Jeffery Schwartz
Harvard Business Review

1988
"Where is Hospital Leadership Coming From"
By David Kinzer
Frontiers of Health Services Management

1989
"The Uninsured: Response and Responsibility"
By Gail Wilensky, Ph.D., and Kala Ladenheim
Frontiers of Health Services Management

1990
"A Radical Prescription for Hospitals"
By Jeff C. Goldsmith, Ph.D.
Harvard Business Review

1991
"Improving Hospital Board Effectiveness: An Update"
By Anthony R. Kovner, Ph.D.
Frontiers of Health Services Management

1992
"The Quest for Quality and Productivity in Health Services"
By Vinod K. Sahney, Ph.D., and Gail L. Warden, FACHE
Frontiers of Health Services Management

1993
"Health Care Leadership in the Public Interest"
By Bruce C. Vladeck, Ph.D.
Frontiers of Health Services Management

EDGAR C. HAYHOW AWARD*

1960
"Motivation and Morale"
By Oswald Hall, Ph.D.

1961
"Problem-oriented Administration"
By Warren G. Bennis, Ph.D.

1962
"The Qualities of an Administrator"
By Ralph N. Traxler, Jr., Ph.D.

1963
*"The Dynamics of Professionalism:
The Case of Hospital
Administration"*
By Harold L. Wilensky, Ph.D.

1964
*"The Spontaneous Development of
Informal Organization"*
By E. Jackson Baur, Ph.D.

1965
*"The Impact of the Hospital on the
Physician, the Patient and the
Community"*
By George Rosen, M.D., Ph.D.

1966
*"The Administrator and Policy
Processes"*
**By John W. Hennessey, Jr.,
Ph.D.**

1967
*"A Philosophical Dimension of
Administration"*
By Leonard A. Duce, Ph.D.

1968
*"When Occupations Meet:
Professions in Trouble"*
By Edward Gross, Ph.D.

1969
*"Applying Economic Concepts to
Hospital Care"*
By Paul J. Feldstein, Ph.D.

1970
*"The Social Responsibility of
General Hospitals"*
**By Bright M. Dornblaser,
FACHE**

1971
*"Professional Development Needs in
Hospital Administration"*
By Louis E. Davis, Ph.D.

---

*The Edgar C. Hayhow Award was established in 1960 to recognize outstanding articles published in the journal *Hospital & Health Services Administration*. The award was named in tribute to Edgar C. Hayhow, chairman of the College, 1947–1948, and the first practicing administrator to have earned a doctoral degree.

Note: The Certified Healthcare Executive designation (CHE) was first authorized for use in August, 1993.

1972
"Conflicting Economic Pressure in Health Care"
By James R. Jeffers, Ph.D.

1973
"An Emerging Medical Staff Organization"
By Everett A. Johnson, Ph.D., FACHE

1974
"Conflict of Interest: Ethical Dilemma"
By Charles M. Ewell, Jr., FACHE

1975
"The Crisis in Health Care System: A Contrary Opinion"
By S. David Pomrinse, M.D., FACHE

1976
"The Ashland Plan: An Ambulatory Care Outreach Alternative for a Community Hospital"
By John N. Simpson, FACHE

1977
"Evaluation of Administrative and Organizational Effectiveness in Hospitals"
By Charles M. Ewell, Jr., Ph.D., FACHE

1978
"Old and New Thinking About Hospital Payments"
By Everett A. Johnson, Ph.D., FACHE

1979
"Evaluating the Performance of the Chief Executive Officer"
By James D. Harvey, FACHE

1980
"The Management of Disruptive Conflicts
By Robert Veninga, Ph.D.

1981
"What Motivates People To Work Effectively"
By David Babnew, Ph.D., FACHE

1982
"Administrative Linkages: Management Issues and Implications"
By Austin Ross, FACHE

1983
"Hospital Administration and Medicine at the Crossroads"
By James W. Summers, Ph.D.

1984
"Physician-Centered Marketing: A Practical Step to Hospital Survival"
By Daniel A. Koger, Ph.D., and Frankie L. Perry, R.N., M.A.

1985
"Doing Good and Doing Well: Ethics, Professionalism and Success"
By James W. Summers, Ph.D.

1986
"Improving Hospital Productivity Under PPS: Managing Cost Reductions"
By Stephen R. Eastaugh, Ph.D.

1987
"In Search of Social Enterprise: A Fable"
By David Starkweather, Ph.D., FACHE

1988
"Decision Points for Hospital-Based Health Promotion"
By Eileen Malo and Laura E. Leviton, Ph.D.

1989
"Voluntary Hospitals: Are Trustees the Solution?"
By John R. Griffith, FACHE

1990
"The Keys to Successful Diversification: Lessons from Leading Hospital Systems"
By Stephen Shortell, Ph.D., FACHE
Ellen Morrison, Ph.D., and Susan Hughes

1991
"Coping with Unbalanced Information about Decision-Making Influence for Nurses"
By Robert H. Schwartz

1992
"The Power of Health Care Value-Adding Partnerships: Meeting Competition through Cooperation"
By Stephen E. Foreman and Robert D. Roberts

1993
"Outcomes Measurement in Hospitals: Can the System Change the Organization?"
Jane C. Lindner, D.B.A.

James A. Hamilton Award*

1958
Administrative Behavior
Herbert A. Simon, Ph.D.
The Macmillan Company

1959
Personality and Organization
Chris Argyris, Ph.D.
Harper & Row

1960
Managerial Psychology
Harold Leavitt, Ph.D.
University of Chicago Press

1961
Men Who Manage
Melville Dalton, Ph.D.
John Wiley & Sons

1962
The Human Side of Enterprise
Douglas McGregor, Ph.D.
McGraw-Hill Book Company

1963
New Patterns of Management
Rensis Likert, Ph.D.
McGraw-Hill Book Company

1964
The Community General Hospital
**Basil S. Georgopoulos, Ph.D.,
and Floyd C. Mann, Ph.D.**
The Macmillan Company

1965
*The Theory and Management of
Systems*
**Richard A. Johnson, Ph.D.,
Fremont E. Kast, Ph.D., and
James E. Rosenzweig, Ph.D.**
McGraw-Hill Book Company

1966
My Years With General Motors
Alfred P. Sloan, Jr.
Doubleday & Company, Inc.

1967
*Men, Management and Morality:
Toward a New Organizational
Ethic*
Robert T. Golembiewski, Ph.D.
McGraw-Hill Book Company

1968
*The Social Psychology of
Organizations*
**Daniel Katz, Ph.D., and Robert
Kahn, Ph.D.**
John Wiley & Sons

---

*The James A. Hamilton Award for book of the year was established in 1958 to identify books of exceptional merit in the field of healthcare or general management. The award is underwritten by the Alumni Association of the Graduate Program in Health Services Research and Policy and Administration of the University of Minnesota in tribute to its course founder and director, James A. Hamilton, Chairman of the College, 1939–40.

Note: The Certified Healthcare Executive designation (CHE) was first authorized for use in August, 1993.

1969
Organization and Environment
**Paul R. Lawrence, Ph.D., and
Jay W. Lorsch, Ph.D.**
Harvard University Press

1970
The Exceptional Executive
Harry Levinson, Ph.D.
Harvard University Press

1971
*Ethos and Executive Values in
Managerial Decision Making*
Clarence C. Walton, Ph.D.
Prentice-Hall, Inc.

1972
*Management Behavior,
Performance and Effectiveness*
**John P. Campbell, Ph.D.,
Marvin D. Dunnette, Ph.D.,
Edward E. Lawler III, Ph.D.,
and Karl E. Weick, Jr., Ph.D.**
McGraw-Hill Book Company

1973
*Health Care in Transition:
Directions for the Future*
Anne Ramsay Somers
Hospital Research and
Education Trust

1974
*Organization Research on Health
Institutions*
Basil S. Georgopoulos, Ph.D.
ISR-The University of Michigan

1975
*Management: Tasks,
Responsibilities, Practices*
Peter F. Drucker, Ph.D.
Harper & Row Publishers

1976
The Achieving Enterprise
William F. Christopher
AMACOM

1977
*Management Control in Nonprofit
Organizations*
**Robert N. Anthony, Ph.D., and
Regina E. Herzlinger, Ph.D.**
Richard D. Irwin

1978
*The Managerial Choice: To Be
Efficient and To Be Human*
Frederick I. Herzberg, Ph.D.
Dow Jones-Irwin

1979
Management Policy and Strategy
**George A. Steiner, Ph.D., and
John B. Miner, Ph.D.**
Macmillan Publishing Company

1980
The New Managerial Grid
**Robert Blake, Ph.D., and Jane
Mouton, Ph.D.**
Gulf Publishing Company

1981
*Leadership: What Effective
Managers Really Do . . . and
How They Do It*
Leonard R. Sayles, Ph.D.
McGraw-Hill Book Company

1982
Managing in Turbulent Times
Peter F. Drucker, Ph.D.
Harper & Row

1983
The Change Resisters: How They Prevent Progress and What Managers Can Do About Them
George S. Odiorne
Prentice-Hall

1984
The Social Transformation of American Medicine
Paul Starr, Ph.D.
Basic Books

1985
Managing Strategic Change in Hospitals: Ten Success Stories
Joseph P. Peters, FACHE, and Simone Tseng
American Hospital Publishing

1986
CEO: Corporate Leadership in Action
Harry Levinson, Ph.D., and Stuart Rosenthal, M.D.
Basic Books

1987
Corporate Pathfinders: Building Vision and Values into Organizations
Harold J. Leavitt
Dow Jones-Irwin

1988
The Well-Managed Community Hospital
John R. Griffith, FACHE
Health Administration Press

1989
The Leadership Challenge
James M. Kouzes and Barry Z. Posner, Ph.D.
Jossey-Bass, Inc.

1990
In Sickness and in Wealth: American Hospitals in the Twentieth Century
Rosemary Stevens, Ph.D.
Basic Books, Inc.

1991
What Kind of Life: The Limits of Medical Progress
Daniel Callahan, Ph.D.
Simon and Schuster

1992
Transforming Healthcare Organizations: How to Achieve and Sustain Organizational Excellence
Ellen Gaucher and Richard J. Coffey
Jossey-Bass

1993
Cornerstones of Leadership for Health Services Executives
Austin Ross, FACHE
Health Administration Press

AFFILIATED GROUP AWARD*

1993
*The Metropolitan Health
Administrators' Association
(MHAA) New York, New York*

---

*The Affiliated Group Award was established in 1993 to recognize out-standing healthcare executive groups and women's healthcare executive networks affiliated with ACHE.

HILL-ROM MANAGEMENT ESSAY COMPETITION IN HEALTHCARE ADMINISTRATION*

1989
"Confidentiality Issues for Health Care Administrators"
Sylvia A. Small
University of Texas—Medical Branch

"Legal Issues in Neonatal Intensive Care"
Barry M. Zajac
University of Michigan

1990
"Total Quality Management in Health Care"
Robert F. Casalou
University of Michigan

"Right to Refuse Medical Treatment"
Carol Lea Moody
University of Texas—Medical Branch

1991
"Hospital Turf Battles: The Manager's Role"
Stephanie Lin Bloom
The George Washington University

"The Significance of Transactional and Transformational Leadership Theory on the Hospital Manager"
Douglas B. Matey
University of New Hampshire

1992
"The Implications of Advance Directives on the Healthcare Institution"
Julie Pachmayer
Governors State University

"Organ Donation and Transplantation: The Need for a Multi-Pronged Approach for Equitable Allocation."
Mimi Modarress
University of Minnesota

1993
"Health Care Coalitions: An Emerging Force for Change"
Karen Lowe Johnson
Trinity University

"Management Implications of Physician Practice Patterns—Strategies for Managers"
Kristin O'Connor
University of New Hampshire at Durham

---

*This competition was introduced in 1989 by the College with the support of Hill-Rom, Batesville, Indiana. The competition is open to students enrolled in those graduate and undergraduate health management programs in Canada and the United States that sponsor Student Chapters of the College.

HEALTH MANAGEMENT
RESEARCH AWARD*

1988
"The Work of Middle Managers in Health Care Organizations"
Linda Roemer, Ph.D.
Simmons College

1989
"Discovering and Evaluating the Tactics Used by Top Health Care Executives to Carry Out Organizational Design"
Paul C. Nutt, Ph.D.
The Ohio State University

1990
"Psychological Type, Health Care Management, and the Myers-Briggs Type Indicator: A Proposal for Research"
Stephen J. O'Connor
University of Wisconsin at Milwaukee
Daniel J. Raab
Memorial Medical Center

1991
"Diffusion and Adoption of Total Quality Management"
Kit N. Simpson, Dr.P.H.
University of North Carolina at Chapel Hill
Curtis McLaughlin, D.B.A.
University of North Carolina at Chapel Hill

1992
"Evaluating Hospital-Physician Integration Strategies"
James B. Goes, Ph.D.
University of Minnesota

1993
"Hospital Board Effectiveness: Board Composition as a Predictor"
Carol Molinari, Ph.D.
University of Kentucky at Lexington

---

*The Health Management Research Award was introduced in 1988 to enhance managerial effectiveness and career opportunities in health services administration. The award is supported through monies left to the Foundation of the American College of Healthcare Executives by Foster G. McGaw, founder of the American Hospital Supply Corporation. The award is granted only to affiliates of the College.

Note: The Certified Healthcare Executive designation (CHE) was first authorized for use in August, 1993.

Stuart A. Wesbury, Jr. Postgraduate Fellowship*

1992
Ronald N. Feldman

1993
Marie A. Rule

2001
Jana M. Meyer

---

*The Stuart A. Wesbury, Jr. Postgraduate Fellowship was established in 1991 to further postgraduate education in healthcare and professional society management. The fellowship was named in honor of Stuart A. Wesbury, Jr., Ph.D., FACHE, president of the College from 1979 to 1991. Student Associates of the College who have earned a graduate degree in health administration from a program accredited by the Accrediting Commission on Education from Health Services Administration are eligible.

ARTHUR C. BACHMEYER
MEMORIAL ADDRESSES*

1949
"Mankind Is Your Concern"
Stuart Chase
Economist, Author
Georgetown, Connecticut

1950
"The Challenge of Liberty"
William F. Russell, Ph.D.
President
Teachers' College
Columbia University
New York, New York

1951
"The Significance of Maturity"
James F. Bender, Ph.D.
Director
National Institute of Human
 Relations
New York, New York

1952
*"Education and Man's Quest for
 Freedom"*
Clark G. Keubler, Ph.D.
President
Ripon College
Ripon, Wisconsin

1953
*"Principles of Effective
 Administration"*
Paul S. Weaver, Ph.D.
President
Lake Erie College
Fainesville, Ohio

1954
"Perspective for Administration"
A. A. Suppan, Ph.D.
*Professor of Literature and
 Philosophy*
Wisconsin State Teachers'
 College
Milwaukee, Wisconsin

1955
"The Administrator Reconsidered"
Robert M. Hutchins, Ph.D.
President
Fund for the Republic
New York, New York

1956
*"What It Means To Be an
 Administrator"*
Marshall E. Dimock, Ph.D.
Dean
Department of Government
New York University
New York, New York

---

*These addresses are underwritten by alumni of the Graduate Program in Hospital Administration of The University of Chicago in tribute to their former director, Dr. Bachmeyer. There was no address in 1960, the year the site of the lecture was changed from the College's Annual Meeting to its educational program, the Congress on Administration.

1957
*"A Practical Philosophy of
Administration"*
Elmore Petersen, Ph.D.
Dean Emeritus
School of Business
University of Colorado
Boulder, Colorado

1958
*"Reflections on the Art of
Administration"*
Ordway Tead
Vice President
Harper & Brothers
New York, New York

1959
*"The Challenge of Being an
Administrator"*
Ralph C. Davis, Ph.D.
Professor of Management
Ohio State University
Columbus, Ohio

1961
*"A Moral Philosophy for
Management"*
Benjamin M. Selekman, Ph.D.
*Kirstein Professor of Labor
Relations*
Harvard University
Cambridge, Massachusetts

1962
"Ethics in Executive Action"
James C. Worthy
Partner
Cresap, McCormick and Paget
Chicago, Illinois

1963
"Statesmanship in Administration"
J. Martin Klotsche, Ph.D.
Provost
University of Wisconsin-
Milwaukee
Milwaukee, Wisconsin

1964
*"Executives and Their Jobs—
Changing Organizational
Structure"*
Thomas L. Whisler, Ph.D.
Professor of Industrial Relations
University of Chicago
Chicago, Illinois

1965
*"Influences of Government on the
Management Function"*
Carl M. Frasure, Ph.D.
Dean
College of Arts and Sciences
West Virginia University
Morgantown, West Virginia

1966
*"New Trends in the Training of
Administrators"*
Henry A. Singer, Ph.D.
Executive Director
Society for Advancement of
Management
New York, New York

1967
"The Effective Executive"
Peter F. Drucker, Ph.D.
Professor of Management
New York University
New York, New York

1968
"The Challenge of Communication"
Arthur Secord, Ph.D.
Professor of Speech
Brooklyn College
Brooklyn, New York

1969
"Crisis in American Health Care"
Charles E. Odegaard, Ph.D.
President
University of Washington
Seattle, Washington

1970
"Universal Compulsory Health Insurance"
Odin W. Anderson, Ph.D., HFACHE
Associate Director
Center for Health Administration Studies
The University of Chicago
Chicago, Illinois

1971
"The Frontiers of Our Time"
Harold P. Plumier
Author, Lecturer, Consultant
Minneapolis, Minnesota

1972
"Financial Prospects and Competition for Capital"
Henry Kaufman, Ph.D.
Partner
Salomon Brothers
New York, New York

1973
"Training for Health Services Management"
Ray E. Brown, FACHE
Executive Vice President
Northwestern McGaw-Medical Center
Chicago, Illinois

1974
"Graduate Education Confronts the Market Place"
Robert H. Strotz, Ph.D.
President
Northwestern University
Evanston, Illinois

1975
"National Health Insurance and the Hospital Administrator"
George Bugbee, LFACHE
Director
Inter-Agency Institute for Federal Health Care Executives
Chicago, Illinois

1976
"Coercive vs. Representative Government
W. Allen Wallis
Chancellor
University of Rochester
Rochester, New York

1977
"Two Sides of the Same Coin: Voluntary Financing and Voluntary Management"
Walter J. McNerney, FACHE
President
Blue Cross Association
Chicago, Illinois

1978
"Spiritual Values in Hospital Administration"
Reverend Raymond C. Baumhart, S.J.
President
Loyola University
Chicago, Illinois

1979
"Research Monitoring Systems"
J. Robert Clement
President
Trebor Health Associates, Inc.
New York, New York

1980
"Compensation for Health Service Executives"
John F. Sullivan
President
Sullivan & Shook
East Lansing, Michigan

1981
"Self Renewal: A Divine Perspective for Hospitals and Managers"
Leland R. Kaiser, Ph.D.
Director
Division of Health Administration
University of Colorado Medical Center
Denver, Colorado

1982
"American Management: Losing Sight of 'Love of the Product'"
Thomas J. Peters, Ph.D.
Principal
McKinsey & Company
Palo Alto, California

1983
"What's Next?"
Peter B. Laubach, D.B.A.
President
Center for Management Programs
Malibu, California
Richard L. Rand
President
PermaHealth Enterprises
Malibu, California

1984
"Administration and the Groves of Academe"
Hanna Holborn Gray, Ph.D.
President
The University of Chicago
Chicago, Illinois

1985
"Healthcare and the Information Revolution"
Paul Starr, Ph.D.
Professor
Harvard University
Boston, Massachusetts

1986
"Risk Transfer and Other Management Alternatives"
John P. McLaughlin
Managing Director and Chairman
Health Care Industry Practice/Client Industry Committee
Marsh & McLennan, Inc.
Atlanta, Georgia

1987
"Life Through an Elder's Eyes"
Patricia Moore
Gerontologist and Author
Moore & Associates
New York, New York

1988
"Breaking the Glass Ceiling: Can Women Reach the Top of the Corporate Ladder?"
Ann M. Morrison
Director
Center for Creative Leadership
LaJolla, California

1989

"Healthcare: The View from My Window"

The Hon. Lynn M. Martin
(R-Illinois)
U.S. House of Representatives
Washington, D.C.

1990

"Healthcare's Changing Corporate Culture"

Terrence Deal, Ph.D.
Professor of Education and Human Development
Peabody College
Vanderbilt University
Nashville, Tennessee

1991

"Access to Care"

The Most Reverend Joseph M. Sullivan, HFACHE
Auxiliary Bishop
Diocese of Brooklyn
New York, New York

1992

"The Physician's Perspective on the Future of Healthcare Administration"

James Todd, M.D.
Executive Vice President
American Medical Association
Chicago, Illinois

1993

"Leadership Is an Art"

Charles Lauer
Publisher
"Modern Healthcare" and
Corporate Vice President
Crain Communications, Inc.
Chicago, Illinois

MALCOLM T. MACEACHERN MEMORIAL LECTURES*

1961
"The Inquiring Mind"
Cyril O. Houle, Ph.D.
Professor of Education
The University of Chicago
Chicago, Illinois

1962
*"The Dynamics of
Professionalization"*
Harold L. Wilensky, Ph.D.
Associate Professor of Sociology
University of Michigan
Ann Arbor, Michigan

1963
*"Vision and Leadership in the
Professions"*
Eldridge T. McSwain, Ph.D.
Dean, School of Education
Northwestern University
Evanston, Illinois

1964
"The Administrator as Teacher"
Daniel R. Davies, Ph.D.
Professor of Management
University of Arizona
Tucson, Arizona

1965
*"Graduate Education for
Administration: Some Recent
Developments"*
Leonard A. Duce, Ph.D.
Dean, Graduate School
Trinity University
San Antonio, Texas

1966
*"The Relevancy of Professional
Education for Management"*
James H. Lorie, Ph.D.
*Professor of Business
Administration*
Graduate School of Business
The University of Chicago
Chicago, Illinois

1967
*"Education Accreditation: Purposes
and Problems"*
Frank G. Dickey, Ph.D.
Chief Administrative Officer
National Committee on
Accrediting
Washington, DC

1968
*"The Adult Educated: A New
Generation of Pioneers"*
William L. Bowden, Ph.D.
*Chairman, Department of Adult
Education*
The University of Georgia
Athens, Georgia

---

*A yearly feature at the College-sponsored Congress on Administration, this lecture is underwritten by the Alumni Association of the Graduate Program in Hospital and Health Services Administration of Northwestern University in tribute to its former director, Dr. MacEachern.

1969
"Educating for the Future"
Ralph Westfall, Ph.D.
Associate Dean for Academic
Affairs
School of Management
Northwestern University
Evanston, Illinois

1970
"Education for Hospital
Administration"
John A. Barr
Dean
Graduate School of
Management
Northwestern University
Evanston, Illinois

1971
"The Dilemma of Hospitals—Is
Public Utility Status the
Answer?"
Fred P. Morrissey, Ph.D.
Professor of Business Management
Graduate School of Business
The University of California
Berkeley, California

1972
"A Review of Some Major
Administration Health Care
Policies"
Scott Fleming
Deputy Assistant Secretary
Health and Scientific Affairs,
HEW
Washington, DC

1973
"The Challenge to Management of
Today's Health Care World"
John Alexander McMahon
President
American Hospital Association
Chicago, Illinois

1974
"Leadership in Complex
Institutions"
Warren G. Bennis, Ph.D.
President
The University of Cincinnati
Cincinnati, Ohio

1975
"Implications of the Reports on the
Commission on Education for
Health Administration"
James P. Dixon, M.D.
President
Antioch College
Yellow Springs, Ohio

1976
"Health Service Administration—
Yesterday and Today"
James A. Hamilton, FACHE
Consultant
South Duxbury, Massachusetts

1977
"The Changing Nature of Society"
Howard F. Didsbury, Jr.
Executive Director
World Future Society
Washington, DC

1978
"The Manager as a Change Agent"
S. G. Huneryager, Ph.D.
Professor of Management
University of Illinois (Circle
Campus)
Chicago, Illinois

1979
"An Analysis of Governing
Developments: Their Effects on
the Business Community"
Richard R. Salzmann
Editor-in-Chief
Research Institute of America
New York, New York

1980
"Goals of Schools and Management: Positive Self-Image, Hope, and Love"
Zacharie J. Clements, Ph.D.
Associate Professor of Education
University of Vermont, Burlington

1981
"Dealing with the Media During a Crisis"
Stephen C. Rafe
Principal
Dynamic Innovations, Ltd.
New York, New York

1982
"Human Concern in Management"
Dan C. Baker
Bulverde, Texas

1983
"Health Care Ethics"
Joseph Cardinal Bernardin
Roman Catholic Archdiocese of Chicago
Chicago, Illinois

1984
"Healthcare: Past, Present and Future"
S. David Pomrinse, M.D.
President
Greater New York Hospital Association
New York, New York

1985
"Anti-Social Ethics"
Richard Lamm
Governor
State of Colorado

1986
"The Aging of America"
Ken Dychtwald, Ph.D.
President
Age Wave
Emeryville, California

1987
"The New American Organization"
V. Clayton Sherman
President
Management House, Inc.
Inverness, Illinois

1988
"Healthcare—Also a Matter of Trust"
James E. Burke
Chairman/CEO
Johnson and Johnson
New Brunswick, New Jersey

1989
"Assessing the Impact of DRGs on the American Healthcare System"
Stuart H. Altman, Ph.D.
Dean, Heller School of Social Policy
Brandeis University
Waltham, Massachusetts

1990
"The Role of the Non-Profit Sector in Today's Healthcare"
George F. Moody
Chairman
American National Red Cross
Washington, DC

1991
"Financing the Future of Healthcare"
Gail Wilensky, Ph.D.
Administrator
Health Care Financing Administration
Washington, DC

1992
"Managing Cultural Diversity"
Judy Rosener, Ph.D.
*Professor and Former Assistant
  Dean*
Graduate School of
  Management
University of California
Irvine, California

1993
*"Delivering Primary Healthcare:
  Innovative Solutions in Urban
  Settings"*
Ronald Anderson, M.D.
President and CEO
Parkland Memorial Hospital
Dallas, Texas

PARKER B. FRANCIS FOUNDATION
DISTINGUISHED LECTURESHIPS*

1975
Peter G. Peterson
Chairman of the Board
Lehman Brothers, Inc.
New York, New York

1976
Gordon McLachlan
Former Secretary
Nuffield Provincial Hospitals
  Trust
London, England

1977
Howard W. Hiatt, M.D.
Dean
Harvard School of Public
  Health
Cambridge, Massachusetts

1978
Pierre A. Rinfret, Ph.D.
President
Rinfret Associates, Inc.
New York, New York

1979
Richard S. Schweiker
United States Senator
State of Pennsylvania
Philadelphia, Pennsylvania

1981
Herbert A. Simon, Ph.D.
Professor of Computer Science &
  Psychology
Carnegie-Mellon University
Pittsburgh, Pennsylvania

1982
Peter Francese
Publisher
American Demographics
Ithaca, New York

1983
Jane Bryant Quinn
Financial Analyst and Commentator
New York, New York

1984
William C. Freund, Ph.D.
Senior Vice President and Chief
  Economist
New York Stock Exchange
New York, New York

1985
Lawrence R. Miller
Partner
L. M. Miller & Company
Atlanta, Georgia

---

*Introduced by the College in cooperation with the Puritan-Bennett Corporation of Kansas City, Missouri, in memory of Parker B. and Mary Francis, for the purpose of presenting outstanding executives from the worlds of commerce, education and government to the health service field. No lecture was given in 1980.

1986
Amitai Etzioni
Professor
George Washington University
Washington, DC

1987
Nancy K. Austin
President
Nancy K. Austin, Inc.
Capitola, California

1988
F. G. (Buck) Rogers
Former Senior Vice President-
Marketing
IBM
Armonk, New York

1989
Lee Sherman Dreyfus
Former Governor
State of Wisconsin
Madison, Wisconsin

1990
Rosemary A. Stevens, Ph.D.
Professor and Chairman
Department of History and
Sociology of Sciences
University of Pennsylvania
Philadelphia, Pennsylvania

1991
Frances Hesselbein
President & CEO
Peter F. Drucker Foundation
For Nonprofit Management
New York, New York

1992
Kevin Phillips
Author and Political Analyst
Bethesda, Maryland

1993
Gloria Borger
Chief Congressional Correspondent
"U.S. News & World Report"
Washington, D.C.

LEON I. GINTZIG
COMMEMORATIVE LECTURES*

1986
*"Health, Healthcare Executives and
their Communities"*
Bruce C. Vladeck
President
United Hospital Fund
New York, New York

1987
"Leadership for Changing Times"
Gerald Greenwald
Chairman
Chrysler Motors Corporation
Detroit, Michigan

1988
"Marketing Warfare in Healthcare"
Jack Trout
President
Trout and Ries Advertising
New York, New York

1989
*"Information Systems as a Strategic
Asset"*
Frank A. Metz, Jr.
Senior Vice President—Finance
IBM
Armonk, New York

1990
"Reevaluating Healthcare Illusions"
Sen. John Kitzhaber, M.D.
President
Oregon State Senate
Salem, Oregon

1991
*"Creating the Future of
Healthcare"*
Leland R. Kaiser, Ph.D.
President
Kaiser and Associates
Brighton, Colorado

1992
*"Delivering Healthcare: Costs and
Questions"*
Richard Morrow
Former Chairman and CEO
Amoco Corporation
Chicago, Illinois

1993
"Leadership and Moral Purpose"
Max De Pree
Chairman
Herman Miller, Inc.
Zeeland, Michigan

---

*A yearly feature at the College-sponsored Congress on Administration, this lecture is underwritten by The George Washington University Alumni Association for Health Services Administration in tribute to the program's former professor and chairman, Dr. Gintzig.

Bibliography

BIBLIOGRAPHIC SOURCES

ACHE Archives and Library (Richard Stull Resource Center), Chicago, IL.

Asa Bacon Library of the American Hospital Association, Chicago, IL.

Center for Hospital and Health Care Administration History, Stuart Wesbury, Malcolm MacEachern, John Mannix Collections, Lewis Weeks Oral History Series. Interviews with John Mannix, Richard Stull, Gerhard Hartman, Stuart Wesbury.

National Library of Medicine, Bethesda, MD.

Allen Memorial Library, Cleveland, OH.

Countway Library, Harvard University, Codman Papers.

AUPHA Library, Arlington, VA.

American College of Surgeon's Archives.

Author's Personal Library.

Interviews: College Staff, Dewey Lutes, John Mannix, George Bugbee, Richard Stull, Stuart Wesbury, Thomas Dolan, Gerhard Hartman, Daphne Grew, Gary Filerman, and others.

ACHE Minute Books, Vol. 1–Vol. 5, 1932–1961.

BIBLIOGRAPHY

American College of Healthcare Executives

(Repeated and Periodical Publications)

Meetings:
Annual Institute for Hospital Administrators 1938–1943
Chicago Institute for Hospital Administrators 1944–1957
Chicago Basic Institute for Hospital Administrators 1958–1961
Chicago Institute on Hospital Administration 1962
The Midwest Institute for Hospital Administration 1941
The Minnesota Institute for Hospital Administration 1939
The New York Institute for Hospital Administration 1941
Western Institute 1940–1964

The Roster
1945, 1949–1959, 1961, 1965.

Membership Directories, Directory
1938, 1941, 1944, 1948, 1964, 1966, 1968, 1969, 1970, 1972, 1974, 1977, 1979, 1981; continuing . . . 1994.

Regional Rosters, Geographic Membership Rosters
Aug. 1, 1937; Aug. 1, 1938; Aug. 1, 1939, 1940, 1941, 1942, 1943, 1945, 1949, 1950, 1951, 1952, 1953, 1954, 1955, 1956, 1957.

Constitution and Bylaws, Articles of Incorporation, and Bylaws
1933, 1934, 1936, 1938, 1939, 1947, 1949, 1951, 1952, 1953, 1955, 1956, 1960, 1966, 1979.

Administrators Digest
Vol. 2, 1960, 1961.

Education Schedule
1960–1973, annual.

Assemblies on Hospital Administration
1965.

Administrative Briefs
Vol. 1, No. 1, April 1966 through Vol. 14, Jan. 1980.

Hospital Administration (Quarterly)
Vol. 1, No. 1, Fall 1956 to Vol. 20, No. 4, Fall 1975 (retitled).

Hospital & Health Services Administration
Vol. 21, No. 1, Winter 1976, continuing.

Annual Reports
  1957 "Annual Report"
  1964 "Annual Report"
  1965 "Progress Report"
  1971 "An Interim Progress Report"
  1972–73 "Progress Report"
  1973–74 " '73–'74 ACHA Report"
  1974–75 "The Year in Review"
  1975–76 "The Year in Review"
  1976–77 "The Year on File"
  1977–78 "Annual Report"
  1979–80 "ACHA Annual Report"
  1980–81 and continuing "Annual Report"
  1991–92 and continuing "Annual Report and Reference Guide"

Bulletin of The American College of Hospital Administrators
  Vol. 1, probably three issues No. 1, 1934 or 1935, No. 2, 1936, No. 3, 1937.

ACHA News
  Jan. 1938, Vol. 1, No. 1 to Vol. 46, 1982–85; and continuing.

Reports to Regents ("A Review of Current Activities of the College")
  Vol. 1, No. 1, Nov. 1965 through Vol. 13, No. 2, April 1977.

Code of Hospital Ethics Approved and Adopted by the American Hospital Association and the American College of Hospital Administrators
  1941 (also published in ACHA News Feb. 1942, pp. 2–41). Revisions 1947, 1958, 1964. The college published its own code in 1970; revised 1973, 1980, 1992.

The Administrative Internship in the Hospital
  Paul B. Gillen and Charles E. Prall. Joint Commission on Education, 32 pages, 1947 and *The Administrative Residency in the Hospital,* 1953, 1954, 1956, 59 pages.

The Administrative Residency
  1965, 51 pages.

Objectives, Membership, Programs
  (variations on this title), 1957, 1960, 1962, circa 1965, 1967, 1972.

Regulations Governing Admission and Advancements
  1966, 1982, 1992, 1993.

Preparing for Advancement
  1980, 1981.

Report to Regents
    1965 and continuing.

Congress on Administration, Announcements
    Annually. First Congress, 1958. Thirty-sixth Congress on Administration, March 1–5, 1993.

Professional Continuing Education Catalog, Seminars on Executive Skills
    1970 and later.

Educational Audio Cassette Catalog

A Brief Description
    1967, 1978, 1982, 1989.

Convocation
    Annual

Programs in Health Administration
    1984, 1985, 1986, 1991, 1992.

Directory of Postgraduate Fellowships and Management Development
    1984, 1985, 1986, 1991–1992.

Executive News
    Vol. 48, No. 8, Vol. 50, No. 1 (March 1987).

Healthcare Executive
    (Bimonthly), Vol. 1, No. 1, Jan./Feb., 1986, continuing.

ACHEvements
    Employee Newsletter, Vol. 1, No. 1, July 23, 1990.

Council of Regents Agenda Materials
    1991.

Professional Development Catalog
    1991, 1992.

Health Administration Press, Catalog of Publications
    1986, continuing.

American College of Healthcare Executives

(Non-periodic Publications, listed by date of publication)

"American College of Hospital Administrators," 1933.

"Articles of Incorporation," March 26, 1934.

"The Hospital Administrator: An Analysis of His Duties, Responsibilities, Relationships, and Obligations," by the 1934–1935 Study Committee of the ACHA, 1935, Fred G. Carter, M.D., chairman.

"A Survey of the Hospital Administrator," 1936.

MacEachern, Malcolm. "Institutes for Hospital Administrators," presented before the meeting of the ACHA, Sept. 13, 1937.

"University Training for Hospital Administration Careers," a report by the Committee on Educational Policies of the ACHA, 1937.

Carter, F.G. "Progress in the Training of Hospital Administrators," ACHA report from *Hospital Management*, June 1938.

Contracts for Hospital Administators, Sept. 26, 1938.

Davis, Michael. "Some Experiences in the Education of Administrators," 1938, reprinted by the College for *Hospitals*, Jan. 1938.

Goldwater, S.S. "The Future of Hospital Administration," reprinted by the College from *Hospitals*, Nov. 1938.

Hayhow, Edgar. "Training Program for Hospital Executive Personnel," ACHA, 18 pages (circa 1938).

"Hospital Administration Reference Library," *ACHA News*, April 1938, 2 pages.

"Opinions Here and There," *ACHA News*, Jan. 1938, pp. 4–11.

"The Administrator's Library," *ACHA News*, Sept. 1939, 3 pages.

Hamilton, James A. "Need for Adequate Education and Training for Hospital Executives," ACHA Reprint from *Hospitals*, Jan. 1939.

Hardgrove, Arden. "Adequate Education and Training for Hospital Administrators," ACHA reprint from *Hospitals*, March 1939.

"Instituto Inter-Americano Par Administradores de Hospitales," San Juan, Puerto Rico, 1940.

Munger, Claude. "Practical Experience for the Administrative Career," 1940.

"Code of Hospital Ethics," *ACHA News*, Feb. 1942, pp. 2–4.

"Educational Session Addresses with a Message from the President," Annual Meeting, Buffalo, 1943.

Hartman, Gerhard. *Hospital Malpractice Insurance*, ACHA special reprint from *The Journal of Business*, University of Chicago, Vol. 16, No. 4, Part 2, Oct. 1943.

"The General Educational Session and the Report of the President," Annual Meeting, Cleveland, 1944.

"A Statistical Survey Based on the 1944 Directory of Membership" (prepared under the direction of the Central Committee on Institutes), Aug. 1944.

Program for the 13th Chicago Institute for Hospital Administrators, Sept. 17–28, 1945.

The Hospital Administrative Internship: A Conference Report, Joint Commission on Education of the AHA and ACHA, held at Columbia University, New York, 1947.

"Students Graduated in Hospital Administration," *ACHA News*, June-July 1947, pp. 2–7.

"Accent on Leadership: Addresses of the 14th Annual Meetings, Sept. 19–20, 1948, Atlantic City, New Jersey."

"At the Helm of the Hospital: The Story of a New Profession," 1948.

"The College Curriculum in Hospital Administration," The Joint Commission on Education of the ACHA and AHA, Charles E. Prall, director, 1948.

"Hospital Administration: A Life's Profession," 1948.

The Hospital Administrative Internship, Joint Commission on Education, reports of the second and third conferences held at Washington University, St. Louis, Jan. 31–Feb. 1, 1948, and at the University of Minnesota, Minneapolis, April 2–4, 1948.

"Mankind Is Your Concern," 1949.

"Trusteeship: A Symposium on the Governing Board and the Administrator, Addresses of the 15th Annual Meeting, Sept. 25–26, 1949, Cleveland, Ohio."

"The ACHA: Basic Information about its Objectives, Program, Membership," 1950.

"Addresses of the 16th Annual Meeting and the Second Annual Bachmeyer Address, Sept. 17–18, 1950, Atlantic City, New Jersey."

Brown, Ray, and Johnson, Richard L. *Hospitals Visualized*, 1952 first edition, 1957 second edition, reprinted 1961. (There is also a Spanish translation.)

"Board of Regents Conference on Future Program and Policy: The Proceedings, Dec. 9–11, 1955," Dewey Lutes, presiding, 1955.

Kipnis, Ira A. *A Venture Forward. A History of the American College of Hospital Administrators*, 1955, 145 pages.

"The Administrative Residency in the Hospital," 1956.

"Accomplishments and Plans for the Future," 1960.

"Questions and Answers: Some Facts about the Proposed Organizational Plan for the College," 1962.

"Regulations Governing Admission and Advancement," 1962.

"ACHA Objectives, Membership Program," 1965.

"A Brief Description, Objectives, Structure, Membership Program," 1967.

"The British National Health Service," 1969, 161 pages.

Chester, T.E. *Graduate Education for Hospital Administration in the United States: Trends*, 1969, 31 pages.

Houle, Cyril O. "The Lengthened Line of Education," foreword by Richard J. Stull, June 1969, reprinted from *Perspectives in Biology and Medicine*, Vol. II, No. 1, Autumn 1967.

"Remarks Made by Richard J. Stull at the Annual Meeting of the Council of Regents, Sept. 16, 1969, Atlantic City."

Starkweather, David B., and Taylor, Shirley J. *Health Facility Combinations and Mergers: An Annotated Bibliography*, 1970.

"So Many People Know So Many Things That Have Not Been Put into Writing," 1971.

"The Swedish Health Services System," 1971, 255 pages.

"The Chief Executive's Role and Responsibility for Administrative Development," Task Force IX, May 4, 1972.

"ACHA Research Cassette Quarterly," 1973.

"The Delivery of Health Services in Australia," 1973, 254 pages.

"Principles of Appointment and Tenure of Executive Officers," Task Force V, 1973, 34 pages.

"Providing Primary Care in Community Hospitals," Task Force VIII (circa 1973).

"Regent's Role in Medical Care Leadership," Task Force III, 14 pages (circa 1973).

"The Role of the ACHA in the Legislative Process," 1973.

"Specialized Management in Hospital Administration," Task Force VI (circa 1973).

"A Statement of the Productivity of Group Medical Practices," Task Force IV, p. 16 (circa 1973).

"The ACHA Congress on Administration Is . . .," 1974.

"An Examination of Shared Services," Task Force X, 1974, pp. 51.

"National Health Insurance: Principle Essential to a Successful Program," report of the Board of Governors Special Study Commission on National Health Insurance, Peter B. Terenzo, chairman, 1974, pp. 54.

"Recommendations on Standards to the Joint Commission on Accreditation of Hospitals," May 24, 1974.

"The Role of the American College of Hospital Administrators in the Legislative Process," Board of Governor's Special Task Force, Everett A. Johnson, chairman (circa 1974).

"Health Services in the European Economic Community," U.S. Department of Health, Education and Welfare, U.S. Public Health Service, Health Resources Administration, DHEW Publication (HRA) 76–638, Washington, DC, 1976. Published in cooperation with the ACHA and the Health Resources Administration.

"Proposed Program of Self Development and Recertification," prepared by the Division of Membership for review by the Board of Governors, April 30, 1976.

"Manual for Interviewers," 1977.

McLachlan, Gordon. "The Universality of Health Problems," 1977.

"The Role of the Governor," report of the Special Task Force on the Role of the Governor, William N. Wallace, chairman, Oct. 1977.

"Report of the Joint Meeting of the ACHA Board of Governors/Task Force on the Report of the Commission on Education for Health Administration," Aug. 10, 1977.

"The Report of the Task Force on the Report of the Commission on Education for Health Administration," 1978, and "Compilation of Reactions of Officers and Governors," May 4, 1977, 15 pp.

"Creating Effective Interaction between Administrative Practice and Academia through Constructive Exchanges of Ideas for Educational Program Development and Instructional Strategy," *Final Report*, July 1978, 58 pages.

Executive Briefing Series—Trends and Issues '78, 1978.

Hepner, James O., ed. *Case Studies in Health Administration*, Vol. I, *Health Planning for Multi-Hospital Systems*, St. Louis: C.V. Mosby, 1978.

The Role of the Regent. A Guide to the Responsibilities of a Regent of the ACHA, revised edition, 1978; annual.

Stull, Richard J. "A Summary Report on a Proposal for Developing the Self-Assessment Component of a College-Based Program with a Goal of Continuing Education, Authentication, and Enhancement of Individual Capacity for Administrative Performance through Life-Long Learning—Including the Board of Governors' Action at the April 29, 1978 Meeting." (This contains several documents, dated April 14, April 17, April 29, May 3, May 5, and May 1978).

A Selected Bibliography for the Well-Read Health Services Manager, Jan. 25, 1979, 50 pages.

"Your Career in Health Services Administration," 1979.

"Accord on the Roles and Responsibilities of the American Hospital Association and the American College of Hospital Administrators in the Development and Implementation of Public Policy," approved July 1980.

Hepner, James O., ed. *Case Studies in Health Administration*, Vol. II, *Hospital Administrator-Physician Relationships*, St. Louis: C.V. Mosby, 1980.

"Statement of the ACHA on Deferred Compensation to the Subcommittee on Select Revenue Matters of the Committee on Ways and Means, United States House of Representatives," April 24, 1980.

"Enhancing Executive Competence: Educational and Practice Perspectives," May 1981.

"Health Services in New Zealand," Oct. 9, 1981.

"Report of the Task Force on Public Information and Marketing," Donald Newkirk, chairman, Feb. 1981.

Wesbury, Stuart A. "Background Information Concerning the Proposal to Change the Name and Objects of the American College of Hospital Administrators," April 1981.

Wesbury, Stuart A., Speech, Jan. 28, 1981, North Carolina Hospital Association, ACHA Breakfast.

ACHA Publications Catalog, Summer 1982.

Brown, Ray E. *Judgment in Administration*, commemorative edition in honor of the 50th anniversary of the ACHA (reprint of 1966 book, New York: McGraw Hill), Chicago: Pluribus Press, 1982.

Contracts for Hospital Chief Executive Officers, 1982, 59 pages.

"Contracts for Hospital Chief Executive Officers," a report of the Ad Hoc Committee on Contracts for Hospital Chief Executive Officers, 1982.

Foundations for Excellence, 23 award-winning articles from *Hospital & Health Services Administration*, Chicago: Pluribus Press, 1982.

"Healthcare Executives Must Prepare for 'Serious Ethical Conflicts,'" and "Ethics: A Critical Factor in Healthcare," Nov. 23, 1982.

Commemorative Edition (boxed set), Brown, Ray E. *Judgment in Administration*; *Foundations for Excellence*; *Challenging the Profession*; *Coming of Age*, 1983.

Joseph Cardinal Bernardin, MacEachern Lecture, March 4, 1983, 10 pages.

"Evaluating the Performance of the Hospital Chief Executive Officer," 1984, 72 pages.

"The Evolving Role of the Hospital Chief Executive Officer," 1984, 108 pages.

"Health Care in the 1990s: Trends and Strategies," 1984 (with Arthur Andersen & Co.), 42 pages.

Darr, Kurt, ed. *Ethics for Health Services Managers*, Vol. 4, Case Studies in Health Administration, 1985, 148 pages.

Hicks, Lanis L., and Boles, Keith (editors). *An Economic Approach to Rationing Healthcare Resources*, Vol. 5, Case Studies in Health Administration, 1985, 134 pages.

White, Elizabeth. "The History of the American College of Hospital Administrators and Public Policy," March 1985.

"Access to Care Survey," packet of five press releases, 1986.

"ACHE Public Policy Process," June 1987.

"ACHE Strategic Plan" (circa 1987).

"Contracts for Healthcare Executives," second edition, 1987, 51 pages.

"The Future of Healthcare: Changes and Choices" (with Arthur Andersen & Co.), 1987, 46 pages.

Hepner, James O., ed. *Hospital Labor Relations*, Vol. 6, Case Studies in Health Administration, 1987, 177 pages.

"Hospital-Sponsored Child Care: A 1988 National Survey" (with American Association of Healthcare Consultants), 1988, 26 pages.

Levey, Samuel, and Hill, James, eds. *Alternative Delivery Systems: Approaches for the Health Care Executive*, Vol. 7, Case Studies in Health Administration, 1988, 95 pages.

"Hospital Chief Executive Officer Role Study 1989" (with AHA, Heidrick and Struggles, Inc.), Research Series No. 2, 1989.

"Hospital Chief Executive Officer Turnover: National Trends and Variations (1981–1987)," 1989.

Arrington, Barbara, ed. *The Evolution of Strategy*, Vol. 8, Case Studies in Health Administration, 1990, 153 pages.

"1989 Survey on Allocating Healthcare Resources," Research Series No. 1, June 1990, 37 pages.

Public Policy Statement: "Enhancing Minority Opportunities in Healthcare Management," 1990.

"Report on Baccalaureate Career Development" (with AUPHA), Jan. 1990, 16 pages.

Ethical Policy Statement: "Impaired Healthcare Executives," 1991.

"The Future of Healthcare: Physician and Hospital Relationships" (with Arthur Andersen & Co.), 1991, 50 pages.

"Gender and Careers in Healthcare Management" (with the Graduate Program in Hospital and Health Administration, The University of Iowa), Research Series No. 3, 1991, 47 pages.

"Hospital Chief Executive Officer Turnover 1981–1990" (with AHA, Heidrick and Struggles, Inc.), 1991, 32 pages.

"Proposed Changes to the Bylaws and Regulations of the ACHE: Official Notice," 1991.

"Strategic Plan, July 1991," 19 pages.

"ACHE Strategic Plan," July 1, 1992.

"Active (Dues-Paying) Affiliates of the ACHE as of January 1, 1992."

"Archives Inventory 1992," 1992, 10 pages.

Dolan, Thomas. "College Update Speech," July 1992, 18 pages.

"Evaluating the Performance of the Hospital CEO in a Total Quality Management Environment," internal document, 1992, published in 1993, 36 pages.

"Examination Outline 1992," 8 pages.

"Report of the Task Force on Beginning and Early Career Development" (with AUPHA), 1992, 39 pages.

Spaeth, Ronald. "Credentials Task Force Recommendations for Changes to the Regulations Governing Admission, Advancement and Re-certification," Oct. 26, 1992, 5 pages.

"Strategic and Operational Overview," Feb. 24, 1992.

Weil, Peter. "Results of the 1991 Directory Update Study," July 21, 1992.

Other References

Abbott, Andrew. *The System of Professions*. Chicago: University of Chicago Press, 1988.

Abel-Smith, Brian. *The Hospitals 1800–1848*. London: Heinemann, 1964.

Accrediting Commission on Education for Health Services Administration. "Sundre Names ACEHSA Executive Secretary." Washington, DC, Dec. 1982.

"ACHA Expands Mission, Wants Clout." *Modern Healthcare*, Oct. 1981, pp. 76–78, 80, 84 (see LaViolette, Suzanne).

"Adminstration Congress to Mark ACHA's 25th Anniversary." *Hospital Topics*, Vol. 36, Jan. 1958.

Agho, Augustin, and Cyphert, Stacey T. "Problem Areas Faced by Hospital Administrators." *Hospital & Health Services Administration*, Vol. 37, No. 1, Spring 1992, pp. 131–135.

Agnew, G. Harvey. "Training in Hospital Administration." *Hospitals*, July 1939.

"AHA, ACHA Approve Revised Ethical Codes." *Hospitals*, Vol. 31, Oct. 16, 1957, pp. 124–127.

Aikens, Charlotte. *Hospital Management*. Philadelphia: W.B. Saunders Co., 1911.

Amberson, J. Burns; McMahon, B.T.; and Pinner, Max. "A Clinical Trial of Sanocrysin in Pulmonary Tuberculosis." *American Review of Tuberculosis*, Vol. 24, 1931, pp. 401–435.

"The American Academy of Medical Administrators." The AAMA Medical Administrative Executive. Southfield, MI: The Academy, Vol. 19, No. 6, Aug. 1982.

American and Canadian Hospitals. Chicago: Physicians Record Company. 1st ed., 1933; 2nd ed., 1937.

American College of Medical Group Administrators. "So Now You're a Nominee." Denver, CO: The College, May 1981.

American College of Medical Group Administrators. "Admission Advancement Criteria." Denver, CO: The College, Jan. 1982.

American College of Osteopathic Hospital Administrators. *1981 Directory* and *Report 1980.* Park Ridge, IL.

American College of Surgeons. "Hospital Standardization." *ACS Bulletin*, March 1918; Jan. 1924; and April 1925.

American College of Surgeons. *Manual of Hospital Standardization.* Chicago: ACS, 1938, 96 pages.

American College of Surgeons. *Imago Chirurgii 1913–1963.* Chicago: ACS, 1963.

American Foundation. *American Medicine: Expert Testimony Out of Court.* New York: The Foundation, 1937.

American Hospital Association. *The Changing Role of the Hospital.* Chicago: AHA, 1980.

American Hospital Association. *Data Book on Multihospital Systems 1980–1981.* Chicago: AHA, 1981.

American Hospital Association. *Ethical Conduct and Relationships for Health Care Institutions.* Chicago: AHA, 1981.

American Hospital Association. *Guide to the Health Care Field.* Chicago: AHA, 1982, 1992.

American Hospital Association. "Hospitals Save Millions and Shared Services Mushroom." Washington, DC: AHA, Feb. 5, 1979.

American Hospital Association. *Hospital Statistics 1982 Edition; 1990–1991 Edition*; *1992–1993 Edition.* Chicago: AHA, 1982, 1992.

American Society for Hospital Food Service Administrators of the American Hospital Association. "Twenty-Five Years of Exceptional Performance in Health Care Food Services Administration." Chicago: The Society, 1992. "Take the Future Into Your Own Hands." Chicago: The Society, circa 1990.

American Society for Hospital Personnel Administration of the American Hospital Association. "Innovations in Human Resources." Chicago: AHA, circa 1982.

American Society for Hospital Purchasing and Materials Management of the American Hospital Association. Brochure. Chicago: AHA, circa 1982.

American Society of Nursing Service Administrators. "Our Role Strengthens Your Many Roles." Chicago, circa 1982.

Anderson, O.W. *Blue Cross Since 1929*. Cambridge, MA: Ballinger, 1975.

Anthony, Robert N., and Herzlinger, Regina. *Management Control in Nonprofit Organizations*. Homewood, IL: Richard D. Irwin, 1975.

Argyris, Chris. *Executive Leadership*. New York: Harper and Bros., 1953.

Argyris, Chris. *Personality and Organization*. New York: Harper and Bros., 1957.

Arrow, K.J. "Uncertainty and the Welfare Economics of Medical Care." *American Economic Review*, Vol. 53, No. 5, pp. 941–973, 1963.

Association for Volunteer Administration. Boulder, CO. Pamphlets, undated manuscript, and personal correspondence, circa 1982.

Association of American Medical Colleges. "Graduate Medical Education: Proposals for the Eighties." *Journal of Medical Education*, Vol. 56, No. 9, Sept. 1981, Part 2.

Association of University Programs in Health Administration. "AUPHA 1948–1993: 25th Anniversary Dinner." AUPHA Library, 1993.

Association of University Programs in Health Administration. *Health Services Administration Education 1979*. Washington, DC: AUPHA, 1979.

Association of Univesity Programs in Health Administration. *Health Services Administration Education 1983–1985, 1989–1991, 1991–1993*. Arlington, VA: AUPHA, 1982, 1989, 1991.

Austin, Charles J. *Information Systems for Health Services Administration*. 4th ed. Ann Arbor, MI: AUPHA Press/Health Administration Press, 1992.

Bachmeyer, Arthur C. "A Course in Hospital Administration." *Transactions of the American Hospital Association*, Vol. 21, 1919, pp. 279–283.

Bachmeyer, Arthur C. "Qualities of a Trustee." *Trustee*, Vol. 4:14, Oct. 1951.

Bachmeyer, Arthur C., and Hartman, Gerhard. *The Hospital in Modern Society*. New York: The Commonwealth Fund, 1943.

Bachmeyer, Arthur C., and Hartman, Gerhard. *Hospital Trends and Developments 1940–1946*. New York: The Commonwealth Fund, 1948.

Bachmeyer, R.W. "Depreciation of Capital Assets." *Hospital Accounting*, Vol. 5, June 1951, pp. 18–19.

Bast, Joseph L.; Rue, Richard C.; and Wesbury, Stuart A. *Why We Spend Too Much on Health Care*. Chicago: The Heartland Institute, 1992.

Bay, Emmet Blackburn. *Medical Administration of Teaching Hospitals*. Chicago: University of Chicago Press, 1931.

Becker, Carl A. *History and Handbook of the American College of Nursing Home Administrators*. ACNHA, 1982.

Becker, Selwyn, and Neuhauser, Duncan. *The Efficient Organization*. New York: Elsevier, 1975.

Beecher, Henry K. "The First Anesthesia Records." *Surgery, Gynecology and Obstetrics*, Vol. 71, 1940, pp. 689–693.

Bellin, Lowell, and Weeks, Lewis. *The Challenge of Administering Health Services: Career Pathways*. Washington, DC: AUPHA Press, 1981.

Bendix, Reinhard. *Work and Authority in Industry*. New York: Harper and Row, 1956.

Berman, Howard J.; Weeks, Lewis E.; and Kukla, Steven F. *The Financial Management of Hospitals*. 7th ed. Ann Arbor, MI: Health Administration Press, 1990.

Berwick, Donald M. "Continuous Improvement as an Ideal in Health Care." *New England Journal of Medicine*, Vol. 320, 1989, p. 53.

Billings, John S. *Description of the Johns Hopkins Hospital*, Baltimore: Johns Hopkins Press, 1890.

Billings, John S. *Ventilation and Heating*. New York: The Engineering Record, 1893.

Billings, John S., and Hurd, Henry M., eds. *Hospitals, Dispensaries and Nursing*. International Congress of Charities, Correction and Philanthropy. Section III. Baltimore: Johns Hopkins Press, 1894.

Billings, John S.; Folsom, Norton; Jones, Joseph; Morris, Caspar; and Smith, Stephen. *Five Essays Relating to the Construction, Organization and Management of Hospitals for the Use of Johns Hopkins Hospital of Baltimore*. New York: William Wood and Co., 1875.

Blake, Robert, and Mouton, Jane. *The New Managerial Grid*. Houston: Gulf Publishing Co., 1964.

Blau, Peter M., and Scott, W. Richard, *Formal Organizations*. San Francisco: Basic Books, 1971.

Block, Louis. *Hospital Trends*, Hospital Topics, circa 1957.

Bowman, John G. "For Hospital Standardization." *Transactions of the American Hospital Association*, Vol. 18, 1916, pp. 288–292.

Bradley, Frank R., Biography. *Hospital Management*, Vol. 85, April 1958, p. 34.

Bradley, Frank R. "How Affiliations Build Up a Great Medical Center, Barnes Hospital and Medical Center, St. Louis." *Hospital Management*, Vol. 76, July 1953, pp. 34–35, 140.

Brines, William S., Biography. *Hospital Topics*, Vol. 36, March 1958, p. 5.

Brines, William S. "Organizations: Annual Administrative Review." *Hospitals*, Vol. 33, April 16, 1959, pp. 100–101.

Brown, Madison B. *History of the Society of Medical Administrators 1967–1984*. Vol. 3. Burlington, VT: The Society, 1984.

Brown, Montague. "An American Version of Theory Z." *Health Care Management Review*, Vol. 7, No. 4, Fall 1982, pp. 23–26.

Brown, Montague, and Lewis, H.L. *Hospital Management Systems—Multi-Unit Organization and Delivery of Health Care*. Germantown, MD: Aspen Systems, 1976.

Brown, Montague, and McCool, Barbara P. *Multi-Hospital Systems*. Germantown, MD: Aspen Systems, 1980.

Brown, Ray E., Biography. *Hospital Management*, Vol. 80, Sept. 1955, p. 32. *Hospital Topics*, Vol. 33, Sept. 1955, p. 3.

Ray E. Brown: Lectures, Messages and Memoirs. Mary M. Blanks; William E. Corely; and Douglas S. Smith, eds. Ann Arbor, MI: Health Administration Press, 1991.

Brown, Ray E., ed. *Graduate Education for Hospital Administration: Proceedings of a National Symposium, Dec. 12–13, 1958*. Chicago: Graduate Program in Health Administration, University of Chicago, 1959.

Brown, E. Richard. *Rockefeller Medicine Men.* Berkeley, CA: University of California Press, 1979.

Buerki, Robin C., M.D., Biography. "HM Salutes." *Hospital Management*, Vol. 88, Dec. 1959, p. 16.

Buerki, Robin C., M.D. "Education in the Evening." *The Modern Hospital*, Vol. 52, No. 6, June 1939.

Buerki, Robin C., M.D. "Responsibilities in Hospital Construction." *Journal of the American Medical Association*, Vol. 147, Dec. 8, 1951, pp. 1414–1416.

Bugbee, George. "New Curriculum Developments: A Two-Year Program." *Hospital Administration*, Vol. 12, No. 4, Fall 1967, pp. 74–81.

Bugbee, George. *Reflections of a Good Life: An Autobiography.* Chicago: The Hospital Research and Educational Trust, American Hospital Association, 1987.

Burdett, Henry C. *The Cottage Hospital.* London: J and A Churchill, 1877.

Burdett, Henry C. *Hospitals and Asylums of the World.* 4 vol. London: J and A Churchill, 1891–1893.

Burkett, Norman. "Perpetual Inventory System." *Hospital Management*, Vol. 87, Feb. 1959, pp. 108–110.

Bureau of the Census, U.S. Department of Commerce. *Historical Statistics of the United States.* 2 vol. Washington, DC: U.S. Government Printing Office, 1975.

Burling, Temple; Lentz, Edith M.; and Wilson, Robert N. *The Give and Take in Hospitals.* New York: Putnam's, 1956.

Burrow, James G. *Organized Medicine in the Progressive Era: The Move Toward Monopoly.* Baltimore: Johns Hopkins University Press, 1977.

Caldwell, Bert W. "American Hospital Association," pp. 11–35 in *American and Canadian Hospitals.* 2nd ed. Chicago: Physicians Record Company, 1937.

Canadian College of Health Service Executives. Toronto, Ontario, Canada, Feb. 1975.

Carper, Wilham B. "A Longitudinal Analysis of the Problems of Hospital Administrators." *Hospital & Health Services Administration*, Vol. 27, No. 3, pp. 82–95.

Carr-Saunders, A.M., and Wilson, P.A. *The Professions.* London, 1933.

Carter, Fred G., M.D. "Administrative Leadership." *Hospitals JAHA,* June 1936, pp. 67–69.

Carter, Fred G., M.D. "Award of Merit." *Hospitals,* Vol. 26, July 1952, p. 51.

Carter, Fred G., M.D. "Hospital as a Health University: A Realistic Approach to Education." *Hospitals,* Vol. 27, Aug. 1953, pp. 65+.

Center for Hospital and Health Care Administration History. "Annual Reports." Chicago: AHA Resource Center.

Center for Hospital and Health Care Administration History. Lewis Weeks Oral History Series. Chicago: AHA Resource Center, 1980s to the present.

Center for Hospital and Health Care Administration History. "United States Hospital Histories." Chicago: AHA Resource Center, 1992, 37 pages.

Chandler, Alfred D. *Strategy and Structure.* Cambridge, MA: MIT Press, 1962.

Chapman, Frank Elmo. *Hospital Organization and Operation.* New York: Macmillan, 1924.

Chester, Theodore E. *Graduate Education for Hospital Administration in the United States: Trends.* Chicago: ACHA, 1969.

Clipson, Colin W., and Wehrer, Joseph J. *Planning for Cardiac Care.* Ann Arbor, MI: Health Administration Press, 1973.

Codman, Ernest A. "Comments." *Transactions of the American Hospital Association,* Vol. 15, 1913, p. 180.

Codman, Ernest A. *A Study in Hospital Efficiency.* Boston: Privately Printed, circa 1917.

Codman, Ernest A. *The Shoulder.* Boston: Privately Printed, 1934.

Commission on Education for Health Administration. James P. Dixon, chairman. *Education for Health Administration,* Vol. I and Vol. II, 1975; *A Future Agenda,* 1977; and *Summary of the Report of the Commission on Education for Health Administration.* Ann Arbor, MI: Health Administration Press, 1974.

Commission on Hospital Care. *Hospital Care in the United States.* Cambridge, MA: Harvard University Press, 1957.

Commission on University Education in Hospital Administration. Herlof V. Olsen, director. *University Education for Administration in Hospitals.* Washington, DC: American Council on Education, 1954.

Committee for the Study of Nursing Education (The Goldmark Report). *Nursing Education in the United States.* New York: Macmillan, 1923.

Committee on the Costs of Medical Care. *Final Report of the Committee, Adopted October 31, 1932.* Chicago: University of Chicago Press, 1932.

Committee on the Grading of Nursing Schools (Final Report). *Nursing Schools Today and Tomorrow.* New York: Privately Published, 1934.

"Committee on Training of Hospital Executives Issues Momentous Report." *Modern Hospital,* Vol. 19, No. 1, July 1922, pp. 1–6.

Conley, Dean, Biography. *Hospital Management,* Vol. 101, March 1966, pp. 53+.

Conley, Dean. "A Career in Hospital Administration." *Bios,* Vol. 20, No. 1, March 1949.

Conley, Dean. "Professional Education in Hospital Administration." *Higher Education,* Vol. 9, No. 17, May 1, 1953 (U.S. Department of Health, Education, and Welfare), pp. 193–199.

Conley, Dean. "What Is Hospital Administration?" *Hospital Management,* Vol. 80, No. 1, July 1955, pp. 30–34.

Cope, Zachary. *The Royal College of Surgeons of England.* London: Anthony Blond, 1959.

Cordes, Donald W. *Hospital Management,* Vol. 35, July 1957, p. 3.

Cordes, Donald W. "Proliferation of Hospital Professions Is a New Challenge to Management." *The Modern Hospital,* 1965.

Corwin, E.H.L. *The American Hospital.* New York: Commonwealth Fund, 1946.

Coyne, Joseph, and Young, Leslie. "Multihospital Bed Transfers." *Health Care Management Review,* Vol. 8, No. 1, Winter 1983, pp. 25–37.

Crozier, Michel. *The Bureaucratic Phenomenon.* Chicago: The University of Chicago Press, 1964.

Cullen, Thomas S. *Henry Mills Hurd, The First Superintendent of The Johns Hopkins Hospital.* Baltimore: Johns Hopkins Press, 1920.

Cyert, Richard M., and March, James G. *A Behavioral Theory of the Firm.* Englewood Cliffs, NJ: Prentice Hall, 1963.

Davis, Loyal. *Fellowship of Surgeons*. Springfield, IL: Charles C. Thomas, 1960.

Davis, Michael M. *Clinics, Hospitals and Health Centers*. New York: Harper & Brothers, 1927.

Davis, Michael M. *Hospital Administration: A Career*. New York: Privately Published, 1929.

Davis, Michael M. "Studies in Hospital Administration at the University of Chicago." *Hospitals*, March 1936.

Michael M. Davis: A Tribute. Chicago: Center for Health Administration Studies, University of Chicago, 1972.

Davis, Michael Marks, and Rorem, Clarence Rufus. *Crisis in Hospital Finance and Other Studies in Hospital Economics*. Chicago: University of Chicago Press, 1932.

Davis, Michael M., and Warner, Andrew R. *Dispensaries: Their Management and Development*. New York: The Macmillan Co., 1918.

Deming, W. Edwards. *Out of the Crisis*. Cambridge, MA: MIT Center for Applied Engineering Studies, 1986.

Dickinson, Robert. "Hospital Organization as Shown by Charts of Personnel and Powers Functions." *Bulletin of the Taylor Society*, Vol. 3, Oct. 1917, pp. 1–11.

Dickinson, Robert. "Standardization of Surgery: An Attack on the Problem." *Journal of the American Medical Association*. Vol. 63, No. 9, August 1914, pp. 763–765.

Dolson, M.T. "How Administrators Rate Different Tasks." *The Modern Hospital*, Vol. 104, No. 6, 1965, pp. 94–97, 166.

Dore, Ronald. *British Factory–Japanese Factory*. Berkeley, CA: University of California Press, 1973.

Dowling, Harry F. *City Hospitals*, Cambridge, MA: Harvard University Press, 1982.

Dowling, Harry F. *Fighting Infection*. Cambridge, MA: Harvard University Press, 1977.

Drew, Charles A. "The Standardization of Hospitals." *Modern Hospital*, Vol. II, No. 1, July 1918, p. 57.

Drucker, Peter F. *Management: Tasks, Responsibilities, Practices*. New York: Harper and Row Publishers, 1974.

The Duke Endowment. *The Small General Hospital Organization and Management.* Charlotte, NC: Duke Endowment, Bulletin No. 3, Feb. 1928, Jan. 1933, revised March 1945.

Echenhoff, Edward, and Harasymirv, Stefan. "Contributors to Research Literature 1948–1973." *Hospital & Health Services Administration,* Vol. 24, No. 3, Summer 1979, pp. 11–20.

Eckert, Anthony W. "Partners in Crisis: Hospitals and the Press." *Hospitals,* Vol. 25, Sept. 1951, pp. 47–50.

Education for Health Services Administration at the University of Michigan, Proceedings of the Workshops. Ann Arbor, MI: University of Michigan, 1972.

Eisenberg, John M., M.D. *Doctors' Decisions and the Cost of Medical Care.* Ann Arbor, MI: Health Administration Press, 1986.

Emerson, Haven, M.D. *Administrative Medicine.* New York: T. Nelson & Sons, 1941.

Emerson, Haven, M.D. *Report of The Hospital Survey for New York.* Vol. I, Summary, 1937; Vol. II, Description of Institutions, 1937; Vol. III, Analysis of Costs, 1938. New York: United Hospital Fund.

Erickson, E.I. Professional Status of Hospital Administration. *Southern Hospitals,* Vol. 20, June 1952, pp. 29–32.

Eyler, John M. *Victorian Social Medicine.* Baltimore: Johns Hopkins Press, 1979.

Faxon, Nathaniel W. *The Massachusetts General Hospital 1935–1955.* Cambridge, MA: Harvard University Press, 1959.

Fayol, Henri. "Administration industrielle et générale." Bulletin of the Société de l'Industrie Minérale 1916. *Industrial and General Administration.* Geneva: International Management Institute, 1929 (first English translation), and London: Pitman, 1967.

Felch, William C., and Greene, Clyde C., Jr. *Aspiration and Achievement, The Story of the American Society of Internal Medicine 1956–1981.* Washington, DC: The Society, 1981.

Feldstein, Martin. *Economic Analysis for Health Services Efficiency.* Amsterdam: North Holland Publishing Co., 1967.

Feldstein, Paul J. *Health Associations for the Demand for Legislation.* Cambridge, MA: Ballinger, 1977.

Flexner, Abraham. "Is Social Work a Profession?" *School and Society,* Vol. 1, 1915, p. 904.

Flexner, Abraham. *Medical Education in the United States and Canada.* New York: The Carnegie Foundation for the Advancement of Teaching, 1910.

Foley, Matthew O. *Handbook of Hospital Management.* Downers Grove, IL: Privately Published, 1933.

Foote, A. E. "Simplification and Standardization." *Transactions of the American Hospital Association,* 1926, pp. 228–239.

Forbes, W. J. "Standardization and Purchase Agreements: Through a Central Hospital Bureau." *Transactions of the American Hospital Association,* Vol. 13, 1911, pp. 288–300.

Freidson, Eliot. *The Hospital in Modern Society.* Glencoe, IL: Free Press, 1963.

Freidson, Eliot. *Profession of Medicine.* New York: Dodd Mead & Co., 1970.

Freidson, Eliot. *Professional Dominance.* New York: Atherton Press, 1970.

Friedlander, Walter J. "Oaths Given by U.S. and Canadian Medical Schools, 1977: Profession of Medical Values." *Social Science and Medicine,* Vol. 16, 1982, pp. 115–120.

Fulton, John F. *Harvey Cushing, A Biography.* Springfield, IL: Charles C. Thomas, 1946.

Gabriel, Sister John, R.N. *Through the Patient's Eyes: Hospitals, Doctors, Nurses.* Philadelphia: Lippincott, 1935.

Galton, Douglas. *On the Construction of Hospitals.* London: Macmillan & Co., 1869.

George, Claude S., Jr. *The History of Management Thought.* Englewood Cliffs, NJ: Prentice Hall, 1968.

Georgopoulos, Basil S. *Organization Research on Health Institutions.* Ann Arbor, MI: The Institute for Social Research, The University of Michigan, 1972.

Georgopoulos, Basil, and Mann, Floyd. *The Community General Hospital.* New York: Macmillan, 1962.

Giedion, Sigfried. *Space, Time and Architecture.* 3rd ed. Cambridge, MA: Harvard University Press, 1956.

Gilbreth, Frank B. "Scientific Management in the Hospital." *Transactions of the American Hospital Association,* 1914, pp. 483–492.

Gilbreth, Frank B. "Motion Study in Surgery," *Canadian Journal of Medical Surgery*, Vol. 40, No. 1, July 1916, pp. 22–31.

Gilbreth, Frank B., Jr., and Carey, Ernestine G. *Cheaper by the Dozen.* Reprint of 1948 edition. Mattituck, NY: Amereon Ltd., 1982.

Gilbreth, Lillian. "Efficiency in the Care of the Patient." *Transactions of the American Hospital Association*, 1914.

Goldsmith, Jeff Charles. *Can Hospitals Survive?* Homewood, IL: Dow Jones-Irwin, 1981.

Goldwater, S.S. "Hospital Planning—A Study of Its Economic Problems." *Modern Hospital*, Aug. and Sept. 1929.

Goldwater, S.S. *On Hospitals.* New York: Macmillan, 1949.

Goldwater, S.S. "A Plan for the Construction of Ward Buildings in Crowded Cities." *Transactions of the American Hospital Association*, Vol. 12, 1911, pp. 178–190.

Goldwater, S.S. "Self Education for Hospital Executives." *Modern Hospital*, Sept. 1920.

Goodrich, Annie W. "How Shall the Superintendents of Small Hospitals Be Trained?" *Transactions of the American Hospital Association*, Vol. 18, 1916, pp. 356–367.

Gordon, Paul. "Top Management Triangle." *Hospital Administration*, Vol. 9, No. 2, Spring 1964.

Gordon, Paul. "The Top Management Triangle in the Voluntary Hospital." *Hospitals*, 1964.

Gorgas, Nellie. "The Storage and Issuance of Hospital Supplies." *Journal of Business*, Vol. 13, No. 2, April 1940. University of Chicago.

Gottlieb, Mark. *The Lives of University Hospitals of Cleveland.* Cleveland: Wilson Street Press, 1991.

Graham, Fred E., and Wright, Robert J. "The American College of Medical Group Administrators: Twenty-Five Years in Brief Perspective." *Medical Group Management*, Sept./Oct. 1981, pp. 60–66.

Greenwood, Ernest. "Attributes of a Profession." In Nosow, Sigmund, and Form, William, eds. *Man, Work and Society.* New York: Basic Books, 1962.

Groner, Frank S., Biography. *Hospital Management*, Vol. 85, Jan. 1958, p. 36.

Groner, Frank S. "Distinguished Service Award to Frank S. Groner." *Hospitals*, Vol. 40, May 16, 1966, pp. 66–70.

Groner, Frank S. "Essentials of Administration: Board Relations." *Trustee*, Vol. 7, Jan. 1954, pp. 14–17.

Groner, Frank S. "What is the ACHA?" *Texas Hospitals*, Vol. 7, No. 4, Sept. 1951, p. 7.

Gulick, L., and Urwick, L., eds. *Papers on the Science of Administration.* New York: Columbia University, Institute of Public Administration, 1937.

Haber, Samuel. *Efficiency and Uplift.* Chicago: University of Chicago Press, 1964.

Hague, James E. *The American Hospital System.* Papers Presented at the Dedication Program of the Baptist Memorial Hospital, Union East Unit, Memphis, Tennessee, Feb. 19, 1968. Pensacola, FL: Hospital Research and Development Institute Inc., 1968.

Hall, Oswald. "Motivation and Morale." *Hospital Administration,* Vol. 1, No. 1, Fall 1956.

Hamilton, James A., Biography. *Hospital Management*, Vol. 84, Dec. 1957, p. 36.

Hamilton, James A. "The College of Hospital Administrators—Its Significance." *Hospitals,* Aug. 1938, pp. 43–48.

Hamilton, James A. "Has the College Come of Age?" *Hospitals,* Vol. 13, No. 11, Nov. 1939, pp. 13–17.

Hartman, Gerhard. "The Administrator's Professional Library." *The Modern Hospital*, Vol. 54, No. 2, Feb. 1940.

Hartman, Gerhard. "Current Institute Development." *The Modern Hospital*, Vol. 52, No. 6, June 1939.

Hartman, Gerhard. "Graduate Education for the Management of Clinics: The Iowa Program." *Group Practice*, Vol. 13, No. 5, May 1964, pp. 295–300.

Hartman, Gerhard. "Graduate Education in Hospital Administration 1934–1937." *Journal of Business of the University of Chicago*, Vol. XI, No. 4, pp. 1–13, Oct. 1938.

Hartman, Gerhard. *Problems and References in Hospital Administration.* Chicago: University of Chicago Press, 1938.

Hartman, Gerhard, and Patrick, Floyd. "The Status of Professionalization in Hospital Administration." *The Medical Journal of Australia*, Feb. 25, 1961, pp. 287–290.

Hartman, Gerhard; Levey, Samuel; and McCarthy, Thomas. "The Graduate Programs and Their Alumni." *Hospitals*, Feb. 16, 1962, pp. 54–57.

Hartman, Gerhard, and Levey, Samuel. "Doctoral Study in an Emerging Profession: Hospital Administration." *Journal of Medical Education*, Vol. 37, No. 4, April 1962.

Hartman, Gerhard, and Weaver, John C. "Role Diversification: Hospital and Health Administration Graduates of the Iowa Doctoral Program." *Hospital Administration*, Vol. 10, No. 3, Summer 1965, pp. 42–48.

Hartman, Gerhard, with others. "The Impact of Graduate Programs in Hospital Administration." *Hospital Administration*, Vol. 7, No. 2, Spring 1962, pp. 41–54.

Hayes, John H. "A History of the Hospital Bureau of Standards and Supplies," *Hospitals*, Vol. 12, No. 2, Aug. 1938, p. 48.

Hayhow, Edgar C., Biography. *Hospital Management*, Vol. 82, Dec. 1956, p. 28.

Hayhow, Edgar C. *Hospital Topics*, Vol. 34, Nov. 1956, p. 3.

Hayhow, Edgar C. "Chronic Care: If Chronic Patients Cannot Pay, Who Should? The Government?" *Hospital Progress*, Vol. 33, Jan. 1952, pp. 55–57.

Hayt, Emanuel, and Hayt, Lillian R. *Legal Aspects of Hospital Practices.* New York: Hospital Textbook Company, 1938.

Health Insurance Institute. *Source Book of Health Insurance Data 1979–1980, 1991.* Washington, DC: Health Insurance Institute, 1980, 1991.

Healthcare Financial Management Association. *HFMA.* Oak Brook, IL: The Association, circa 1982.

Herzberg, Frederick I. *The Managerial Choice: To Be Efficient and To Be Human.* Homewood, IL: Dow Jones-Irwin, Reprinted. Salt Lake City, UT: Olympus Publishers, 1982.

Herzlinger, Regina; Moore, Gordon; and Hall, Elizabeth. "Management Control Systems in Health Care." *Medical Care*, Vol. II, No. 5, Sept.-Oct., 1973. Also Chapter 13 in Anthony Kovner and D.

Neuhauser, eds. *Health Services Management: Readings and Commentary.* Ann Arbor, MI: Health Administration Press, 1978.

Hornsby, John A. "Proposed Inspection and Standardization of Hospitals." *Modern Hospital,* Vol. 1, No. 3, Oct. 1913, p. 100.

Hornsby, John A. "Standardization of Hospitals." *Transactions of the American Hospital Association,* Vol. 15, 1913, pp. 175–190.

Hornsby, J.A., and Schmidt, Richard E. *The Modern Hospital: Its Inspiration, Its Architecture, Its Equipment, Its Operation.* Philadelphia: W.B. Saunders Co., 1913.

Hosick, June E., and Steele, Merrill F. "On the Value of Modern Personnel Policies: Job Attitude Influences Quality of Service." *Hospitals,* Vol. 25, May 1951, pp. 32+.

"How Business Schools Began." *Business Week.* Oct. 12, 1963, pp. 114–116.

Information Please Almanac 1981. 35th ed. New York: Simon and Schuster.

International Association of Hospital Central Service Management. "What Is IAHCSM?" Chicago: The Association, circa 1982.

Jackson, Henry X. "The Agony of Choice." May 21, 1980, Commemorative Fifth Annual Malcolm T. MacEachern Commemorative Lecture, Hospital and Health Services Management Program, Northwestern University, Evanston, IL.

Jaeger, Jon. "Education for Health Administration: A Reconceptualization." Chicago, Center for Health Administration Studies, University of Chicago, Health Administration Perspectives Series No. A10, Dec. 1972.

Johnson, Everett A., and Johnson, Richard. *Hospitals in Transition.* Rockville, MD: Aspen, 1982.

Johnson, Richard A.; Kast, Fremont E.; and Rosenzweig, James E. *The Theory and Management of Systems.* NY: McGraw-Hill, 1963.

Julius Rosenwald Fund. *Negro Hospitals. A Compilation of Available Statistics* (introduction by Michael M. Davis). Chicago: The Fund, Feb. 1931.

Kakar, Sudhir. *Frederick Taylor: A Study in Personality and Innovation.* Cambridge, MA: MIT Press, 1970.

Kalisch, Philip, and Kalisch, Beatrice. *The Advance of American Nursing.* Boston: Little Brown, 1978.

Katz, Daniel, and Kahn, Robert L. *The Social Psychology of Organizations.* New York: John Wiley & Sons, 1966.

Katzive, J.A. "The Vanishing Medical Hospital Adminstrator." *Hospital Topics,* Vol. 43, Feb. 1965, p. 41.

W.K. Kellogg, Foundation. *The First Twenty-Five Years.* Battle Creek, MI: Privately Printed, 1955.

Kerlikowske, Albert C., Biography. *Hospital Topics,* Vol. 33, Jan. 1955, p. 2.

Kerlikowske, Albert C. "On Major Problems Facing Hospitals: Biggest Problem of Hospital Is Concern with People." *Hospitals,* Vol. 27, Feb. 1953, p. 36.

Kidd, Gene, Biography. *Hospital Topics,* Vol. 33, Aug. 1955, p. 3.

Kipnis, Ira A. *A Venture Forward: A History of the American College of Hospital Administrators.* Chicago: ACHA, 1955.

Koontz, H., and O'Donnell, C. *Principles of Management.* New York: McGraw-Hill, 1955.

Kouzes, James M., and Posner, Barry Z. *The Leadership Challenge.* San Francisco: Jossey-Bass, Inc., 1987.

Kovner, Anthony R., and Neuhauser, D., eds. *Health Services Management: Readings and Commentary.* 4th ed., Chapter 3, "ACHE Code of Ethics," pp. 56–70. Ann Arbor, MI: Health Administration Press, 1990.

Lapp, John Augustus, and Ketcham, Dorothy. *Hospital Law.* Milwaukee: Bruce Publishing Co., 1926.

LaViolette, Suzanne. "ACHA Broadens Its Mission in Search for Expanded Clout." *Modern Healthcare,* Oct. 1981, pp. 76–78, 80, 84.

Lawrence, Paul R., and Dyer, Davis. *Renewing American Industry.* New York: The Free Press, 1983.

Lawrence, Paul, and Lorsch, Jay. *Organization and Environment.* Boston, MA: Division of Research, Harvard Business School, 1967.

Leavitt, Harold J. *Managerial Psychology.* Chicago: University of Chicago Press, 1958, 1964.

Leavitt, Harold J. *Corporate Pathfinders: Building Vision and Values into Organizations.* Homewood, IL: Dow Jones-Irwin and New York: Viking, 1987.

Lerner, Monroe, and Anderson, Odin W. *Health Progress in the United States 1900–1960*. Chicago: University of Chicago Press, 1963.

Letourneau, Charles V. *The Hospital Administrator*. Chicago: Starling Publications, 1969.

Letourneau, Charles V., and Letourneau, Jacqueline E. "Evolution of the Hospital Administrator." *The Modern Hospital*, March 1966.

Levenson, Harry. *The Exceptional Executive*. Cambridge, MA: Harvard University Press, 1968.

Levenson, Harry, and Rosenthal, Stuart. *CEO: Corporate Leadership in Action*. New York: Basic Books, 1984.

Levey, S., and McCarthy, T. "What Administrators Worry About: Money." *The Modern Hospital*, Vol. 98, No. 2, 1962, pp. 90–92.

Likert, Rensis. *New Patterns of Management*. New York: McGraw-Hill, 1961, 1967.

Lindsey, Almont. *The Pullman Strike*. Chicago: University of Chicago Press, 1942, 1964.

Lutes, J. Dewey, Biography. *Hospital Management*, Vol. 82, Feb. 1956, p. 32.

Lutes, J. Dewey. *The Hospital Governing Board*. Augusta, GA: Tidwell Printing Co., April 1949.

Lutes, J. Dewey. "Why the College of Hospital Administration?" *Hospital Management*, Nov. 1933.

MacEachern, Malcolm T., M.D., Biography. *Hospital Management*, Vol. 80, Aug. 1955, p. 26.

MacEachern, Malcolm T., M.D., Biography. *Hospital Management*, Vol. 82, Aug. 1956, p. 52.

MacEachern, Malcolm T., M.D., Biography. *Hospitals*, Vol. 30, Feb. 16, 1956, p. 88.

MacEachern, Malcolm T., M.D. *Hospital Organization and Management*. Chicago: Physicians Record Company, 1935.

MacEachern, Malcolm T., M.D. *Medical Records in the Hospital*. Chicago: Physicians Record Company, 1937.

Mackintosh, Donald J. *Construction, Equipment and Management of General Hospitals*. London: Hodge & Co., 1916.

MacLean, Basil C., Biography. *Hospital Management*, Vol. 84, July 1957, p. 34.

MacLean, Basil C. "On General Hospital Bed Capacity: Shorter Bed Stay Seen in Hospital of the Future." *Hospitals*, Vol. 24, May 1950, pp. 24–26.

"Management Stressed at ACHA Congress." *Modern Hospital*, Vol. 90, No. 3, March 1958, pp. 49–50, 144–148.

March, James G., and Simon, Herbert A. *Organizations*. New York: John Wiley & Sons, 1958, 1966.

Martin, Franklin H. "The Catholic Hospital Association as a Factor in Standardization." *Hospital Progress*, Vol. 7, Aug. 1926, p. 303.

Matzick, Kenneth J. *A National Survey to Evaluate Continuing Education in the Field of Hospital Administration*. Health Care Research Series Number 5. Graduate Program in Hospital and Health Administration, The University of Iowa, 1967.

Mayo, George Elton. *The Human Problems of an Industrial Civilization*. Boston: Division of Research, Harvard Business School, 1933.

Maysent, Harold W. "Guide to Budget Management." *Modern Hospitals*, Vol. 86, June 1956, pp. 81+; Vol. 87, July 1956, pp. 72+; Aug. 1956, pp. 70+.

McGregor, Douglas. *The Human Side of Enterprise*. New York: McGraw-Hill, 1960.

McNeill, William H. *Plagues and Peoples*. Garden City, NY: Anchor Press, Doubleday, 1976.

McNerney, Walter J. with others. *Hospital and Medical Economics*. 2 vol. Chicago: Hospital Research and Educational Trust, 1962.

Medical Group Management Association. "Dedicated to Improving Medical Group Practice." Denver, CO: The Association, 1982.

Mills, Alden B. *Hospital Public Relations*. Chicago: Physicians Record Company, 1939.

Mills, Alden B. "How to Write for Publication." *The Modern Hospital*, Vol. 56, No. 1, Jan. 1941.

Mooney, Fraser D. "On the Shortage of Practical Nurses: Preparation and Acceptance Essential for the Practical Nurse." *Hospitals*, Vol. 25, Dec. 1951, p. 28.

Mooney, James D., and Reiley, A.C. *Onward Industry!* New York: Harper & Brothers, 1931.

Morrill, Warren P. *Hospital Manual of Operation*. New York: Lakeside Publishing Co., 1934.

Morris, Richard B., ed. *Encyclopedia of American History.* New York: Harper & Brothers, 1953.

Mouzelis, Nicos. *Organization and Bureaucracy.* Chicago: Aldine, 1968.

Munger, Claude W. "Administrative Intern." *Modern Hospital,* Vol. 53, Sept. 1939, pp. 61–63.

Dr. Claude Munger, Biography. *Modern Hospitals,* Vol. 74, March 1950, p. 88.

Mushkin, Selma. *Biomedical Research: Costs and Benefits.* Cambridge, MA: Ballinger, 1979.

National Executive Housekeepers Association, Inc. *The First 50 Years 1930–1980.* Gallipolis, OH: The Association, 1980.

National HMO Census 1982. Excelsior, MN: Interstudy, June 30, 1982.

Neff, Robert E. "Practical Use of an Isolation Ward in a General Hospital for the Treatment of Tuberculosis." *Drs.' Chest,* Vol. 20, Nov. 1951, pp. 557–563.

Neuhauser, D. "Cost Effective Clinical Decision Making and the Medical Care Manager." *Hospital & Health Services Administration,* Vol. 25, No. 3, Summer 1980, pp. 55–61.

Neuhauser, D. "Ernest Amory Codman and the End Result of Medical Care." *International Journal of Technology Assessment in Healthcare,* Vol. 6, No. 2, 1990, pp. 307–325.

Neuhauser, D. "Organizational Behavior Literature in Health Administration Education." Washington, DC: AUPHA, May 1972.

Neuhauser, D. *The Relationship between Administrative Activities and Hospital Performance.* Chicago: Center for Health Administration Studies, The University of Chicago, June 1971.

Newkirk, Donald R. "Public Relations Annual Administrative Review." *Hospitals,* Vol. 33, April 16, 1959, pp. 117+.

Newsholme, Sir Arthur. *Fifty Years in Public Health: A Personal Narrative with Comments.* London, 1935.

Newsholme, Sir Arthur. *Health Problems in Organized Society.* London: P.S. King & Son, 1927.

Newsholme, Sir Arthur. *International Studies on the Relationship between the Private and Official Practice of Medicine.* London: Allen & Unwin. Baltimore: Williams and Wilkins, 1932.

Newsholme, Sir Arthur. *Medicine and the State.* London: Allen & Unwin. Baltimore: Williams and Wilkins, 1932.

Nightingale, Florence. *Introductory Notes on Lying-In Institutions.* London: Longmans, Green, Longmans, Roberts & Green, 1871.

Nightingale, Florence. *Notes on Hospitals.* 3rd ed. London: Longmans, Green, Longmans, Roberts & Green, 1863.

Norby, Joseph G., Biography. *Hospitals,* Vol. 29, Part 1, Aug. 1955, pp. 82–83.

Norby, Joseph G. "Is a Job in Hospital Administration More or Less Stable than Most Administrative Jobs? Adequate Security in Hospital Administration." *Hospitals,* Vol. 26, Feb. 1954, pp. 52–54.

Ochsner, A.J. "Hospitals Are Standardizing Themselves." *Modern Hospital,* Vol. 3, No. 1, July 1914, p. 38.

Ochsner, A.J. "Hospitals of the U.S. to be Standardized." *Modern Hospital,* Vol. 9, No. 6, Dec. 1917, p. 424.

Ochsner, Albert J., and Sturm, Meyer J. *The Organization, Construction and Management of Hospitals.* Chicago: Cleveland Press, 1907.

O'Connor, Edwin. *The Last Hurrah.* Boston: Little Brown, 1956.

Olsen, Herluf V., Commission on University Education in Hospital Administration. *University Education for Administration in Hospitals.* Washington, DC: American Council on Education, 1954.

Ouchi, William G. *Theory Z.* Reading, MA: Addison-Wesley, 1981.

Parsons, Talcott. "Suggestions for a Sociological Approach to the Theory of Organizations." *Administrative Science Quarterly,* Vol. 1, No. 1, 1956, pp. 63–85, 224–239.

Peabody, Francis Weld. *The Care of the Patient.* Cambridge: Harvard University Press, 1927. Also, *Journal of the American Medical Association,* Vol. 88, 1927.

Peabody, Francis Weld. *Doctor and Patient, Papers on the Relationship of the Physician to Men and Institutions.* New York: Macmillan, 1930.

Peebles, Allon. A *Survey of Statistical Data on Medical Facilities in the United States.* Report No. 3 of the Committee on the Costs of Medical Care. Washington, DC, Nov. 1929.

Pennell, Elliott; Mountin, Joseph W.; and Pearson, Kay. *Business Census of Hospitals 1935 General Report.* Supplement No. 154 to the

Public Health Reports, U.S. Public Health Service, Washington, DC: U.S. Government Printing Office, 1939.

Peters, Thomas, and Waterman, Robert H. *In Search of Excellence.* New York: Harper and Row, 1982.

Ponton, Thomas Ritchie, M.D. *The Medical Staff in the Hospital.* Chicago: Physicians Record Company, 1939. 2nd ed. revised by Malcolm MacEachern, 1953.

Porter, Glenn. *The Rise of Big Business 1860–1910.* New York: Thomas Crowell, 1973.

Powell, Boone, Biography. *Southern Hospitals*, Vol. 23, June 1955, p. 23.

Prall, Charles E. *The College Curriculum in Hospital Administration.* Chicago: Physicians Record Company, 1948. (Also see under ACHA.)

Prall, Charles E. *Problems of Hospital Administration.* Chicago: Physicians Record Company, 1948.

Puestow, Charles B. "A Tribute to Malcolm T. MacEachern." *Bulletin of the American College of Surgeons*, May-June, 1956, pp. 151–152.

Quatrano, Louis A. *Health Services Administration Education 1979.* Washington, DC: AUPHA, 1978.

Radiology Management (American Hospital Radiology Administrators), Vol. 4, No. 3, June 1982.

Rankin, W.S.; Hannaford, H.E.; and Van Arsdall, H.P. *The Small General Hospital.* Charlotte, NC: Trustees of the Duke Endowment, 1928 (revised March 1945).

Rappleye, Willard C. *Principles of Hospital Administration and the Training of Hospital Executives.* Report of the Rockefeller Committee on the Training for Hospital Executives, 1922.

Reader, W.J. *Professional Men.* London: Weidenfeld and Nicolson, 1966.

"Regents Rebel, Veto Name Change Proposal." *Modern Healthcare*, Oct. 1981, pp. 77–78.

Reiser, Stanley. *Medicine and the Reign of Technology.* Cambridge, MA: Cambridge University Press, 1978.

Reverby, Susan. "The Search for the Hospital Yardstick: Nursing and the Rationalization of Hospital Work," Chapter 11 in Susan Reverby and David Rosner, eds. *Health Care in America: Essays in Social History.* Philadelphia: Temple University Press, 1979.

Risse, Guenter B. *Hospital Life in Enlightenment Scotland: Care and Teaching at the Royal Infirmary of Edinburgh.* Cambridge, England: Cambridge University Press, 1986.

Rivett, Geoffery. *The Development of the London Hospital System: 1823–1982.* London: King Edward's Hospital Fund for London, 1986.

Roethlisberger, F.J., and Dickson, W.J. *Management and the Worker.* Cambridge, MA: Harvard University Press, 1939.

Rorem, Clarence Rufus. *The Public's Investment in Hospitals.* Chicago: University of Chicago Press, 1930.

Rosenberg, Charles E. *The Care of Strangers. The Rise of America's Hospital System.* New York: Basic Books, 1987.

Rosett, Richard N. "Business Education in the United States." Selected Paper No. 59. Graduate School of Business, University of Chicago, 1982.

Rosner, David. *A Once Charitable Enterprise: Hospitals and Health Care in Brooklyn and New York 1885–1915.* Cambridge, England: Cambridge University Press, 1982.

Sawyer, Albert E. "Problems of Hospital Management with Special Reference to the University of Michigan Hospital." *Michigan Business Studies,* Vol. II, No. 2, April 1929. Ann Arbor, MI: University of Michigan, School of Business Administration, Bureau of Business Research, 1929, 83 pages.

Sayles, Leonard R. *Leadership: What Effective Managers Really Do . . . and How They Do It.* New York: McGraw-Hill, 1979.

Senge, Peter M. *The Fifth Discipline: The Art and Practice of the Learning Organization.* New York: Doubleday, 1990.

Shanahan, Robert J. *The History of the Catholic Hospital Association 1915–1965.* St. Louis, MO: The Catholic Hospital Association of the United States and Canada, 1965.

Shortell, Stephen M. "Theory Z: Implications and Relevance." *Health Care Management Review,* Vol. 7, No. 4, Fall 1982, pp. 7–22.

Shortell, Stephen, with others. "The Effects of Management Practices on Hospital Efficiency and Quality of Care." Chapter 6 in Stephen M. Shortell and Montague Brown, eds. *Organizational Research in Hospitals.* Chicago: Blue Cross Association, 1976.

Simon, Herbert A. *Administrative Behavior.* New York: Macmillan, 1947, 1957.

Sims, Stanley L. *LaCrosse Lutheran Hospital: A History 1899–1979.* LaCrosse, WI: Lutheran Hospital Foundation, 1981.

Smith, George D., and Steadman, Laurence E. "Present Value of Corporate History." *Harvard Business Review,* Nov.-Dec. 1981, pp. 164–173.

Society of Medical Administrators. "A History of the Society of Medical Administrators and the Medical Superintendents Club," 1920–1955 (64 pages) and 1920–1955, 1956–1967 (96 pages). These two versions were privately published in 1958 and 1967 by the Society.

Soderstrom, Lee. *The Canadian Health System.* London: Croom Helm, 1978.

Southwick, Arthur F. *The Law of Hospital and Health Care Administration,* 2nd ed. Ann Arbor, MI: Health Administration Press, 1988.

Starkweather, David B. "The Classicists Revisited." *Hospital Administration,* Vol. 12, No. 3, Summer 1967, pp. 69–80.

Starr, Paul. *The Social Transformation of American Medicine.* New York: Basic Books, 1982.

Steele, M.F., Biography. *Hospital Management,* Vol. 84, Sept. 1957, p. 36.

Steinberg, S.H. *Historical Tables 55 BC–AD 1945.* 3rd ed. London: Macmillan, 1949.

Steiner, George A., and Miner, John B. *Management Policy and Strategy.* New York: Macmillan Publishing Co., 1986.

Steinwald, Bruce and Neuhauser, Duncan. "The Role of the Proprietary Hospital." *Journal of Law and Contemporary Problems,* Vol. 35, No. 4, Autumn 1970, pp. 817–838.

Stephenson, George W. *American College of Surgeons at 75.* Chicago: American College of Surgeons, 1990.

Stevens, Edward B. *The History of the Medical Group Management Association 1926–1976.* Denver, CO: The Association, 1976, 135 pages.

Stevens, Edward F. *The American Hospital of the Twentieth Century.* New York: The Architectural Record Company, 1918, revised ed., 1921; 3rd ed., 1928.

Stevens, Rosemary. *American Medicine and the Public Interest.* New Haven, CT: Yale University Press, 1971.

Stevens, Rosemary. *In Sickness and In Wealth: American Hospitals in the Twentieth Century.* New York: Basic Books, 1989.

Stevens, Rosemary. "'A Poor Sort of Memory': Voluntary Hospitals and Government Before the Depression." *Milbank Memorial Fund Quarterly,* Vol. 60, No. 4, Fall 1982, pp. 551–584.

Stimson, Ruth, and Taylor, Shirley, eds. *Executive Development for Graduates of Master's Degree Programs in Hospital and Health Care Administration.* Berkeley, CA: Graduate Program in Hospital Administration, University of California, 1973.

Stone, Captain J.E. *Hospital Organization and Management.* London: Faber & Gwyer, 1927.

Sutton, Frank C. "An Administration Develops a Service Report for Trustees." *Hospitals,* Vol. 25, April 1952, p. 82.

Swanson, A.J. *Hospital Management,* Vol. 82, Oct. 1956, p. 31.

Swanson, A.J. "On Asking the Board for Higher Rates: Showing Added Expenses Justifies Higher Rates." *Hospitals,* Vol. 25, March 1951, pp. 24–26.

Taylor, Frederick W. *The Principles of Scientific Management.* New York: Harper & Bros., 1911.

Taylor, Frederick W. *Shop Management.* New York: Harper & Bros., 1903.

Terenzio, Peter B. "Should Nurses Do Venipuncture?" *American Journal of Nursing,* Vol. 51, Oct. 1951, pp. 603–604.

Terrel, Tol, Biography, *Hospital Management,* Vol. 84, Nov. 1957, p. 34.

Terrell, Tol. "How Small Hospitals Can Organize for Efficiency and Good Service." *Hospital Management,* Vol. 73, April 1952, 44 pp.

Thomas R.Z. "Telling Hospitals' Story to the Public." *Southern Hospitals,* Vol. 25, Dec. 1957, p. 70.

Thompson, John D., and Golden, Grace. *The Hospital: A Social and Architectural History.* New Haven: Yale University Press, 1975.

The Timetable of Technology. New York: Hearst Books, 1982.

Toner, J.M. "Statistics of Regular Medical Associations and Hospitals of the United States." *Transactions of the American Medical Association,* Vol. 24, 1873, pp. 314–333.

U.S. Department of Health and Human Services. *Health United States 1981, 1990.* Washington, DC: U.S. Government Printing Office, 1981, 1990.

U.S. Department of Health, Education, and Welfare. *Health in America 1776–1976.* U.S. Public Health Service, Health Resources Administration, Washington, DC: U.S. Government Printing Office, 1976.

U.S. Department of Health, Education, and Welfare. *Health United States 1980, 1990.* Washington, DC: U.S. Government Printing Office, 1980, 1990.

University Education for Administration in Hospitals; see Herluf Olsen.

"The Value to Medical Service Corps Officers of Affiliation with the American College of Hospital Administrators." *U.S. Airforce Medical Service Digest,* Vol. 10, Feb. 1959, p. 27.

Veblen, Thorsten. *The Theory of the Leisure Class.* Macmillan, 1899. Reprinted, New York: Mentor, 1953.

Vogel, Ezra. *Japan as No. 1.* New York: Harper and Row, 1981.

Vogel, Morris J. *The Invention of the Modern Hospital: Boston 1870–1930.* Chicago: University of Chicago Press, 1980.

Vraciu, Robert A., and Zuckerman, Howard S. "Legal and Financial Constraints on the Development and Growth of Multiple Hospital Arrangements." *Health Care Management Review,* Vol. 4, No. 1, Winter 1979, pp. 39–47.

Walter, Frank J. "On Taking a New Hospital Adminstrative Job: An Understanding of Needs and Problems Necessary." *Hospitals,* Vol. 27, May 1953, p. 26.

Walton, Clarence C. *Ethos and Executive Values in Managerial Decision Making.* Englewood Cliffs, NJ: Prentice-Hall, 1969.

Walton, Mary. *The Deming Management Method.* New York: Dodd, Mead and Co., 1986.

Walton, Mary. *Deming Management at Work.* New York: G.P. Putnam's Sons, 1990.

Washburn, Frederic A., and Bresnahan, John F. "Medical and Surgical Efficiency in Large General Hospitals." *Transactions of the American Hospital Association,* Vol. 17, 1915, p. 338.

Washburn, F.A., and Howland, W.B. "The Training of Hospital Administrators." *Transactions of the American Hospital Association,* Vol. 12, 1911, pp. 249–255.

Weber, Joseph John. *First Steps in Organizing a Hospital.* New York: MacMillan & Co., 1924.

Weber, Max. *The Theory of Social and Economic Organization.* Translated by A.M. Henderson and Talcott Parsons. The Free Press of Glencoe, 1964. New York: Oxford University Press, 1947.

Weeks, Lewis. Hospital Administration Oral History Series. Chicago: AHA, Center for Hospital and Health Care Administration History, 1984 to present.

Weeks, Lewis, and Berman, Howard. *Shapers of American Health Care Policy: An Oral History.* Ann Arbor, MI: Health Administration Press, 1985.

Wesbury, Stuart A. "Career Patterns in Health and Hospital Administration." Unpublished doctoral dissertation, University of Florida, 1972.

Wesbury, Stuart A. "Toward a Broader View of Health Care," Chapter 19 in Sloane, Robert M., and Sloane, Beverly L., *A Guide to Health Care Facilities, Personnel and Management*, 3rd ed. Ann Arbor, MI: Health Administration Press, 1992, pp. 211–220.

Wilson, Florence, and Neuhauser, Duncan. *Health Services in the United States.* 2nd ed. Cambridge, MA: Ballinger, 1982.

Wilson, Lucius. "On Major Problems Facing Hospitals: Hospitals Train Nurses Then Lose Them to Other Agencies." *Hospitals*, Vol. 26, Dec. 1952, p. 36.

Witt, John A. *Building a Better Hospital Board.* Ann Arbor, MI: Health Administration Press, 1987.

Wolverton, Charles A. "Dr. Malcolm T. MacEachern Honored by Hospital Administrators." Remarks in the House of Representatives, Aug. 11, 1954. *Congressional Record*, Appendix, Aug. 16, 1954, p. A6048.

"Ray Woodham, A Tribute." *Inside*, Fall 1983, Vol. 15, No. 3. Albuquerque, NM: Southwest Community Health Services.

Woodward, Joan. *Industrial Organization Theory and Practice.* London: Oxford University Press, 1965.

Woolsey, Abby Howland. *Handbook for Hospitals.* State Charities Aid Association. New York: G.P. Putnam's Sons, 1883.

The World Almanac 1991. Mahweh, NJ: World Almanac Books, 1991.

Wren, George R. "An Historical View of Health Administration Education." *Hospital & Health Services Administration,* Vol. 25, No. 3, Summer 1980, pp. 31–42.

Wylie, W. Gill. *Hospitals: Their History, Organization, and Construction.* New York: D. Appleton & Co., 1887.

Yaw, Ronald. "Why Don't You Run the Hospital Like a Business? All Right, Then So Be It." *Hospitals,* Vol. 24, Jan. 1950, pp. 41–42; *Trustee,* Vol. 3, Feb. 1950, pp. 29–32.

Yoshino, M.Y. *Japan's Managerial System: Tradition and Innovation.* Cambridge, MA: MIT Press, 1968.

Photographs

Glimpses of some College activities over the years are found in this collection of both old and recent snapshots.

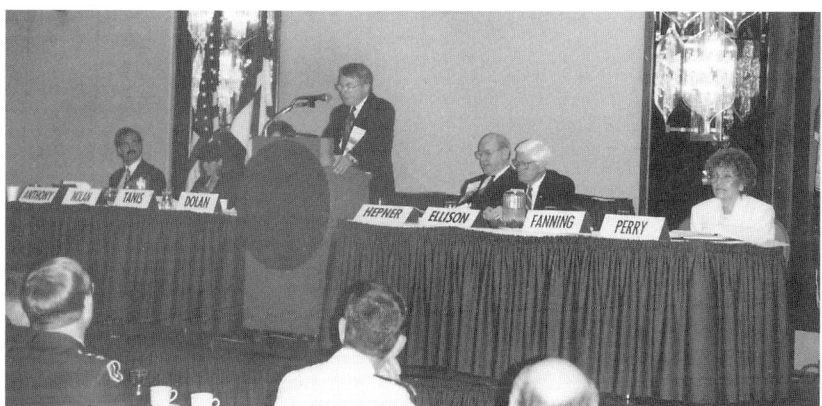

The College's Annual Meeting took place every summer at the location selected for the Annual Convention of the American Hospital Association. In 1992, that was in Denver, with Robert Fanning, FACHE, Chairman, 1992–1993, presiding.

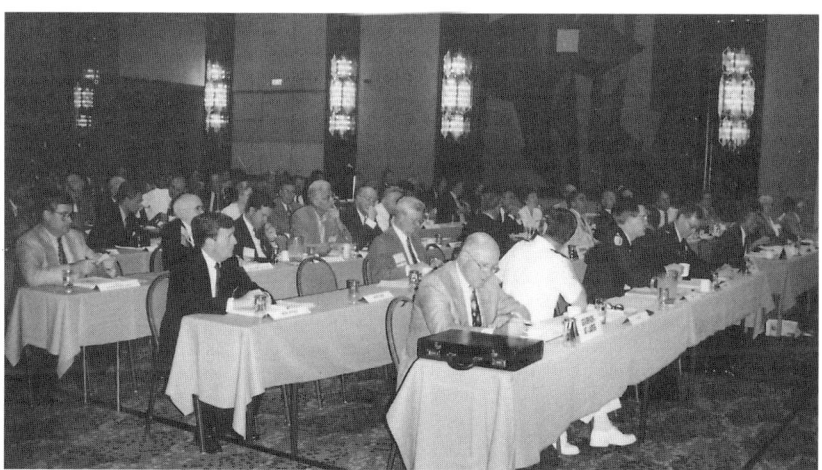

The listeners are attending the Council of Regents meeting which takes place every year at this time.

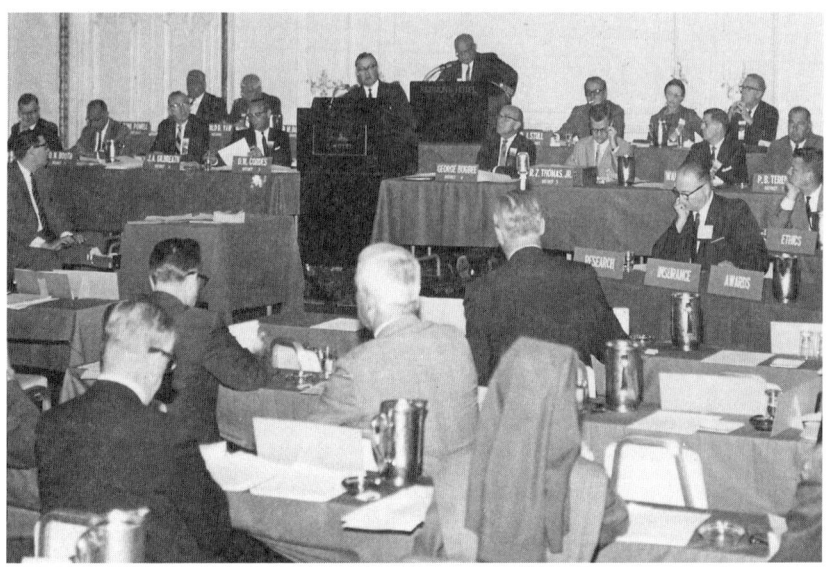

The first Council of Regents meeting was held in 1965 at the 31st Annual Meeting in San Francisco. Robert W. Bachmeyer, LFACHE, presided.

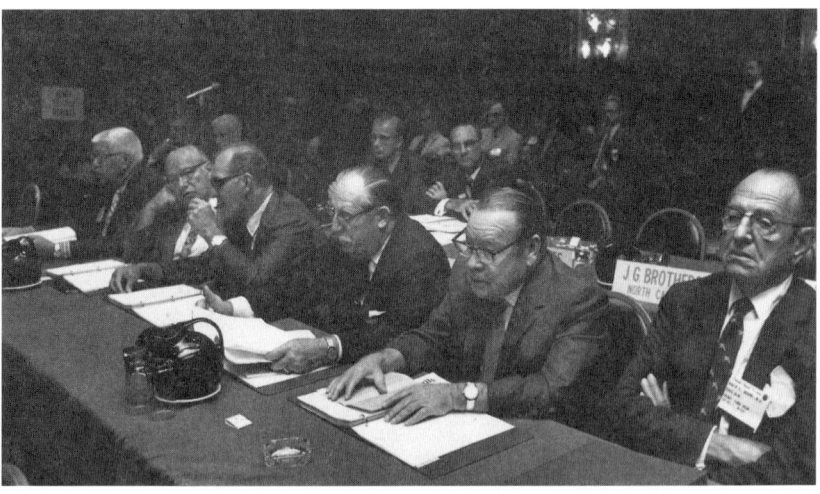

Past Chairmen traditionally attend the Council of Regents meeting at the College's Annual Meeting. Left to right: Ronald D. Yaw, LFACHE, 1964–65; Robert W. Bachmeyer, LFACHE, 1963–64; Tol Terrell, FACHE, 1961–62; James A. Hamilton, FACHE, 1939–40; Frank S. Groner, FACHE, 1957–58; and Robin Buerki, M.D., Charter Fellow, 1938–39.

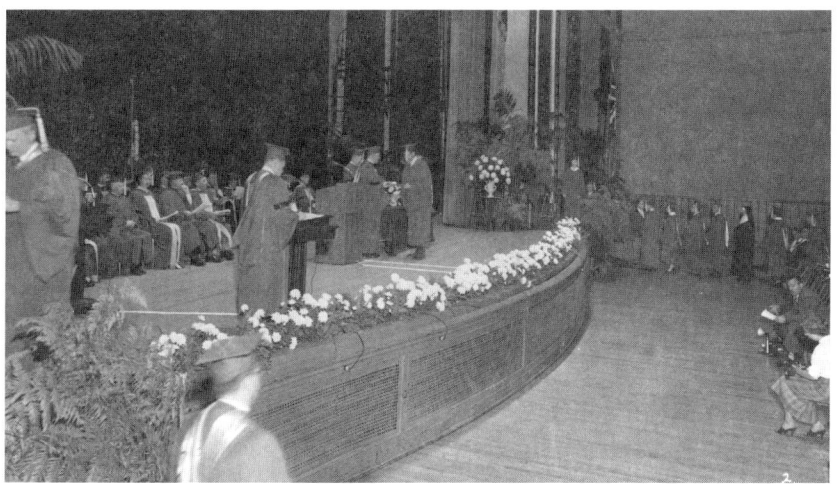

The capstone of the Annual Meeting is Convocation, which honors those who advance in the College each year. The photo shows a Convocation of a number of years ago.

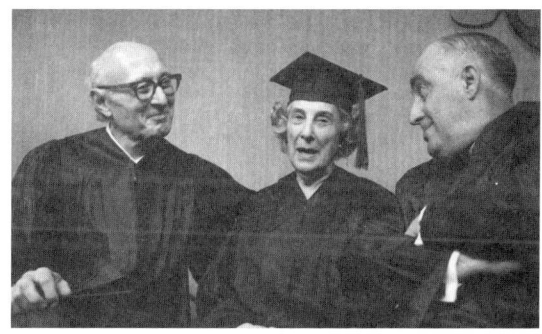

Honorary Fellows at Convocation Ceremonies at the 1964 Annual Meeting: Luther L. Terry, M.D., Viola Pinanski, and Clarence A. Warden, Jr.

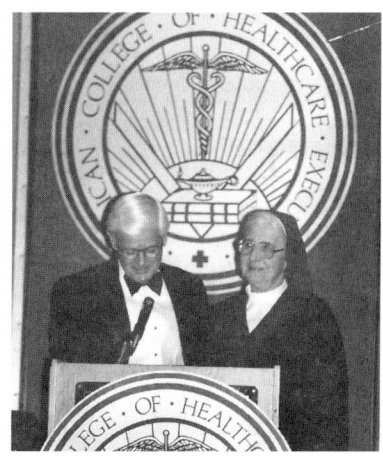

Gold Medal Awards (and in earlier years, the Silver Medal Award) have traditionally been announced at the Sunday evening banquet during the Annual Meeting. In 1991, Sister Irene Kraus, FACHE, received a Gold Medal Award from Paul Ellison, FACHE, Chairman, 1991–92.

Each year the College took advantage of exhibit space provided in conjunction with the Annual Convention of the American Hospital Association. In a photograph of about 1973, a member chats with W. Richard Kirk, FACHE, of the College's staff at the exhibit booth.

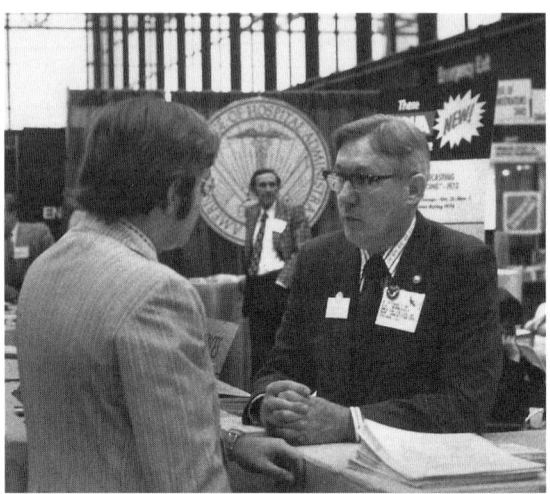

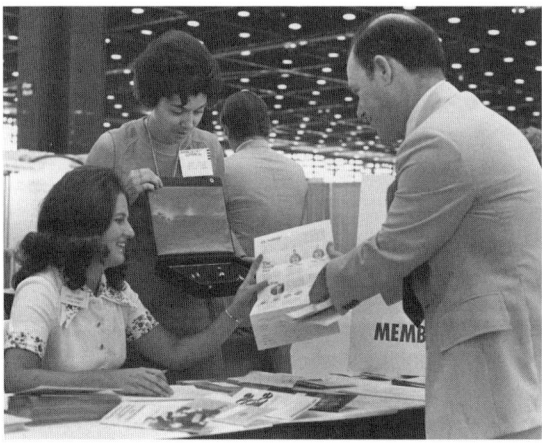

Members can use the opportunity afforded by the Annual Meeting to find out about new programs, services, and publications of the College.

By the late 1980s, the College's exhibit booth had become a portable construction, invitingly open to interested attendees. The separate but adjacent booths of Health Administration Press and Career Decision, Inc. (partially visible in the background of the 1992 photograph) further expanded the College's presence.

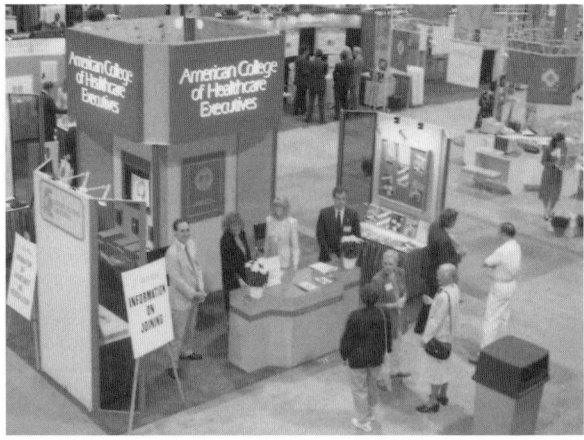

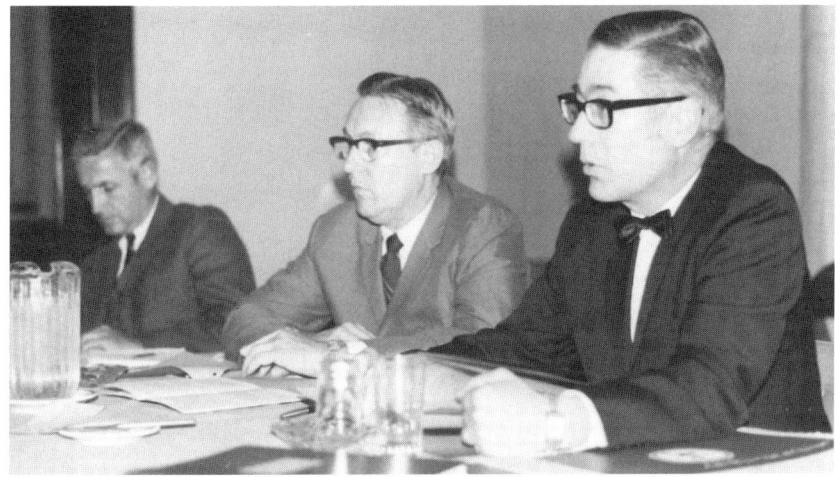

During each year, many College members are active in the work of ACHE committees and editorial boards. The photograph from the early 1980s shows Bernard Lachner, LFACHE, W. Richard Kirk, FACHE, and Vernon Stutzman, LFACHE, in a meeting of the Committee on Membership.

College staff attend educational programs and the meetings of other associations to provide information to members and prospective members.

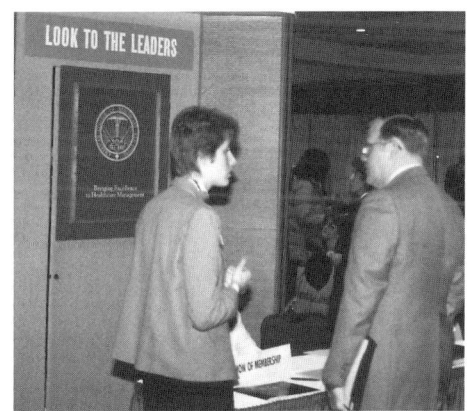

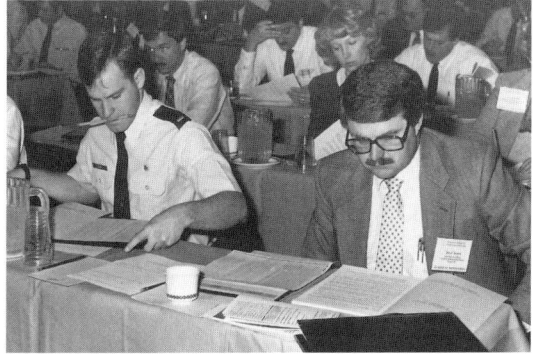

Examinations are scheduled throughout the year at various locations. Here examinations are being taken at one of the cluster programs in the early 1990s.

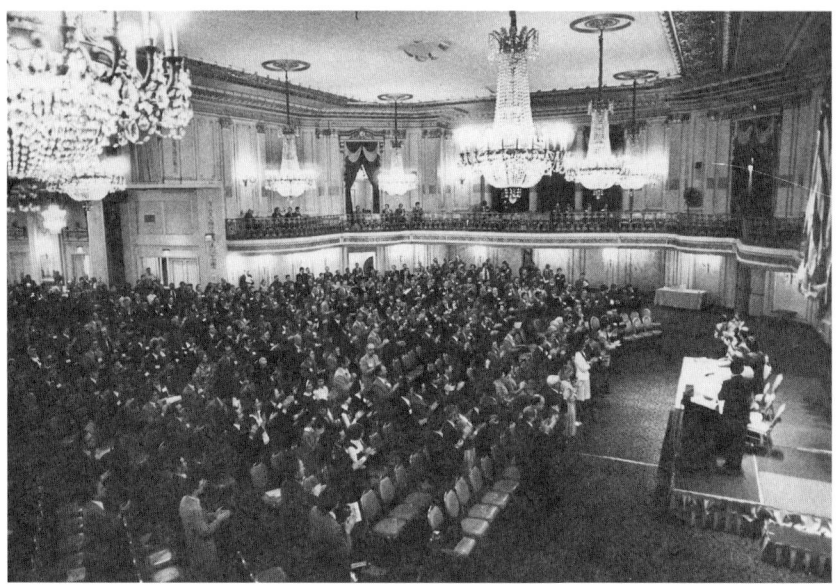

The annual Congress on Administration began in 1958 to mark the College's 25th anniversary. It has always been held in Chicago in February or March and draws over 4,000 attendees, for seminars, lectures, meetings, and other activities. Chicago's Palmer House was the site for many Congress sessions.

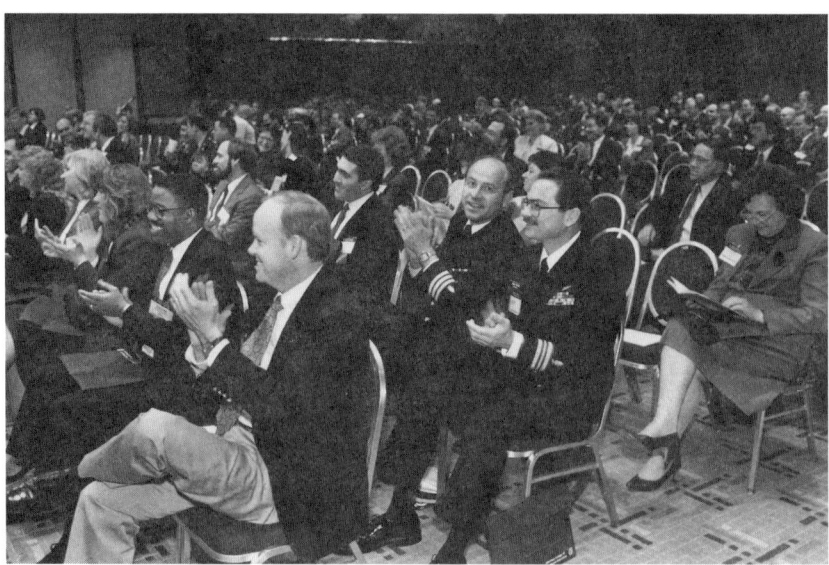

Since the mid-1980s, most sessions have taken place at the Hyatt Regency Hotel.

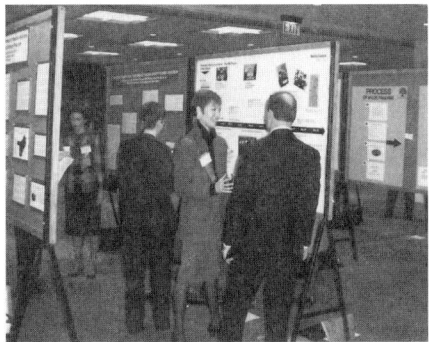

In 1983, the Management Innovations Poster Sessions were begun. Presenters can show the areas in which their organizations excel and discuss their new programs with other leaders.

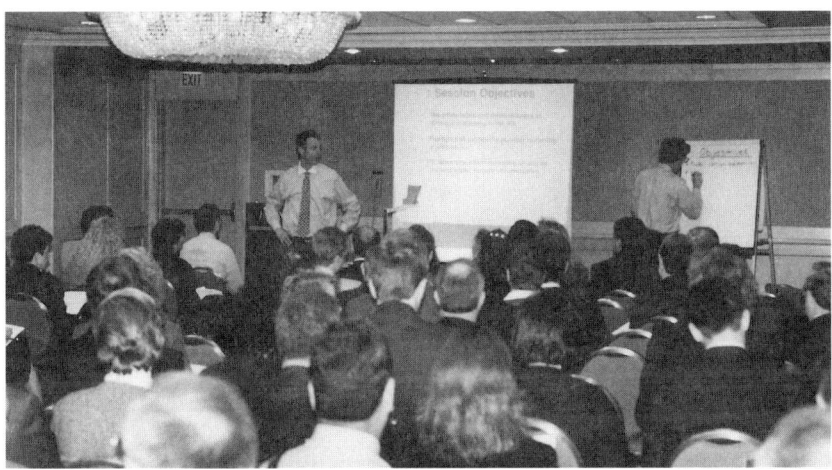

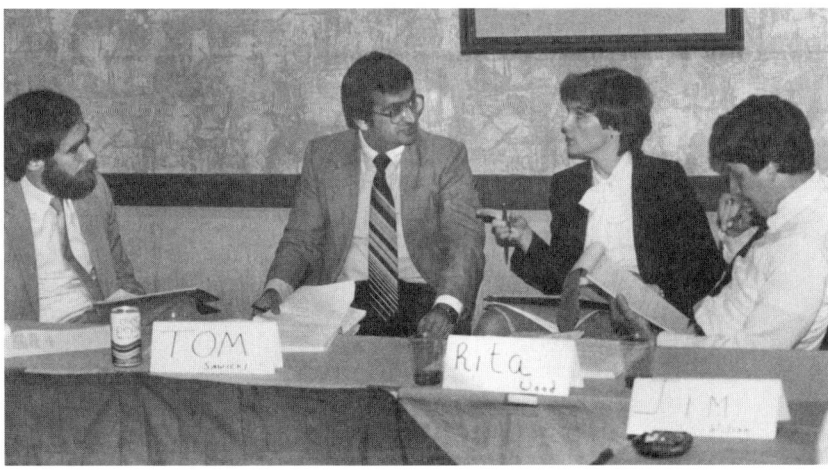

Educational activities are at the center of Congress. In 1993, there were 93 Management Seminars. Typical scenes from these sessions are shown, illustrating the dialogue and interaction typical to these programs.

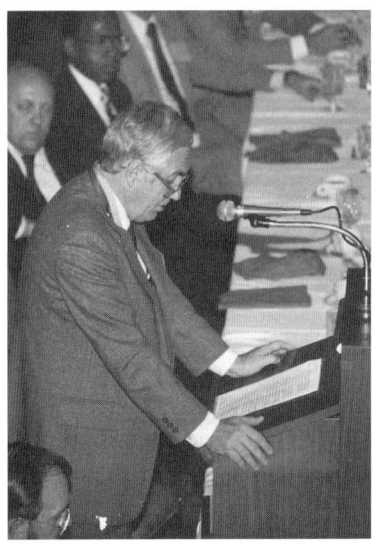

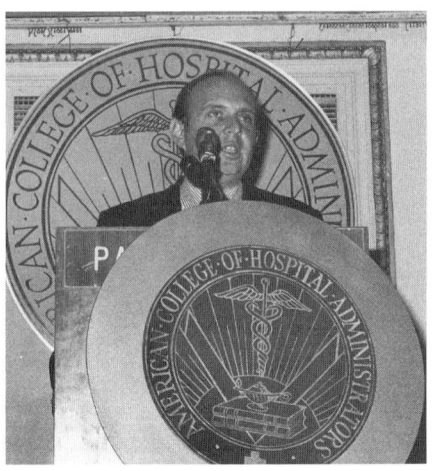

The 23rd Arthur C. Bachmeyer Memorial Address was presented by Henry Kaufman, Ph.D., at the 15th Congress on Administration in 1972, held at the Palmer House.

Memorial Addresses and Awards are featured at Congress. Lecturers and award winners over the years are shown here. Donald R. Newkirk, LFACHE, Chairman, 1980–81, presides at one of the awards luncheon.

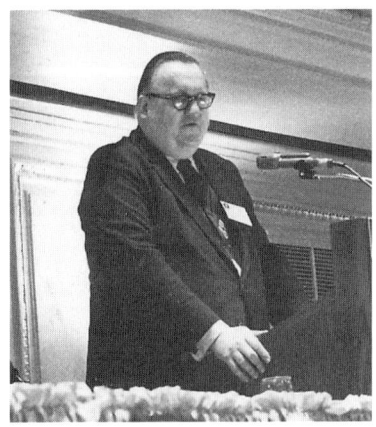

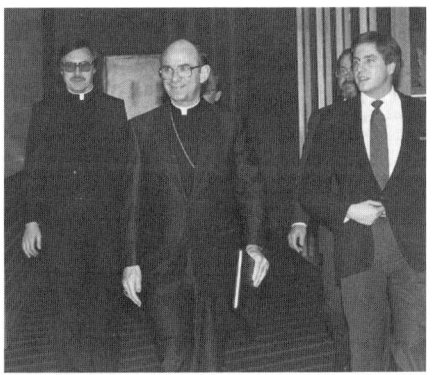

Cardinal Joseph L. Bernadin delivered the Malcom T. MacEachern Memorial Lecture at the 26th Congress.

Gordon L. Lippett, Ph.D., received the 1974 Dean Conley Award for his journal article, "Hospital Organization in Post Industrial Society," published in *Hospital Progress.*

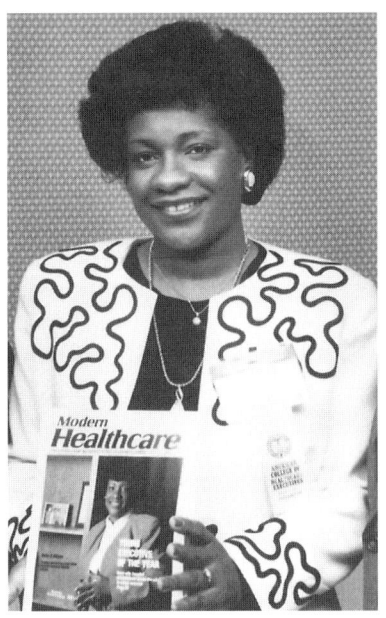

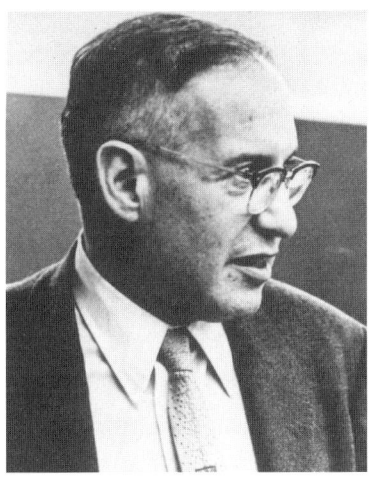

The 1990 Robert S. Hudgens Memorial Award for "Young Healthcare Executive of the Year" was presented to Denise Williams, CHE, President of Roseland Community Hospital in Chicago.

Peter F. Drucker, Ph.D., twice won the College's James A. Hamilton Hospital Administrators' Book Award: in 1975 for *Management: Tasks, Responsibilities, Practices* and in 1982 for *Managing in Turbulent Times.*

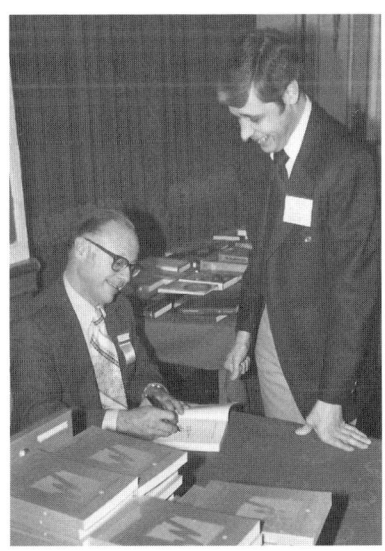

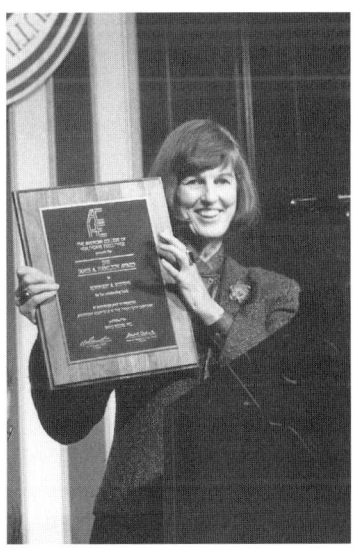

In 1979, the Hamilton Award went to George B. Steiner, Ph.D. and John B. Miner, Ph.D., for their book, *Management Policy and Strategy.* In 1990, it was presented to Rosemary Stevens, Ph.D., for *In Sickness and In Wealth.*

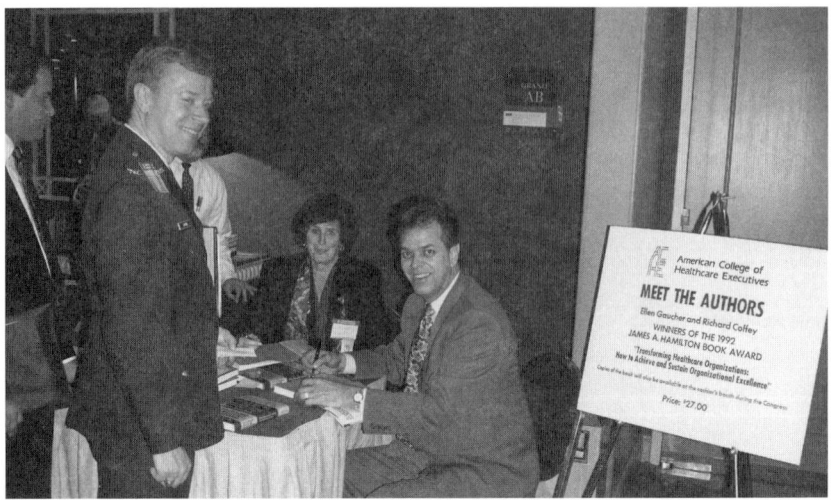

The Hamilton Award was shared again in 1992 by Ellen Gaucher and Richard Coffey for *Transforming Healthcare Organizations: How to Achieve and Sustain Organizational Excellence.*

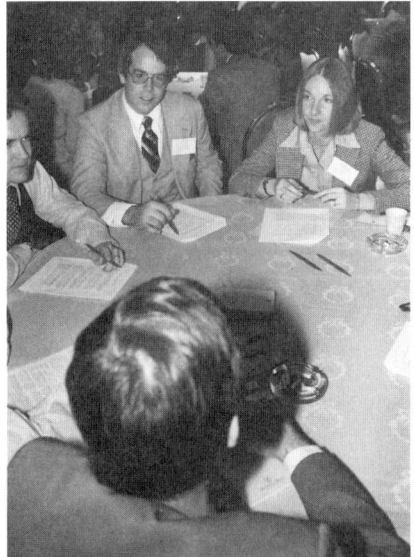

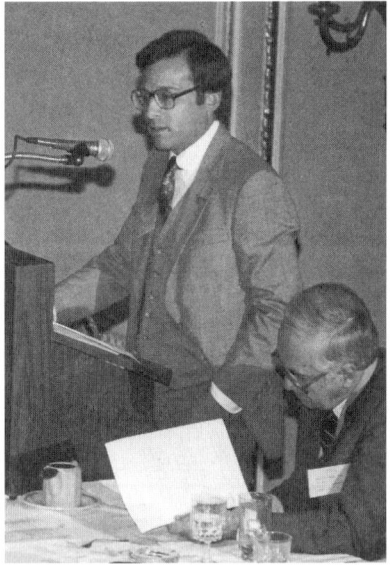

For about fifteen years an important part of the Congress on Administration was the Student Forum. Here and on the next page are photographs from early forums.

In the early 1980s a computer game for students was introduced. Lloyd Morgan of Arthur Andersen & Co., supporter of the computer competition, addressed Congress attendees in 1981.

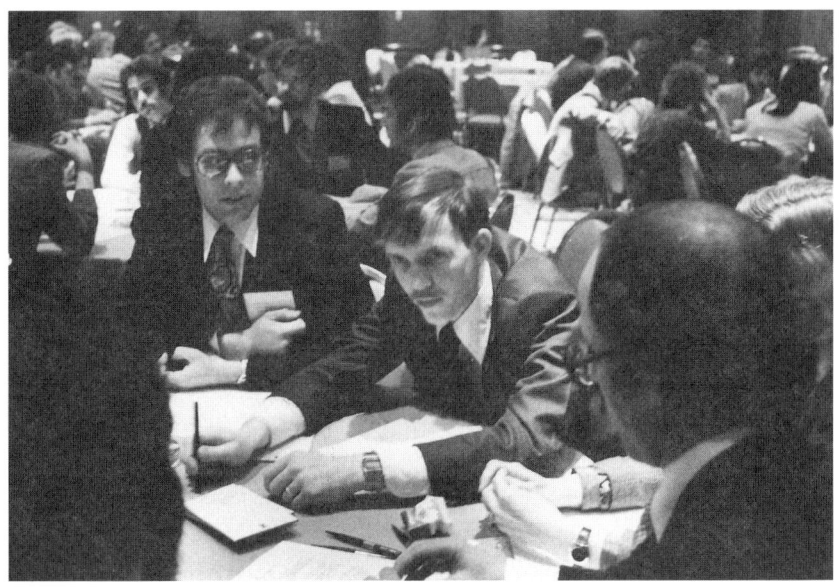

By 1993, over 100 colleges and universities throughout the U.S. and Canada had Student Chapters affiliated with the ACHE. Students representing graduate and undergraduate programs in health services management have an opportunity to attend Congress. These snapshots show students and faculty at a Student Forum in the early 1980s.

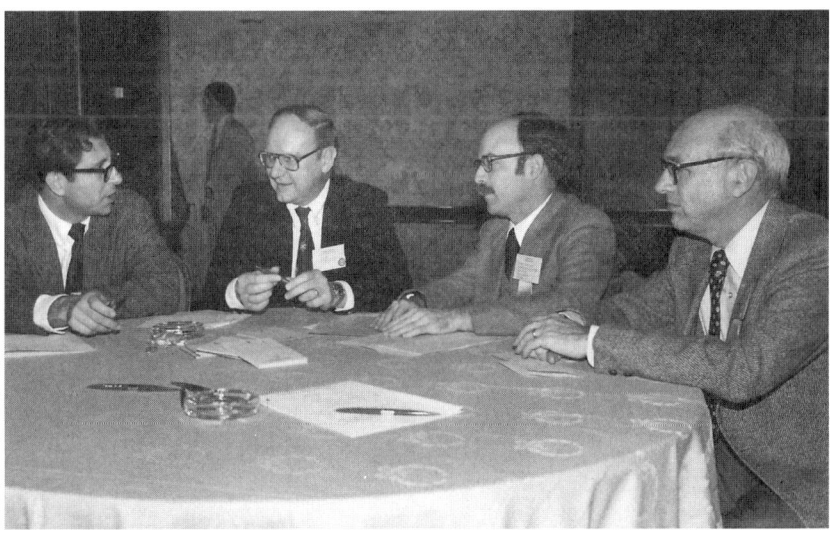

Faculty members, left to right are: B. Jon Jaeger, Ph.D., FACHE, James O. Hepner, Ph.D., FACHE, Chairman, 1990–91; Stephen L. Tucker, D.B.A., FACHE; and Philip N. Reeves, Ph.D., LFACHE. Many academic programs hold alumni meetings on an evening during Congress.

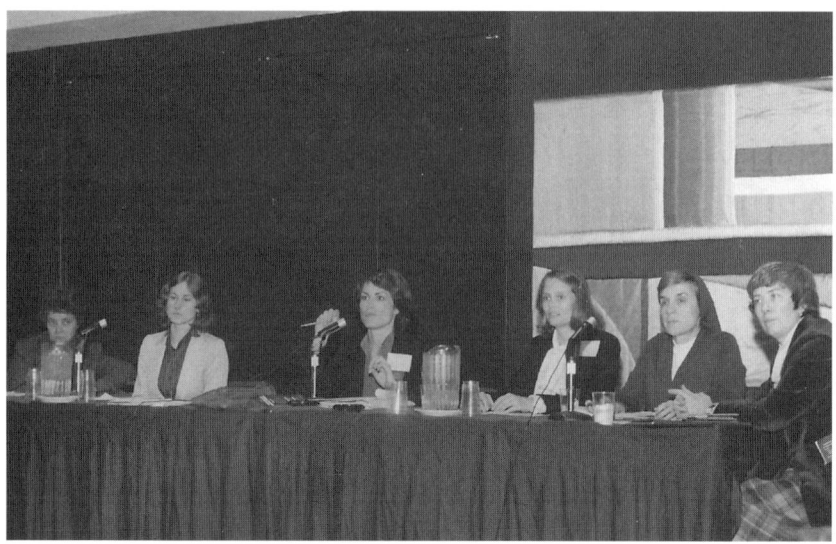

Other activities at Congress concentrate on the Affiliated Groups. Various meetings were well-established by 1982. At that time, Women in Health Administration had a traditional luncheon at Congress. By 1992, they had become the Women Healthcare Executive Networks and had a breakfast meeting.

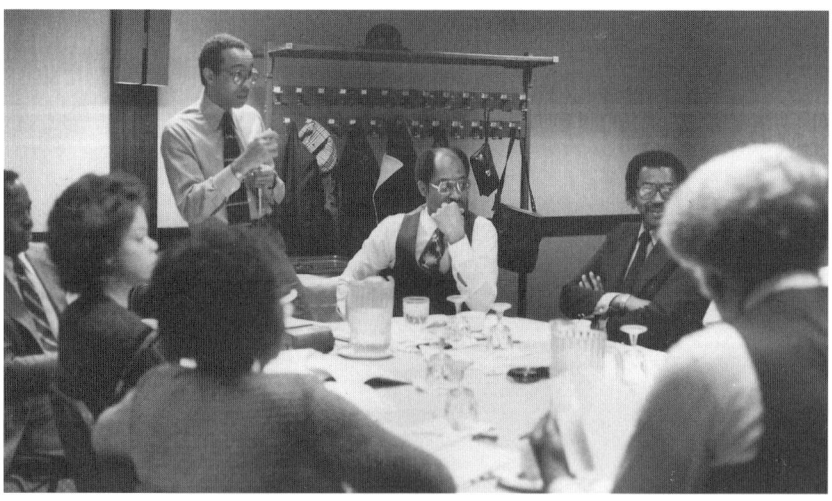

The National Association of Health Services Executives (NAHSE) holds an annual meeting at Congress.

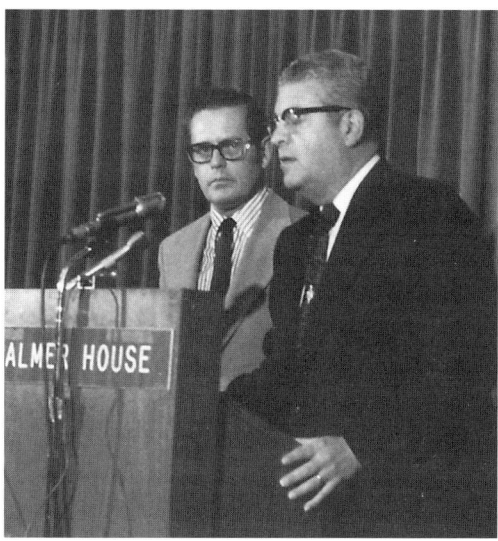

The College has often taken advantage of the Congress on Administration to communicate significant issues and trends to the media. Shown speaking above are, left, Everett A. Johnson, Ph.D., LFACHE, Chairman 1971–72, and Henry X. Johnson, FACHE, Chairman, 1976–77.

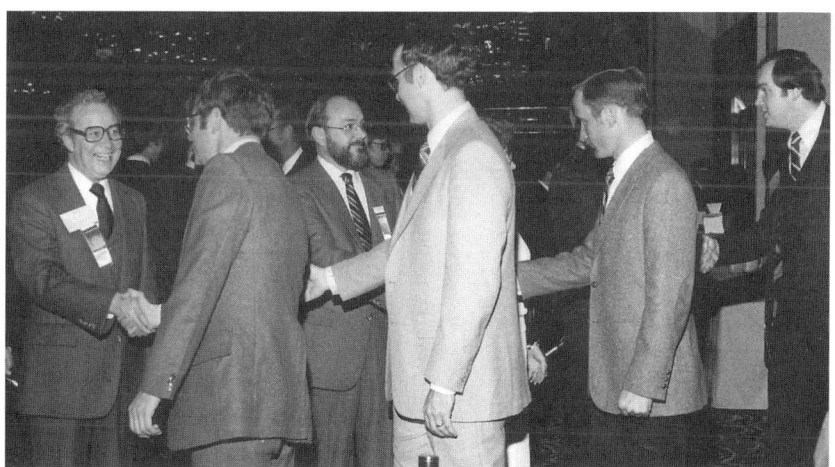

Social activities also form part of Congress. From 1982, a photograph shows Charles T. Wood, LFACHE, Chairman 1981–82, and Stuart A. Wesbury, Jr., Ph.D., FACHE, and then President of the College, greeting members at one of the traditional receptions.

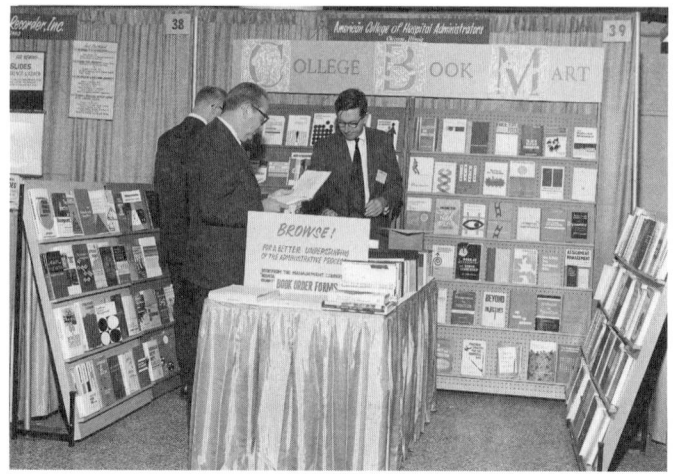

Members find out about the latest publications in the field at the College's Book Mart at the Congress on Administration.

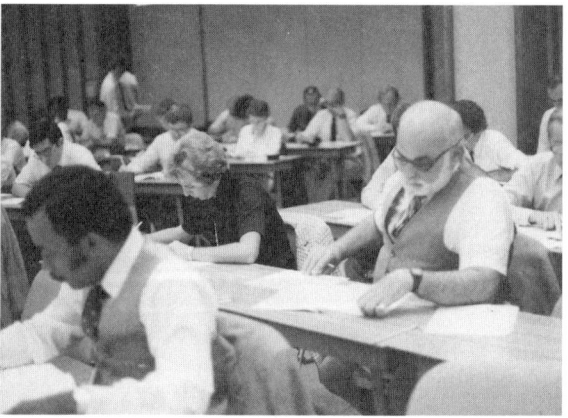

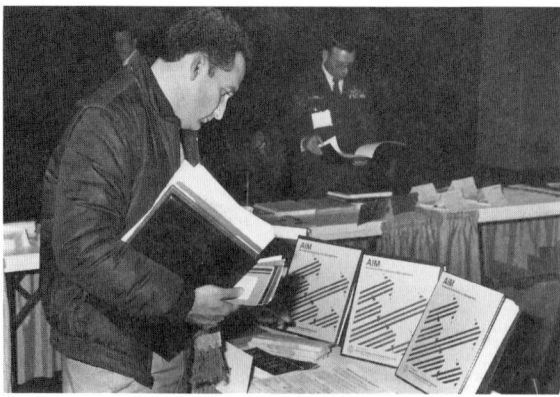

And there are packets to study and exams to take.

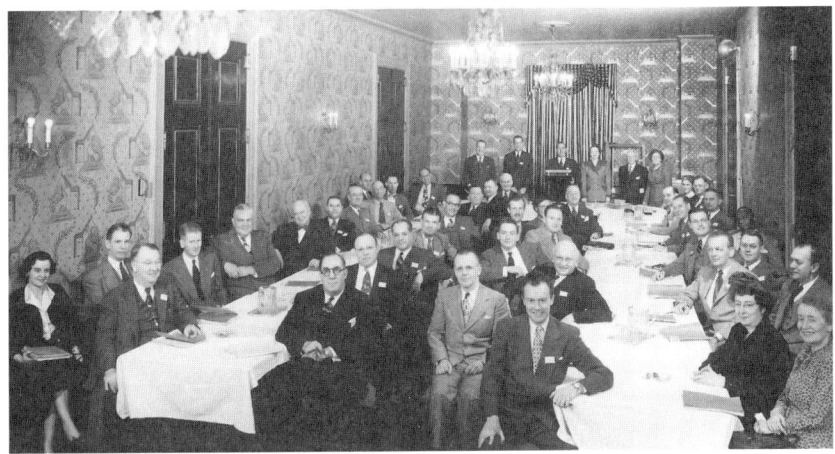

Education was an important activity from the College's earliest days, as can be seen in these old photographs. The first is from a Pilot Study Program for Preceptor Training, held at the Palmer House in Chicago in April 1950.

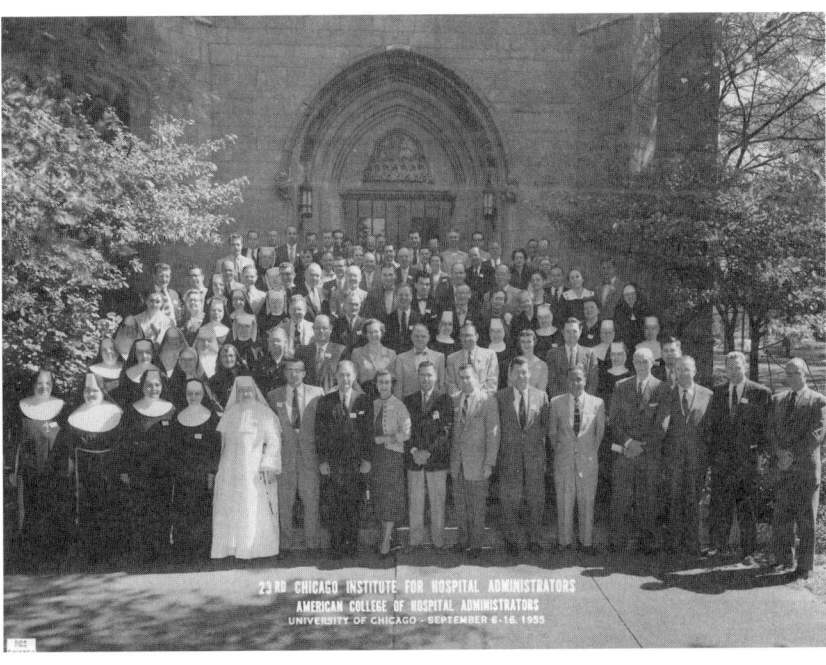

This photo poses the attendees at the 23rd Chicago Institute for Hospital Administrators, in September 1955.

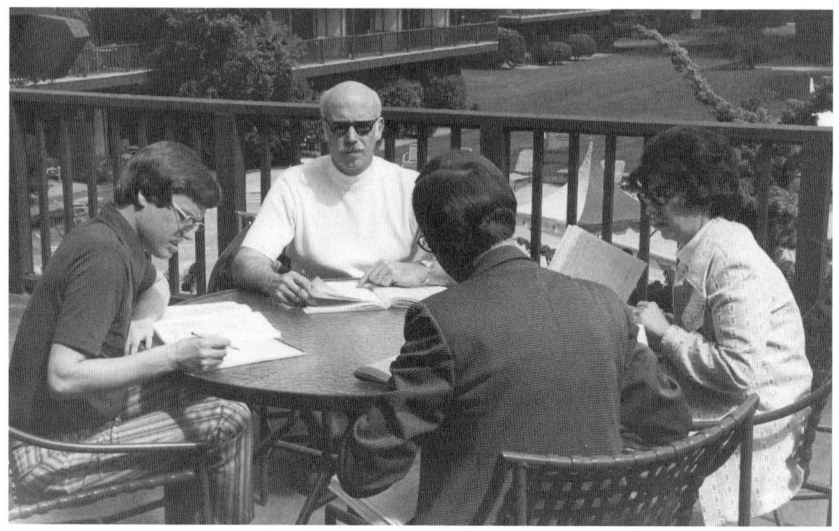

As time went on, these educational programs evolved and increased. Conferences, institutes, and seminars began to take place at many locations and numerous times throughout the year. In 1974 there was a seminar in Monterey, California, and in 1983 one in London, England.

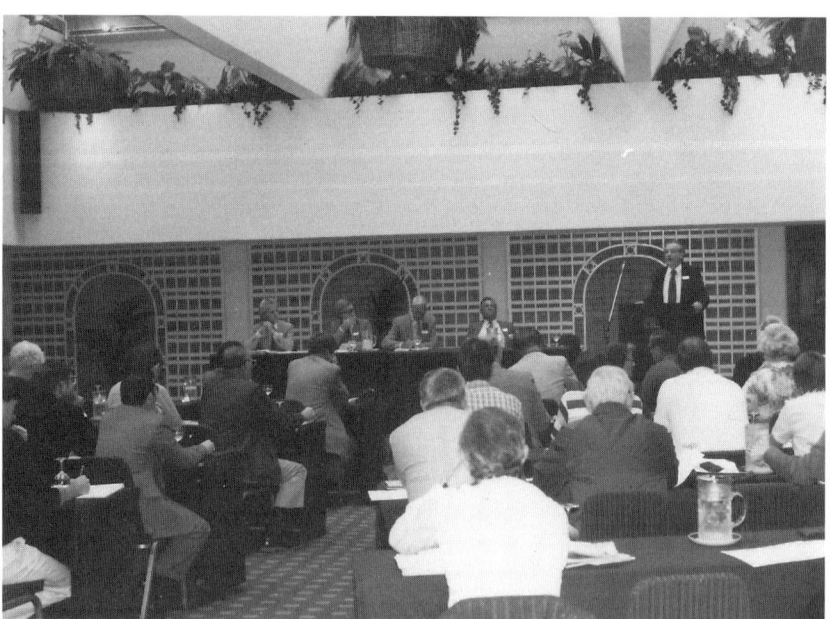

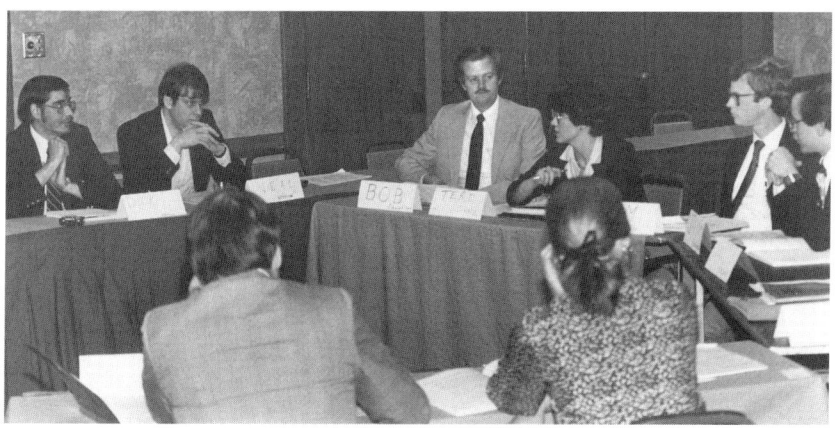

Seminars stressed dialogue, interaction, analysis of case studies, and role playing.

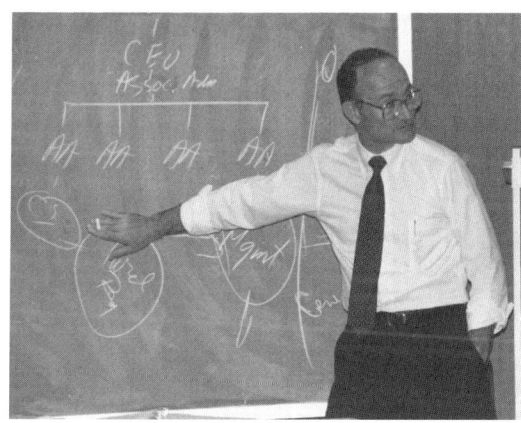

For almost twenty years, Peter Laubach, DBA, HFACHE, taught some of the College's most popular seminars.

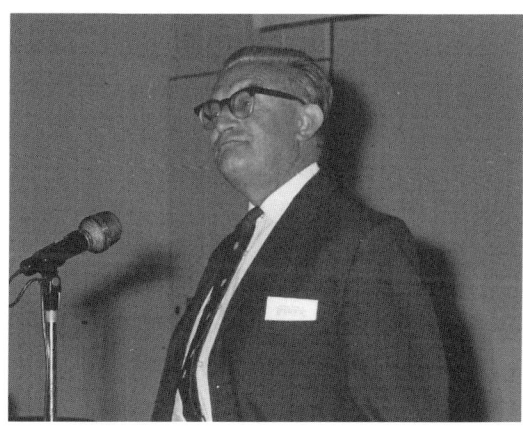

In 1967, the first Fellows' seminar (now an annual affair) was addressed by Theodore Chester, CBE.

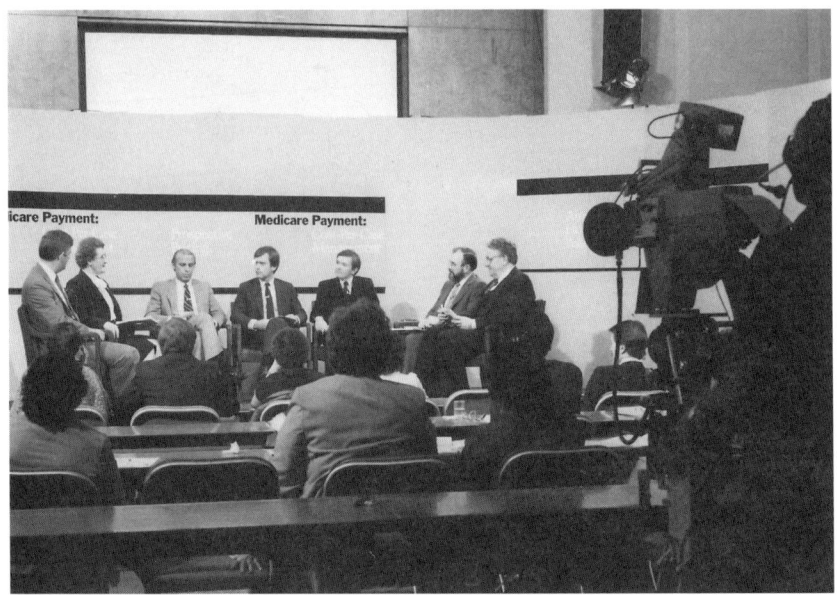

Over the years innovative educational programs have continually been introduced. Among them was the College's first live video teleconference in 1983. Produced in cooperation with the American Hospital Association and featuring Fellows from around the country, the conference discussed practical strategies for coping with prospective pricing.

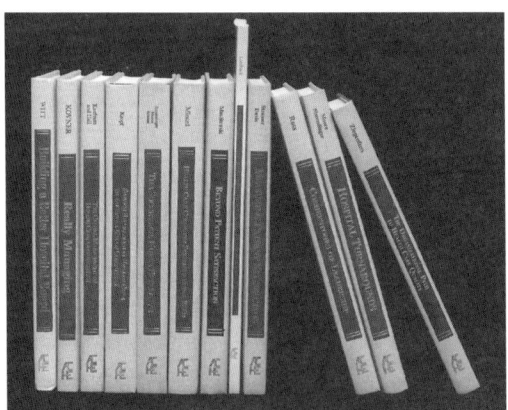
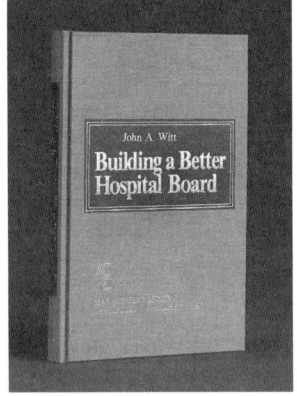

In 1986, the College greatly expanded its publications program by acquiring Health Administration Press and its inventory of books and journals in health services management. A new series of books was initiated, the American College of Healthcare Executives Management Series. *Building a Better Hospital Board*, by John A. Witt was the first book in the series.

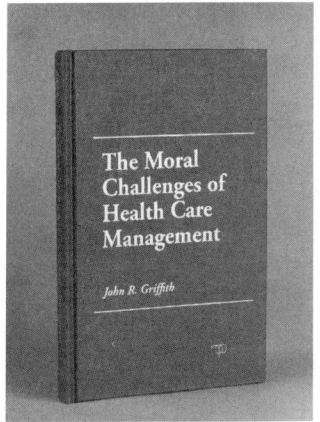

In 1989, Self-Directed Learning Programs based on books from the Press began to appear. Such independent study programs enable members to gain educational credit at their own pace and place. *The Moral Challenges of Health Care Management* is the basis for one of these programs.

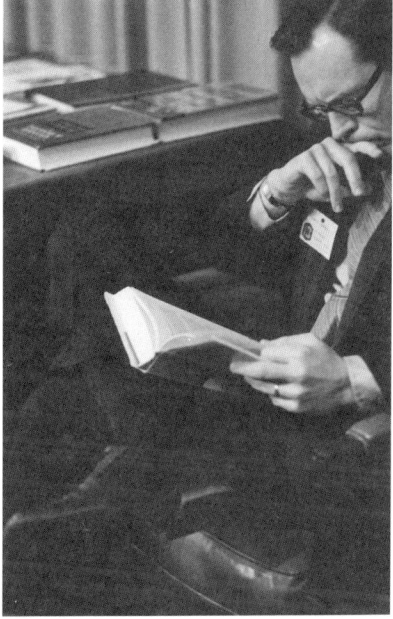

In 1990, the College acquired Pluribus Press, including the manuscript for a book by and about Ray E. Brown, FACHE. Health Administration Press produced the book.

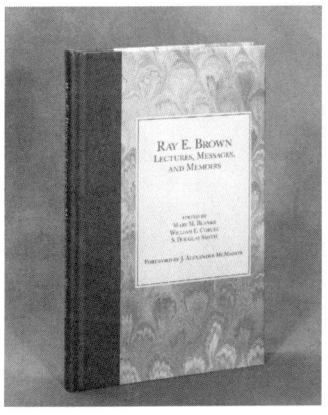

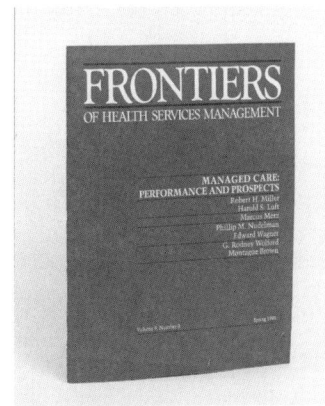

Frontiers of Health Services Management is one of the journals, in addition to *Hospital & Health Services Administration*, the membership journal, and *Healthcare Executive*, the College's magazine, brought out by the College.

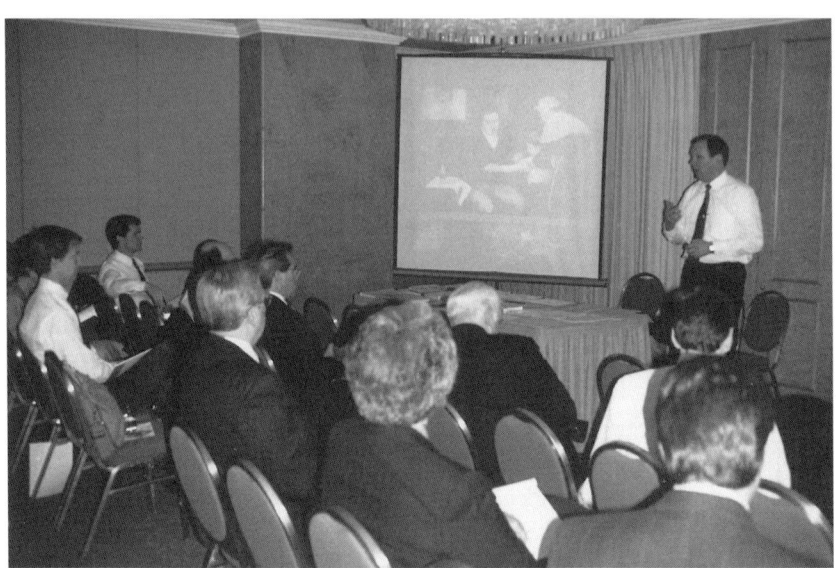

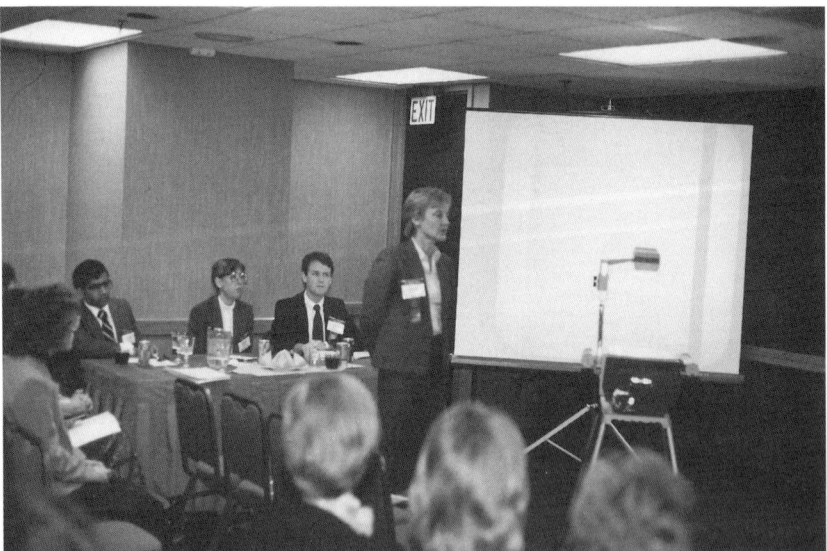

Cluster programs are another innovation. Like the Executive Skill Builders and Self-Directed Learning Programs, they were begun in response to members' concerns about educational funds and the time they can spend away from their home organizations. The clusters provide an opportunity to take up to three different seminars in less than a week.

The snapshots show seminars at cluster programs in 1992.

Name Index

Subject Index